MEDICAL EMERGENCY!

MEDICAL EMERGENCY!

The St. Luke's–Roosevelt Hospital Center

Book of Emergency Medicine

Stephan G. Lynn, M.D.,

with Pamela Weintraub

Hearst Books/New York

Library of Congress Cataloging-in-Publication Data

Medical Emergency! : the St. Luke's–Roosevelt Hospital Center book of emergency medicine / by Stephan G. Lynn, M.D., with Pamela Weintraub
    p.   cm.
   Includes index.
   ISBN 0-688-13679-6
   1. Medical emergencies–Popular works. 2. First aid in illness and injury—Popular works. I. Lynn, Stephan G. II. Weintraub, Pamela. III. St. Luke's–Roosevelt Hospital Center.
   [DNLM: 1. Emergency medicine. 2. Emergencies. WX 215 E562 1996]
   RC87.E254 1996
   616.02'5—dc20

                                                 95-33047
                                                   CIP

Printed in the United States of America

First Edition

1 2 3 4 5 6 7 8 9 10

BOOK DESIGN BY JENNIFER HARPER

To the more than two million patients and their friends and families who have sought out the emergency departments at St. Luke's–Roosevelt Hospital Center on Manhattan's West Side during my career as the director of the Department of Emergency Medicine

Acknowledgments

Emergency Medicine is truly a team effort; it's the "team sport" among all of the medical specialties. The end product of our work every day in the Emergency Department is resolving medical emergencies for our patients—the result of the interaction of a large number of caring professionals—physicians, nurses, social workers, and many others. This book is the result of the caring and concern of those members of the Emergency Medicine Team at St. Luke's–Roosevelt Hospital Center. They include:

Harrison Bloom, MD, Director, Division of Geriatrics in the Department of Medicine at St. Luke's–Roosevelt Hospital Center

Camille Gianarris, Chaplain and faculty member in the Department of Emergency Medicine at St. Luke's–Roosevelt Hospital Center

Amos Grunebaum, MD, Director, Maternal and Fetal Medicine Service, Department of Obstetrics and Gynecology at St. Luke's–Roosevelt Hospital Center

Gregg Husk, MD, Director of the Residency Training Program in Emergency Medicine at St. Luke's–Roosevelt Hospital Center

Ilene Kaufman, MD, Director, Pediatric Emergency Department at St. Luke's–Roosevelt Hospital Center

Ellen Krasnoff, First Aid Instructor, St. Luke's–Roosevelt Hospital Center

David Kroning, MD, Assistant Director, Pediatric Emergency Department at St. Luke's–Roosevelt Hospital Center

Richard Marsella, EMT-P, MBA, Director, Special Programs and the Fast Care Ambulance Service at St. Luke's–Roosevelt Hospital Center

Daniel Mathisen, EMT-P, Director, Pre-Hospital Care, Department of Emergency Medicine at St. Luke's–Roosevelt Hospital Center

Eleanor Mulligan, RN, Clinical Coordinator, Roosevelt Hospital Emergency Department

Gus Pappas, AEMT-P, Division Chief, New York City Emergency Medical Service

Suzanne Pavel, RN, Clinical Specialist, Roosevelt Hospital Emergency Department

Gary Pollino, AEMT-P, Ambulance Supervisor, St. Luke's–Roosevelt Center

Jorge Rey, MSW, Social Worker, St. Luke's Hospital Emergency Department

Wendy Rives, MD, Attending Psychiatrist, Roosevelt Hospital Emergency Department

Adrienne Shiloff, Former Patient Representitive, Roosevelt Hospital Emergency Department

Prentice Steffen, MD, Attending faculty physician and Board Certified Sports Medicine Specialist at the Emergency Department at St. Luke's–Roosevelt Hospital Center

Douglas Wornell, MD, Director, Psychiatric Emergency Department at St. Luke's–Roosevelt Hospital Center

Maurice Wright, MD, Assistant Director, St. Luke's Hospital Emergency Department

Susan Xenarios, CSW, Director, Rape Intervention Program/Crime Victims' services at St. Luke's–Roosevelt Hospital Center

We would also like to thank the following individuals for their help and guidance:

Sean L. Finnerty, EMT-D and Firefighter, New Jersey

Scott Greiff, EMT-P, New Jersey

Anna Moretti, Legal Affairs Coordinator for the New York City–based non-profit group, Choice in Dying

Mark Douglas Obenour, EMT-P, A.A.S

Contents

CONTENTS

Each day I come to work and enter what I call "my special world"—my emergency department at St. Luke's–Roosevelt Hospital Center. Some friends and colleagues ask, "Why do you want to work there? How can you take the stress?" I don't have to think long about the answer; I know why. Every time I enter the emergency department, I am given the opportunity to see life at its ultimate peaks and valleys—to participate in the early arrival of a new baby and to experience the "inner smile" of both the parents and the staff at the prospect of a new life, to stem the flow of blood and relieve the pain and anxiety while stitching a cut hand, to comfort and stabilize a heart attack victim and give the medication that will actually reverse the damage to a living and beating heart, to bring someone back from the brink of death and see his family in the hallway the next day, and, when necessary, to help a family through their first twinges of grief upon the loss of a loved one. These are the everyday joys and challenges of life in the emergency department, and I wouldn't have it any other way. I am an emergency physician.

This book is dedicated to the more than two million patients and their friends and families who have sought out the emergency departments at St. Luke's–Roosevelt Hospital on Manhattan's West Side during my career as director of its Department of Emergency Medicine. To each of those patients who left the emergency department with the reduction of his pain or anxiety, with a sense that she could continue to experience the joys and disappointments that make up our daily lives, and to those who left appreciative and satisfied at the opportunity to have interacted with the emergency medicine team, I am grateful for the opportunity to have offered medical intervention that made a difference. I am grateful to have been there when my patients needed me in so many different ways.

My patients have sustained me; they have given me their trust and allowed me to teach others both the art and science emergency medicine; on occasion, they have put their lives in my hands, and they have inspired me to write this book. I could not have done this without them and to each of them, I am grateful.

Chapter 1

State of Siege: How to Recognize a Medical Emergency

It's just after noon when the ambulance gets the call: A huge sign has toppled from a building, its metal rim snagging a construction worker on a platform below. The worker and sign plummet two stories to the ground, a tangle of cardboard, metal, and flesh.

Rushed by ambulance to the emergency department, the patient is bruised all over and crying in pain. But miraculously, X rays reveal that he has sustained just one major injury. The falling sign has twisted his leg into a straight, clean break immediately below the knee.

Lucky to be alive and to have received such prompt care at his emergency department—the midtown-Manhattan Roosevelt site of the St. Luke's–Roosevelt Hospital Center—this patient will recover use of his leg. But he will have a hard road ahead. He will face major surgery requiring the use of metal screws to hold his bones together, followed by months of rehabilitation. And, as the physician on call in the emergency department comments after viewing the X ray, "He'll set off a buzz passing through metal detectors at airports for the rest of his life!"

Later that afternoon, in the cavernous tunnels of the New York subway system, a social worker on his way home collapses. Transit police summon an ambulance. Within minutes, two paramedics hurry down the subway stairs. They lift the man, strap him to a stretcher, and carry him to the ambulance waiting above. Sirens blaring, they rush him to the bustling Roosevelt emergency department, where he slowly regains consciousness and demands to be released. But after questioning, emergency department nurses find he is unable to relay the date, the place, or even his name. With gentle but insistent prodding, nurses and paramedics convince him to stay. Lucky for him. Doctors find he has had a severe epileptic seizure. And thanks to the diagnosis, appropriate treatment can begin.

■ ■ ■

It's four in the morning when a two-year-old awakens sobbing and burning hot. On vacation in New York, the family has been staying in a midtown-Manhattan hotel. Their pediatrician back home is thousands of miles away. Rushing down to the hotel lobby, they hail a cab to the closest emergency department. After examining the girl and conducting some lab tests, the attending physician diagnoses the problem: dehydration and scarlet fever. The child is given glucose solution intravenously for hydration, Tylenol to bring down the fever, and a prescription for penicillin. A disease that could have wreaked havoc if left to blossom untreated has been nipped in the bud.

A broken leg, an unexplained seizure on a subway train, very high fever in the very young; most of us recognize these dire situations as clearcut emergencies. A trip to the ED—the emergency department of your local hospital—is the only viable response to what could otherwise be fatal or injurious in the extreme. If your leg is crushed in a car crash; if you have fallen from a great height; if you have crushing chest pain that renders you nauseous and takes your breath away; if you have been injured internally by a gun or knife, you must go to the emergency department. It doesn't take years of medical training, after all, to realize that if you are wheezing like a foghorn, bleeding profusely, or unconscious, the emergency department is the place for you.

But visit the emergency department and you'll see other situations as well. A young woman comes in to complain of a mild cough and nervousness. "Why so nervous?" asks the nurse. The reason is riveting: Social Services has taken her children, saying she cannot care for them. Now, wandering the streets at a loss for what to do, too disenfranchised even to find an attorney, she has come to a place of healing—her local ED.

Another patient, a young man new to town without a doctor of his own, was on the job creating layouts for a magazine. Cutting patches of type with his X-Acto knife, he sliced his finger instead. Now, sitting in the emergency department, he watches as a highly trained emergency physician, one able to set broken legs, diagnose rare immunological disorders, and bring cardiac patients "back from the dead," wraps his finger in a state-of-the art dressing. "Leave it alone for two days," the young man is advised with a pat to the shoulder. "Don't get it wet. And be careful next time you use that knife."

Outside in the waiting room is a man with insomnia, a woman with a sprained wrist, and a child with a cold. Meanwhile, talking to the nurse is a man in his twenties who claims to need vitamins. "I need more energy, more vigor," he insists, "I want hormones to make me strong!" After hearing the nurse explain that the ED does not dispense vitamins, he decides to go on his way.

Given the range of complaints seen in the emergency department these days, defining medical emergency is no easy task. Of course, the American College of Emergency Physicians has tried. Red-alert symptoms in that group's list include fainting; chest or upper abominal pain or pressure; sudden dizziness; weakness or change in vision; difficulty breathing or shortness of breath; severe or persistent vomiting; coughing up or vomiting blood; bleeding that won't stop; suicidal or homicidal feelings; or other significant changes in mental status, including confusion or unusual behavior.

Who can argue?

But things are not always that clear. You slip while whirling around the ice at Rockefeller Center one evening, and your ankle is throbbing. Do you really need to go and sit in the ED for an hour, sharing the experience with strangers, and possibly picking up some germs? Or is it a safe bet your ankle is merely sprained—injured, but not so badly that you won't be able to hobble around come morning and go to your family doctor then?

You've had the flu for days, and now your fever soars to 103 degrees Fahrenheit. You feel so lightheaded, you jokingly tell your wife, you might be having an out-of-body experience. Of all the altered states you've experienced since your party days at college a decade ago, this is the most extreme. But go to the emergency department? Hang out with victims of heart attack, stroke, and gun blasts? Please. "I'm drinking liquids. I'm taking an antibiotic. Give it a chance to work," you bargain with your spouse and the Fates. "If the fever goes up to a hundred and six, we'll go to the hospital then."

Your father, age seventy-two, calls you on the phone. He's felt exhausted all day, he tells you. And now he has a fever of 102. He'd call his doctor, but it's long past office hours. Should he go to the ED? You advise him to wait until morning. Logic tells you that's OK. After all, your children have fevers all the time, and the pediatrician usually suggests Tylenol and bed rest, and no antibiotics at all. Still, why can't you shake the nagging feeling that something serious is wrong?

Without a doctor in your family, how do you know if any given injury or illness is urgent, requiring immediate medical attention? When your problems fall into that gray zone, how do you figure out whether they're emergencies or if treatment can wait? It might surprise you to learn that the flu victim with the soaring fever was probably correct in deciding that he should just take his prescribed antibiotic, sip ginger ale, and rest in bed. But the ice skater should have gone to the hospital; his ankle was broken, and he made the injury worse by waiting and trying to use it the next day. As for the seventy-two-year-old man, his fever indicated a severe bacterial infection. He wound up in intensive care. He should have ignored the advice of his well-intentioned daughter, and called an ambulance instead.

Indeed, with all the publicity about overuse of the emergency department by those who lack primary-care physicians, many people don't realize that when it comes to true medical emergencies, the ED is often *underutilized.* In many instances people with urgent or life-threatening medical problems wait and wait—sometimes until it's too late—before they reach out for help.

In the pages that follow, you will learn about the nature of medical emergency. You will learn how to recognize medical emergencies and prepare for them well in advance. You'll learn to aid victims and perhaps even save lives before professional help arrives. You'll get a sense of when it's imperative for you to get to a hospital at once, and when it's OK to stay home. And you'll learn to negotiate the complex world of the modern, high-tech emergency department (a term that is increasingly replacing the designation emergency *room,* suggestive of the old days when interns ran the show) so that you can receive the best possible care.

The ABC's of Emergency Medicine

When doctors, nurses, and paramedics study emergency medicine, their first lessons always revolve around the basics of survival—the vital functions people in the field have dubbed the ABC's. It's simple: A is for *airway;* B is for *breathing;* and C is for *circulation.*

Airway obstruction, in which the throat is somehow blocked, means oxygen cannot reach the lungs for delivery to the body. If the airway remains blocked, death can come in minutes. Obstruction is most often caused by choking—food is the usual culprit—or by swelling so advanced, it has begun to restrict the trachea, also known as the windpipe, the tube extending from the larynx to the lungs. Severe infections of the throat, such as very inflamed strep throat, or epiglotitis (a quick-moving infection most often seen in children) can sometimes block the airway. So can an allergic reaction. And, for those who are unconscious, the most common airway obstruction is the tongue itself (discussed under first-aid tips in Chapter 3).

HOW TO RECOGNIZE **Choking/Airway Obstruction**

Inability to speak or make a sound

Dusky or blue-tinged skin surrounding fingernails and lips

Extreme effort to breathe

Collapsing or passing out

And don't forget the universal choking distress signal in which the victim clutches his/her throat between the thumb and index finger.

Breathing problems may also turn into serious emergencies if untreated. The reason is clear: During the process of breathing (or ventilation) we take in oxygen from the air and exhale carbon dioxide—a fair and useful exchange. Without oxygen the cells of our body cannot survive. Brain and heart-muscle cells are particularly sensitive; deprived of oxygen for as little as five minutes, brain and heart cells will simply die.

Whenever ventilation is threatened our lives are at risk. Those who require immediate care are asthmatics having asthma attacks; pneumonia patients with labored breathing; cardiac patients afflicted by shortness of breath; and drowning victims not breathing at all. In the case of the drowning victim or anyone who has stopped breathing, mouth-to-mouth resuscitation—also known as rescue breathing—is the ticket. For others, an immediate visit to the emergency department is key.

HOW TO RECOGNIZE **Respiratory Distress**

Shortness of breath

Labored, or slow, shallow breathing

Use of abdominal and neck muscles to assist breathing

Blue-tinged skin surrounding fingernails and lips

Even if the airway is clear and breathing unimpaired, another critical function—circulation—is needed to get the oxygen to the body's cells and vital organs, including the brain. If blood cannot reach the lungs to pick up that motherlode of biological gold, oxygen, and if it cannot effectively carry life-giving oxygen throughout the body, then the result could be dire: cardiac arrest, in which the heart stops pumping; or major shock, in which the body's major organs, deprived of oxygen, start to fail.

Signs of circulatory distress may be subtle. Anyone experiencing dizziness, for instance, might be suffering because the heart has not been pumping blood effectively enough to another vital organ—the brain. In one recent instance, notes Nurse Suzanne Pavel, St. Luke's–Roosevelt Hospital's clinical specialist in charge of continuing education for the emergency department, a patient came in with a small knife cut on her finger. "She said she'd cut the finger while making a dinner salad," Pavel reports, "because she was dizzy." Acting on the report of dizziness, doctors ordered an electrocardiogram and discovered the patient had had a heart attack. The symptom of dizziness, a red alert for emergency department doctors, was just one result of the shock caused by the heart.

Circulation will also be compromised by hemorrhage—profuse bleeding internally or externally. You don't need to be a rocket scientist to recognize the possibility of excessive bleeding in an external wound. Often an open, bleeding wound is not as bad as it looks, but to be sure, get to the ED at once.

Recognizing internal bleeding, on the other hand, can be tricky. If you or a loved one are injured, and if you have received a powerful blow to the abdominal or pelvic area, don't assume you're OK just because you don't have an open, bleeding wound. Look for signs of shock: from nausea, vomiting, weakness, and dizziness to extreme thirst and cold, to clammy hands. And if you suspect shock, get to the emergency department at once.

Remember, if you suspect circulation has been impeded, do not waste time driving to the hospital. Instead, summon an ambulance so that medical care can begin at once. And while waiting with a friend or relative, administer basic first aid (outlined in Chapter 3).

HOW TO RECOGNIZE **Shock/ Circulatory Collapse**

Weak and rapid pulse

Confusion, disorientation, dizziness

Cold, clammy hands and pale skin

Extreme thirst

Nausea and vomiting

High anxiety

Fingernails which, when pressed in, turn white and do not return to pinkish hue in two seconds

Remember, you may be at risk for shock if you have been in a traumatic accident, if you have been severely burned, or if you have cancer or diabetes. Internal or external loss of blood can put you in danger of going into shock as well, and the risk is even greater if you are pregnant.

"Our strategy is to hope for the best and plan for the worst," says Nurse Suzanne Pavel, and to continuously assess our patients for the ABC's. "Someone may be bleeding profusely or suffering from severe infection, but if they're not getting oxygen into their lungs, if their heart cannot pump blood to the body's organs and cells, their brain may be damaged, and their ability to live at all is severely compromised." For anyone making a medical assessment in the ED—and for anyone evaluating the urgency of a problem—the ABC's come first.

Medical Red Alert

But after the ABC's have been attended to, other symptoms may signal the need for immediate intervention as well. One of the most prominent signs of danger, notes Dr. Gregg Husk, director of the St. Luke's–Roosevelt Residency Program in Emergency Medicine, is a "disturbance in cognition," an inability to reason, communicate, or identify ordinary things. Such disturbances, says Dr. Husk, tend to be markers for a wide variety of serious medical ills, from epilepsy to stroke to seizure. "The machine up there is so easily wrecked by a variety of insults," he notes. "Disturbances of cognition can be markers for things that are really grave."

Emergency Department personnel also focus on profuse bleeding from external wounds and internal injuries or ills. Generally showing up as bright red or dark and granular (like coffee grounds) blood in vomit or stool might signify internal bleeding or a devastating internal injury; in the case of a pregnant woman, some vaginal bleeding may mean miscarriage. In such instances, immediate intervention, including surgery, is the only way to proceed.

A sharp, torturous pain in the area of the testicles can sometimes signal the condition known as torsion. For young, healthy men, who sometimes experience the condition without any injury or previous symptoms, the problem can be devastating. Indeed, if your friend is moaning, twisting, and grabbing at his crotch, get him to the ED at once. If he has suffered torsion, his testicle is twisted so that its blood supply is cut off. If untreated for anywhere from twelve to twenty-four hours, the cut-off testicle will die.

The list of traumas goes on: severe burns, drug overdoses; poisoning; eye injuries that result in great pain or perhaps blindness; neck and spinal injuries. All require immediate emergency care.

Under the Urgency Umbrella

Outright emergencies are not the only problems to take you to the emergency department. Dr. Husk defines another set of situations: Less dire than life-or-death emergencies, these "urgencies" must nonetheless be treated within twenty-four hours, or by the next day. "If they are not," Husk says, "significant damage to health could result."

In fact, while magazines and newspapers proclaim inappropriate overuse of the ED for mundane aches and pains, those who suffer urgencies often attempt to tough it out. They avoid the emergency department in hopes their problem will go away, and as a result, sometimes make matters worse.

Under the urgency umbrella, Husk places such problems as low-grade fever that fails to go away; nonfacial cuts larger than a half-inch (such cuts on the face must be stitched immediately, or they may leave a scar); blood in the urine; athletic injuries from muscle pulls to ligament tears; and severe pain.

One of the most misunderstood urgencies, notes Husk, is the garden-variety cut. If you sustain a cut long or deep enough to require stitches—anything deep enough to expose tissue inside the body, anything more than a half an inch in length on your face or hands, and anything over an inch in length along the rest of your body—you must obtain urgent care and have stitches as soon as possible. That's because the opening into your body will tend to accumulate bacteria at a rapid rate, and once the cut is too infected (after about twelve hours), it's impossible to sew it together; you'd just be locking the bacteria inside. Without the stitches, of course, you won't die. But you might suffer a debilitating infection and retain an unsightly scar.

Dr. Husk also advises that you get to the ED if there's even a remote possibility you have broken a bone. "People assume if they can use a leg, arm, or wrist, it's not broken, but that's not always true," he points out. "If you use a broken arm or leg, you can make the fracture or break worse. You can also cause swelling, which will then make it virtually impossible to apply a cast until the swelling goes down." If you've fallen on your wrist and suffer wrist pain, he adds, even if you can move your wrist, there's a particularly high chance you've suffered a fracture or a break.

In fact, if you've suffered any injury involving force, do not wait more than twenty-four hours to check it out. If you've been in a car accident or if you've fallen from a height, you may be in more trouble than you think. If, in the aftermath of such a trauma, you suffer pain to the head, chest, abdomen, back, or neck, it's imperative that you get to the hospital at once. Be particularly attuned to neck pain: It may signify something as serious as damage to the bones that support your skull and protect your brain.

Dr. Husk also warns patients not to tough out severe pain. "Pain alone is not lethal," he comments, "but it's sure not good for you." Pain is your body's way of telling you that you may have suffered a serious injury or may have a significant illness. If you have severe ear pain, for instance, you may have an ear infection serious enough to rupture the ear drum or cause an equilibrium problem. If your eye is hurting, you may have suffered a corneal abrasion—a scratch to the cornea, one part of the eye necessary for sight. If the object or grit that caused the abrasion remains in the eye, moreover, it can leave you with a corneal scar that might affect your vision forever.

Should these problems take you to the ED at three in the morning when you can also be treated a few hours later, say at eight in the morning? "If the pain is so severe that you are unable to sleep with simple pain medication," says Husk, "if seconds seem like hours, don't wait. Come on down to the ED at once. After all, emergency physicians consider treating pain part of their job description: Patients passing kidney stones, for instance, often suffer breath-stopping pain, and commonly visit the ED. Most of our energy is spent alleviating discomfort. Why should you suffer? Besides, pain is a powerful signal that something is very wrong. If you let the condition persist too long, it can become increasingly damaging."

To Go or Not to Go: When It's Best to Stay Home

Finally, says Dr. Stephan G. Lynn, director of emergency medicine for St. Luke's–Roosevelt Hospital, there is a whole list of ills for which a visit to the emergency department may not be advisable. Though it's important to listen to your body, Lynn asserts, the first rule of thumb is to seek treatment elsewhere if it's appropriate. The reasons are obvious. If your problem is not truly an emergency—strep throat, for instance, or a cold—you may be asked to wait in the emergency room for many hours, while other, more dire problems are treated first. All the while, you may be exposed to the germs of other patients suffering from flu, virus, or other contagious illness. And your trip to the emergency department will probably cost more than what you would pay your personal physician.

If your problem is relatively minor, your best bet is to contact your family doctor or local clinic. If your illness or injury is serious, but not imminently fatal, you may still need to go to the emergency department, but you could benefit from contacting your own doctor first. He or she may be able to call ahead to inform the emergency staff about your special medical needs—or, knowing your personal situation, may be able to suggest whether or not a trip to the ED is for you.

Dr. Husk also suggests that, if unsure, you should phone the ED. "My guess," says Husk, "is that if I stood in front of a national meeting and suggested patients call the ED, my colleagues would 'kill' me, because we're busy enough as it is. But, in fact, if you're having trouble finding your doctor, and debating whether to come to the emergency department or not, a phone call to the ED might be clarifying. We can give some straightforward first-aid advice, and if your problem is a mosquito bite, we can suggest you may not have to come. If people call Roosevelt, the truth is, we don't have a problem speaking to them at all."

Of course, this does not mean you should avoid the emergency department if it is the best place for treatment, even if you are not at death's door. In some areas, or at some times of the day or night, on weekends, and on holidays, the ED may be the only way to find treatment for a wide variety of ailments often considered the domain of general practitioners. Moreover, your medical history and age may make certain symptoms more urgent for you than for others. For example, if you're a patient with a history of heart trouble, it's especially likely that symptoms of chest pain may signal a heart attack; going to your general practitioner first might waste precious minutes or hours that emergency medicine professionals could have used to save your life.

Personal Emergency

Emergency physicians point out that the decision to visit the emergency department often depends on your personal profile: your age, your condition or health status, your family history, and any other risk factors you may have. Not long ago at Roosevelt, for instance, a forty-six-year-old woman with diabetes came in for an ankle sprain, and while awaiting a physician, developed shortness of breath. Ordinarily, shortness of breath in such a young woman still menstruating would not suggest heart trouble. But diabetes happens to be a strong risk factor for cardiac problems. Aware of this, emergency personnel rushed her to the electrocardiogram machine, where a heart attack in progress was found; and she had come to the ED for a twisted ankle. Other risk factors for heart disease, such as high cholesterol level or lack of exercise might have escaped emergency workers treating a mere sprain, so it's up to patients to communicate and make certain that emergency staff are informed of all of their medical problems.

Age is also a risk factor. For instance, moderately high fever in a forty-year-old may not be dangerous. But, says Dr. Husk, it can be a sign of serious illness in the elderly or the very young. For those over seventy, says Husk, fever can be especially problematic, warranting a trip to the emergency department even when it isn't accompanied by chronic forms of disease.

"It sounds a little ridiculous," Husk explains, "to say that if you have a fever over 100.4 degrees Fahrenheit, taken orally, you need to get yourself to a doctor or the ED, but it's true. Statistics bear it out. While someone in his or her thirties with a fever of, say, 102 degrees, is likely to have a virus that's not too serious, a senior citizen is more likely to be seriously ill. First of all, seniors have been around for a longer time, and have built up immunity to more of the viral illnesses afflicting humans on Earth. They're also not regularly exposed to young children, a source of viral disease. If you study people between the ages of thirty and sixty with a fever greater than 100 degrees, you will find that the vast majority of the time the fever comes from a virus. But if you look at the elderly population, the numbers change. Old folks end up with few of the common illnesses that go away. On the other hand, they are greatly at risk for more serious bacterial illnesses that require antibiotics, including urinary tract infections and pneumonia, among others. What's more, once they've contracted the bacterial infection, they're more at risk of deteriorating as a result. Studies have shown that one out of every five elderly people with fever over 100.4 ultimately dies of the infection that caused the fever. Those numbers should convince these people that they need to be seen by a health practitioner at once."

In the very young, on the other hand, extremely high fevers can cause brain damage or even death. In an infant under two months of age, for instance, where the immune system is not yet highly developed, fever of 104 degrees Fahrenheit or more may signal such bacterial infections as pneumonia and meningitis. In a child under two years of age, high fever may indicate pneumonia or flu. After age two, moderately high fever need not cause as much alarm, though for all of us, the higher a fever gets, the riskier it becomes.

Often, the decision to use the emergency department or to see your private physician amounts to a judgment call. Your decision will depend on your access to rapid primary care; your personal risk factors, including age, weight, and health; and the capabilities of doctors, hospitals, and ambulance transports in your area. For some patients, the decision to use the ED is an economic one: Our troubled society has rendered the emergency department itself part medical care facility, part social services agency, and part safety net for great numbers of people who need to be there because they simply have nowhere else to turn. There's no single equation, but as we will explain in more detail in Chapter 2, to come up with a personal formula, ask your personal physician what might constitute an emergency for you. What's the best course of action if you feel chest pain? If your child has a fever? What should you do if you feel the onslaught of dizziness, numbness, or cramps? Which local hospital is most appropriate, and how should you plan to arrive?

The Patient Defines the Emergency

The list of emergency dos and don'ts, the special conditions and qualifications, may seem overwhelming. After all is said and done, how can you know for sure whether to come to the ED? For Dr. Lynn, one answer works best: "You, the patient, define the emergency. You're the one feeling the pain and anxiety. You know your past medical history, your surroundings and the medical resources of your community. Thus, you are probably best able, at least initially, to judge whether a trip to the emergency department is in order. Your decision is key."

To devoted ED professionals, this is not just the medically appropriate attitude but the politically correct one as well. "A lot of people come to the emergency department and we, as physicians, nurses, and paramedics, with our knowledge and experience, look at the patient and say, 'Why in the world did he come to the emergency department with that little tiny cut on his finger?' " Dr. Lynn explains. "But I know that to that person, the injury is serious. He's not trained in the same way I am. He got nervous, saw blood, felt pain, and didn't know what to do. Because of my training, it's my job to deal with the problem and to educate him about what to do next time around."

Indeed, even though insurance companies don't always get it, when it comes to emergency medicine, Monday-morning quarterbacking is not where it's at. You feel a sharp abdominal pain and rush to the emergency department, only to find constipation is the culprit. You're sent home with a container of milk of magnesia, which you could have picked up easily in the pharmacy across the street. Not only did you waste your time, but, adding insult to injury, your insurance carrier may refuse to cover the visit because a diagnosis of constipation is not on its list of appropriate diagnoses in the emergency department.

But as a sick patient seeking care, second-guessing should not come into play. You must direct your attention toward the symptoms you feel; it is not your responsibility to define the eventual diagnosis, made only after the nurse and physician, with years of training, have taken vital signs, drawn blood, ordered X rays, and conducted a thorough physical exam.

At all times, say emergency workers, it's best to err on the side of caution. Gary Pollino, paramedic supervisor at St. Luke's–Roosevelt Hospital, puts it this way: "As the patient, you've got to play it safe. Anytime you're unsure of what to do, anytime you're scared and fear your life or welfare may be at stake, seek medical help at once. In other words, when in doubt, assume the worst, and call your physician, call the ambulance, or come into the ED. Sure, the ambulance crew that gets there, or the nurse who sees you in the emergency department, may be looking at you a little funny, but you'd rather play it safe. Imagine the alternative: Your husband suffers chest discomfort, but rather than make a fuss over nothing, rather than worry about scorn at the ED, you give him some Maalox and go to sleep, hoping it will pass by morning. Only problem is, when you wake up in the morning, he's dead."

Remember, it's always best to follow your instinct. You know better than anyone in the world how you feel normally and when you just don't feel right. If you're not feeling normal, something has gone wrong and you need to be evaluated. The diagnosis and the treatment, if any, can be determined only after you've gone to professionals.

Focus on the Symptoms, Not the Diagnosis Up the Road

Again and again, emergency physicians emphasize that it is impossible to reproduce four years of medical school, plus three or four more years of emergency medicine training, into a simple guide to this field. No manual can teach you to differentiate pneumonia from the flu, or a badly sprained ankle from a broken one. Indeed, when medical students and interns study diseases and the associated symptoms, they learn to make diagnoses based not only on observations, but also on blood tests, X rays and many other diagnostic techniques. For you, the patient, it's best to look at the palette of symptoms you exhibit—your complaint, in other words—and then decide how to proceed based on what you feel.

You have fallen and experience a sharp, pulsing pain in your left shin; what should you do? Or perhaps what seems like extreme pressure pain suddenly originates in your chest and radiates down your arm; what's the best course of action? You have a paper cut on your index finger and the blood has started to gush. Do you clean with soap and water and apply a Band-Aid or rush to the hospital for stitches?

The answers are not often black and white. Indeed, medical diagnosis is often a gray area based on art as well as science. The art and science of emergency medical diagnosis take years to master; attempting to be your own diagnostician is a mistake. You must learn to exercise simple common sense in deciding what to do in the face of a medical emergency.

How do you differentiate between situations that require the skill and facilities of an emergency department, as opposed to those that can be treated by a primary-care physician, or with the help of your own first-aid kit at home? Dr. Lynn suggests looking at each complaint on an individual basis. For instance, if you've fallen and hurt your head, you must be taken to the emergency department if you lose consciousness. If your head hurts or if you sustain a bump, but you never black out or feel nauseated, a visit to your primary-care doctor on the next business day will often suffice.

If you sustain a cut a quarter of an inch long on your elbow, cleaning and bandaging using your first-aid kit at home may be adequate. If the cut is half an inch long, and on your face, get to the hospital, where immediate cleaning, stitching, and bandaging will prevent the appearance of an unsightly scar.

As for chest pain, it can, of course, signal a heart attack and, possibly, impending cardiac arrest. (Heart attack, or myocardial infarction, involves blockage of an artery by a blood clot and damage to heart muscle; it can cause cardiac arrest, in which the heart stops cold.) How do you know whether your chest pain is the result of heart trouble? Often there's no way you can know for sure, and the symptom is generally sufficiently alarming to take you to the ED at once. But if you are twenty-five years old, in great shape, and suffer momentary chest pain after a hard serve at tennis, common sense might suggest that the cause for the discomfort is a strained muscle rather than the failure of your heart. Statistics and precedence will be on your side.

Feedback on some of the most common complaints brought to the emergency department are in the list that follows.

AN EMERGENCY PRIMER

The following list summarizes the most prevalent ills and injuries seen in the St. Luke's–Roosevelt Emergency Department. Note that a problem may be of tremendous urgency even if it does not appear on this list. If your instinct tells you to obtain emergency medical care, by all means, follow that instinct and get to the ED at once.

Cuts

Though many people with cuts come to an emergency department, cuts do not necessarily require emergency care unless they are bleeding profusely, are more than half an inch long, are on the face, or are on a functionally important part of the body like the hands or feet. In fact, most small cuts on an arm, or a leg can be treated effectively at home with some soap and water, antiseptic, and a Band-Aid. For a cut less than half an inch long, with little blood, it may be appropriate to seek out a primary-care physician. However, if you have an open wound through which you can see internal tissue, or an avulsion, in which a flap of skin has come loose, get to the emergency department at once. You may need stitches to prevent scarring and infection, and, if you have not had a tetanus shot in the past five or ten years, you will need one within about twenty-four hours to prevent a deadly tetanus infection.

Profuse Bleeding

Significant bleeding from any cause or from any source should be considered an emergency. Whether you are vomiting blood, discharging blood in the stool or urine, having prolonged or serious vaginal bleeding, or bleeding from a large open wound, you must see a physician, probably an emergency physician, at once. (Yes, even a nose bleed requires medical attention if it persists.)

Large, Open Wounds

If your wound is large, open, and bleeding profusely, it is possible to lose a lot of blood. What's more, open wounds are subject to bacterial contamination. Cover the wound with gauze or a clean cloth to prevent infection, attempt to control the bleeding according to instructions in Chapter 3 (how to apply pressure), and get to the emergency department at once.

Puncture Wounds

Injuries caused by a stab from a pointed object such as a nail or a knife, may at first seem unalarming because little bleeding is visible externally. However, puncture wounds can cause serious, even deadly, bleeding inside the body, as well as significant infection. Other internal damage can result as well. If you suffer a puncture wound, get to the ED or a doctor at once. But remember, if the object that caused the puncture is still in the wound, do not try to remove it. By doing so, you can cause as much damage on the way out as was done on the way in.

Bruises

Bruises, or closed wounds, result from damage to the soft tissue beneath the skin's surface. Characterized by swelling, black-and-blue marks, or hematomas (blood pooling beneath the skin), small bruises do not require emergency department care. However, if the bruise is large enough, swelling beneath the skin can occur as a result of serious damage to the body, including vital organs, and a visit to the ED is advised.

Amputation

If any part of the body—a limb, a fingertip, a flap of skin—is amputated, preserve the part according to instructions in Chapter 3, and get to the ED at once.

Burns

Many burns caused by an open flame, a hot liquid, or a hot object can be treated at home with first-aid techniques described in Chapter 3. If the burn causes only redness and not blistering; if it involves only a small area of the body; if it is not on the face, hands, feet, or genitalia, it can probably be treated at home. However, the smoke that accompanies the flame that caused the burn can also induce severe respiratory problems, including swelling that blocks the airway, sometimes resulting in death. To prevent this eventuality, particularly in children and infants, look for coughing or hoarseness, wheezing, difficulty breathing, spit or phlegm tinged with soot, or red sores inside the mouth. If any of these symptoms appear; if the burn has affected the face, hands, feet or genitalia; and if the burn covers more than an inch or so of the body, or if the burn is blistered, get to the ED at once. And before you leave, make sure all burning clothing has been extinguished. Emergency department personnel report that a surprising number of burn victims arrive with their clothes still smoldering!

Breaks and Sprains

Injuries to bones and muscles can often be painful and quite dramatic. But to emergency medicine professionals, they are usually considered urgencies

AN EMERGENCY PRIMER

requiring prompt treatment, not emergencies in the truest sense of the word. However, if you believe you may have fractured a bone, a trip to the ED is advised unless you have immediate access to an orthopedist with an X-ray machine in his office. Do not try to diagnose your own injury; sprains may be far less serious than breaks or fractures, but it's often difficult for the layperson to tell the difference. In general, a painful injury that causes obvious deformity to an extremity or to a body part like an ankle or wrist must be X-rayed and promptly evaluated by a physician, usually in the emergency department. Finally, in rare circumstances, broken bones may literally be life-threatening. Dislocation of the hip, which may threaten blood and nerve supply to the legs, requires immediate attention at the hospital. And if a suspected break, especially in the pelvic area, is accompanied by severe pain and lightheadedness, do call an ambulance; there may be some very serious and invisible internal bleeding.

Multiple Injuries

Should you suffer multiple fractures, bruises, or internal injuries in a significant accident, it's crucial to get the highest level of medical attention as quickly as you can. You may have heard of the so-called golden hour—the window of time during which seriously injured patients must reach the operating room before rates of survival drastically decline. If you have been injured in a car accident or in a high fall, call the paramedics so that treatment may begin at once. And remember to ask to be taken to the nearest trauma center.

Joint Pain

Joint pain rarely requires evaluation in the emergency department. The major exception is pain in a single joint that appears red, hot, and swollen, seems infected, and is impossible to move. Such "septic arthritis" can severely damage a joint.

Head Injury

If, after a blow to the head, you observe disorientation or there is a loss of consciousness, a seizure, or difficulty in talking, moving, or thinking, get to the ED at once. Dire results of blows to the head include a bruised or bleeding brain. Any head injury followed by loss of consciousness must be evaluated at the ED, quickly.

Neck Injury

If a neck injury causes significant pain in the neck, "electric" sensations in the arms, or difficulty in moving or feeling, it is crucial to get to the hospital at once. A broken or badly strained neck can cause permanent injury to the spinal cord. Successful recovery can depend on early diagnosis and treatment. Don't attempt to move your neck and expect the ambulance to use very special precautions in doing so.

Chest Injury Caused by Trauma

Anytime the chest has been injured in an accident, be it at a football game or in a multicar pileup on the freeway, evaluation at the ED is important. You will probably need an X ray and an electrocardiogram (EKG) to check the health of your heart, lungs, and rib cage.

Crushing Chest Pain

Chest pains may signal heart attack. Though your chest pain may turn out to be simple indigestion, you should never disregard it. Unexplained chest pain should take you to the hospital at once. The most alarming form of chest pain is the feeling of a crushing weight or a vise pressing on your chest. It is a sure sign that you must call an ambulance immediately. A heart attack is also signaled when chest pain persists for a long period of time; when it's associated with nausea, vomiting, shortness of breath, or sweating, as well as the sensation that pain is radiating down the arm or to the neck.

Milder Chest Pain

Anyone suffering chest discomfort should also be on the lookout for angina, a pain of less intensity and shorter duration but similar in quality to the pain of a heart attack. But signs of angina can sometimes be missed. For instance, you're raking leaves and you get a twinge in your chest. Is it the chest pain of a heart attack or angina, or the ache of a pulled muscle in the chest wall? Never attempt to decide for yourself. If you're unsure or if it's the first time, err on the side of safety and get to the emergency department as quickly as you can. A recent finding of the famed Framingham Heart Study in Massachusettes is instructive. Researchers found that about a quarter of all patients who reported no chest pain but were diagnosed with heart trouble had had previous heart attacks. These heart attacks, of which the patients were completely unaware, were detected only by electrocardiogram; the patients had minimized or forgotten the cardinal sign of heart attack—chest pain.

AN EMERGENCY PRIMER

Difficulty in Breathing

If you've ever had a reason to call the paramedics, it's now. While it may be impossible to diagnose the problem immediately, disruption of the respiratory system is a clearcut violation of your ABC's (*airway, breathing,* and *circulation*) and can be fatal. Your breathing problem may have many explanations: asthma, pneumonia, inhalation of toxic gas or smoke, emphysema, bronchitis, pulmonary edema (often caused when the heart fails, as blood backs up in the lungs), or even choking or airway obstruction. If you detect any signs of respiratory distress, including nostrils that open wide; an Adam's apple that moves up upon inhalation; and use of neck and stomach muscles to aid in the breathing process, get to the ED at once. A word to the wise: Most asthmatics end up in the emergency department because they have failed to take their medication or have allowed their prescription to run out; plan ahead and avoid that unnecessary trip to the ED.

Abdominal Pain

Abdominal pain is one of the most common problems taken to the emergency department today. Most of the time abdominal pain comes from simple indigestion, mild food poisoning, or viral infection, and it may require no emergency intervention. However, there are instances where survival depends on seeking emergency medical care at once. For instance, you might, unbeknownst to you, be bleeding internally, particularly if you suffer from peptic ulcer disease. Your colon may be perforated, or circulation to the intestines may be compromised. You may have appendicitis, which usually presents with pain in the right lower quadrant—the right side of the bottom of the abdomen, just above the groin. Abdominal pain in women of child-bearing age may mean a woman is suffering an ectopic pregnancy, in which a fetus has begun to develop outside of the normal location within the uterine wall. And finally, according to Dr. Lynn, severe, overwhelming, debilitating abdominal pain that covers the entire abdomen, rendering your stomach rigid, is a sure sign of trouble. If acute abdominal pain is accompanied by cold and sweaty skin or a weak or rapid pulse, your condition might be serious, and a trip to the emergency department is a must.

Acute Pain in the Side

If you're suffering acute distress in this area you may be passing a kidney stone. One of the most agonizing problems seen in the ED, kidney-stone pain frequently radiates from the flank around to the groin and down into the area of the genitalia. It may present as back pain as well. In general, the pain comes and goes in waves and is frequently associated with nausea and vomiting. Since kidney-stone pain is often spurred by dehydration, it's more likely to occur in spring and summer than in other seasons. This condition usually requires a trip to the ED, where physicians can manage the pain with medicine until the stone has passed, guard against infection, and watch to make certain the stone has not blocked the ureter, the tube extending from the kidney to the bladder.

Back Pain

Unless back pain is so severe it prevents walking or is associated with loss of control of the bladder, bowel, or leg movements or sensation, it can be treated by physicians in the office or at home. Once your ability to walk or feel becomes impeded, however, hospital evaluation could be critical. Those who suffer back pain as the result of trauma such as a fall from a horse or car crash must get to the ED, since fracture of vertebrae or a spinal-cord injury must be treated at once.

Sudden, Unexpected Pain in the Groin

When this symptom appears inexplicably and without trauma, in a male, especially a young male, it may be a sign of torsion—a twisting of the testicle, which impedes circulation to the area. If not recognized and treated within twelve hours, the testicle dies due to lack of blood supply. A patient with sudden unexpected onset of severe testicular pain should hurry to the emergency department.

Partial Weakness or Numbness

A feeling of numbness or weakness in just part of the body, usually on one side, is often a sign of stroke, which occurs when a clot or hemorrhage in the brain results in neurological problems. A stroke is always sudden, as its name suggests—as in a "stroke of lightning"—a literal bolt from the blue. If you suffer any unexpected neurologic dysfunction, including the inability to move your hand, a sense of numbness in your leg, or problems with vision, you must report to the ED at once to be evaluated for stroke. Remember, the sudden onset of weakness, paralysis, confusion, visual fuzziness, speech disorder, or coma could indicate a stroke.

AN EMERGENCY PRIMER

Loss of Consciousness

Loss of consciousness, either because of fainting, hitting one's head, or being knocked unconscious, is a clarion call for a trip to the emergency department.

Altered State of Consciousness

Someone who seems disoriented and confused should get to a doctor at once. If a friend or family member cannot tell you three specific things—his name, his present location, and the date—he is not what physicians call "oriented times three," and any number of serious medical problems, from diabetes, to stroke, to heart attack, may be at the root. If ingestion of drugs or alcohol is not responsible for this altered state of consciousness, another reason must be found, and evaluation in the ED is important.

Convulsions, Fits, or Seizures

Seizures, caused by the widespread discharge of brain cells, are generally characterized by convulsions, though different types of seizures take different forms. The grand mal seizure includes uncontrollable twitching of the arms and legs and loss of consciousness, sometimes accompanied by tongue biting, confusion, and incontinence. Localized motor seizures are characterized by convulsions in just one part of the body. Though most seizures occur because of failure to take prescribed anti-seizure medication, sufferers must be seen by a doctor, usually in the ED, at once. Repetitive seizures that take place while the sufferer is unconscious constitute an extreme medical emergency, since they may result in permanent brain damage.

Headache

Most headaches don't require emergency care, but sudden, unexpected, severe headache—what you might refer to as "the worst headache of my life"—needs to be seen in an emergency department. A headache that occurs with stiffness of the neck, or with neurologic symptoms—certainly, loss of consciousness—needs to be seen in an emergency department promptly. A headache accompanied by severe, unexpected pain in the eye, where there are no signs of infection and there's no previous disease, is sometimes a sign of glaucoma, and an emergency department visit is necessary.

Violent, Suicidal, and Delusional Behavior

Someone whose mood or behavior is extremely disturbing or physically threatening to himself or others must be seen by a doctor at once. People who are suicidal, violent, or delusional must be treated as soon as possible. If this individual is too resistant to be taken to a doctor or hospital, you must call an ambulance and the police for transport to the ED.

Extreme Allergic Reaction

If, after eating a meal, receiving an injection, taking a medication, or receiving an insect sting, you break out in hives, become flushed and swollen, or feel weakness or respiratory distress, an extreme allergic reaction may be in progress. There is no time to waste. The ABC's could be seriously threatened. You or someone with you must call the paramedics or get you to the local ED. Some of us, knowing we have severe allergies, carry self-injecting epinephrine (adrenaline); this is a time to use it.

Severe Rash or Hives

Rashes, if sudden and extreme, may take you to the ED, especially if you suspect they may be associated with a new medication. A dangerous allergic reaction could be the cause (see above).

Red, Blistering Skin Not Caused by Sunburn

This could be a sign of severe bacterial infection or an allergic reaction, and requires a trip to your doctor or the emergency department at once.

Bites

If you have been bitten by a snake, a raccoon, a dog, a spider, or even a human being, you should seek medical attention at once. If possible, have someone from your town's emergency service isolate the "biter." For instance, if you've been bitten by a rabid dog, you will need rabies injections. To avoid this series of injections, you must test the attacking animal to learn if it is, in fact, rabid itself. Snake and scorpion bites may require specific antivenom to counteract the venom. You will need to describe the snake or spider, or bring the dead animal with you so that the correct antivenom can be prescribed. The human bite might be more dangerous than you think. Because it can transmit innumerable diseases and infections harbored by people, the human bite can be serious, often requiring a tetanus shot and antibiotic treatment as well as careful followup. Seeking treatment through your family doctor or the ED must remain a judgment call, depending on the circumstances of the attack and the availability of your family doctor and the services the doctor's office provides.

AN EMERGENCY PRIMER

Poisoning

If you or someone you know has ingested a potentially poisonous substance, call your regional poison control center for instructions. By giving instructions over the phone, the poison center consultant may be able to help you rid the body of poison before it reaches the internal organs. Then call the ambulance for help from paramedics and transport to the local ED. It's not widely known that many of the most popular ornamental plants are poisonous to humans and should be kept out of the reach of toddlers. (According to the American Red Cross, some garden and household plants that you may not realize are poisonous include azalea, Carolina jessamine and yellow jessamine, elderberry, foxglove, lily of the valley, mountain laurel, mistletoe berries, oleander, nightshade, poinsettia, and rhododendron.) At the St. Luke's–Roosevelt Emergency Departments, we call the New York City Regional Poison Center at 212-P-O-I-S-O-N-S. You may call it, your local regional Poison Center, or the telephone operator.

Drug Overdose

If a friend or relative has suffered a drug overdose, accidental or intentional, get that person to the ED as soon as possible. Treatment and the use of a medical antidote may be lifesaving.

Alcohol-Related Disease

Merely drinking a bit too much, of course, is generally not cause for a visit to the emergency department. However, alcohol in large quantity or over a long enough period of time may engender a host of medical emergencies requiring immediate intervention. If the blood alcohol level goes over 400 milligrams per deciliter (possible if you drink half a pint of, say, 80-proof rye in ten minutes) then sudden death through depression of respiration is possible. In extreme intoxication, the ABC's of survival are at risk. Life-threatening seizures or delirium tremens (DTs) can result when an alcoholic stops drinking, cold turkey. In these instances, a trip to the emergency department is advised as well.

Problems in Pregnancy

If you or someone near to you suffers unexpected bleeding, strong contractions, labor pains, or pain in the lower abdomen during pregnancy, go to the emergency department at once.

Fever

Most of the time, fever can be treated by a primary-care physician or local clinic. Go to the ED for fever only when a primary-care physician is unavailable; when the fever is more than 105 degrees Fahrenheit; or when the patient is an infant or senior citizen.

Severe Flu-like Symptoms

If your symptoms include some combination of headache, dizziness, weakness, disorientation, cough, and fever, you might think you have the flu. And you very well could. If so, aspirin, chicken soup, and some TLC will see you through. But how do you know if you have a simple case of the flu, potentially deadly pneumonia, or meningitis? You don't. If your symptoms are intense and if they persist, don't wait it out. Get to your doctor. And if your doctor is unavailable, get to the ED. If you have pneumonia, Legionnaires' disease, or meningitis, you may have to be hospitalized. And a word of caution: Don't give aspirin to a child or to anyone at risk for bleeding when flu-like symptoms occur.

Chapter 2

On the Advance Team: How to Prepare for a Medical Emergency

Picture this: A woman is home with her husband, age forty-two, as he mows the backyard. He expresses a feeling of numbness radiating down his left arm, then he collapses to the ground. The woman spends about five minutes trying to revive him before realizing he's unconscious, and nothing she does helps. She'd better call the ambulance, she decides, and dials 911. But the couple have just moved to a new town, and though 911 is the emergency number for most areas of the country it is not here. She calls information, gets the number, and dials again. She frantically begs the paramedics to come. But anxious to get back to her ailing spouse, hangs up before the operator has had the chance to ask for certain crucial information. For instance, the dispatcher never records the cross street for the couple's address, or a description of the house. This is especially problematic because the house number is not prominently displayed on the front door or mailbox and she and her husband are not visible from the street. What's more, in the rush to get back to her stricken husband the woman doesn't clearly communicate some of the most distressing symptoms, which the dispatcher would have recognized as a sign of possible cardiac arrest. Nor does she stay on the phone long enough to receive vital first-aid information. Specifically, she could have been given on-the-spot instructions in cardiopulmonary resuscitation, providing her spouse with minutes of extra survival time through a flow of blood and oxygen to his failing brain and heart.

By the time the paramedics figure out where the couple live and arrive at the door, essential time has been wasted. Since emergency workers were not given a complete description of the symptoms, they leave the defibrillator, needed to give the heart a jump start, in the ambulance.

The defibrillator is retrieved and used, the patient is given supplementary oxygen, and the urgent race to the hospital begins. Hearing the paramedics plan to go to a facility nearby, the woman argues that at the hospital five miles farther up the road her second-cousin moonlights on Thursdays. His influence, she insists, could help.

Crucial seconds pass before the paramedics simply ignore this plea and go to the first facility, noted for excellence in cardiac care. A nurse rushes the patient into the room set inside for heart emergencies, and alerts the crack cardiac team on call. Despite the sophistication and training provided in this case, chance of survival is poor. The reason: This husband-and-wife team never considered the eventuality of a medical emergency. They never learned how to call an ambulance. They failed to assess the medical facilities in their area. In short, when push came to shove as it did here quite suddenly and unexpectedly, valuable minutes were wasted through mistakes that could have been avoided had they been prepared.

In many cases those minutes mean the difference between life and death. Victims badly injured in auto accidents have the best chance of survival if they make it to the ED and the operating room within the first "golden hour," enabling surgeons to stabilize their vital signs, stem the loss of blood and protect their vital organs. Emergency departments are asked to give suspected heart patients an electrocardiogram (EKG) within ten minutes of entering the hospital, and, if indicated, to provide clot-dissolving thrombolytic medication as soon as possible. In cases of severe allergic reaction, poisoning, hemorrhaging during pregnancy, and other conditions, time is of the essence if a patient is to survive. A dramatic example of the need for immediacy is when it comes to medical emergency is the rare, highly virulent, flesh-destroying streptococcal bacteria that has gotten so much publicity of late in the British and American press. While rare, this bacterial illness can kill a victim within a day. It's safe to say that getting to the ED on time *can* be a death-defying act.

The key to rapid response in the face of medical emergency—the difference, in many cases, between life and death—is a state of preparedness. Before you ever have a medical problem you must educate yourself as to the various emergencies most likely to occur, and establish clearcut plans of action in advance. When it comes to your health, you are on the advance team.

A Talk with Your Own MD

A first step, says Dr. Lynn, is sitting down with your personal physician during a routine visit and asking as simply as possible, "What do I do if I need to go to the emergency department?" This is a multipart question, Dr. Lynn emphasizes, and the first issue you must take up is what your doctor can and cannot handle in her or his own office.

Do not assume that your doctor can handle "everyday" emergencies. You must ask. One paramedic remembers being called to a doctor's office for an asthmatic. "Well, you figure she's in the doctor's office—certainly the doctor has already given her a shot of adrenaline (accepted protocol for severe asthma attack) and some oxygen," he relates. "We walk into the doctor's office, and the doctor is standing at the front door. 'Come on, hurry up,' he says to us. 'She's having trouble breathing.' We go in there, and there's this girl who's an asthmatic, as white as the sheets on my bed, gasping for air. The internist, who should have been qualified to treat her until we arrived, seemed unsure about what to do. I was stunned. We had to start from square one, just as we would if we'd gone to her apartment. We had to start the IV, we had to give her the shot of adrenaline, we had to give her oxygen, and by the time we arrived she was so severely ill that we had to pass a breathing tube down her trachea."

In another instance, a St. Luke's–Roosevelt ambulance team was dispatched to a local physician's office, where a patient had come in with chest pains. Having suffered a minor heart attack, the man needed an intravenous line, and he required oxygen because his breathing was labored, probably due to edema (water on the lungs). Despite the patient's obvious condition, the doctor had initiated none of these treatments, thus wasting the patient's precious time—first by having him come to the office in the first place, and then by having him sit in his reception room awaiting his turn to be seen. This patient would have improved his chance of full recovery quite drastically had he just called the ambulance to take him to the ED.

On the same day, a young boy with a temperature of 101 degrees Fahrenheit and a hacking cough sat waiting in the emergency department. After examining the boy in triage (an initial evaluation), it took the nurse a minute to reach a conclusion: The problem was probably an upper respiratory infection. The child needed treatment that day. But his condition was what the hospital called an urgency—just not as crucial as the heart attacks, asthma attacks, and head injuries also coming through the door. When the emergency physician saw the boy later that evening, he did what any competent doctor would have done: prescribed bed rest, plenty of fluids, and a cough medicine and decongestant to relieve the child's symptoms. A visit to the boy's pediatrician would have provided the same level of care in a shorter time for less money. And because of the child's personal relationship with his pediatrician, he would also have received a much-needed dose of TLC.

Had these patients spoken with their respective physicians beforehand, it is likely that the boy would have gone to his doctor's office, while the asthma and heart patients would have rushed to the ED.

When exploring conditions your doctor feels require special attention by the emergency department, make sure you review the usual suspects: chest pain, breathing problems, abdominal pain, fever, disturbances in consciousness, injuries—including cuts, bruises, sprains, and broken bones—childhood sicknesses, and more. When does your doctor want you to come to her office, and when does she want you to call in before rushing off to the ED? There are certain medical rules that apply to everyone.

You should also explore your doctor's technical capabilities. For instance, can he perform laboratory tests at the office? Can he suture a wound? Can he take and read X rays on the spot? Can she deliver oxygen or provide important medications through an intravenous line? (Don't assume your doctor can do all these things, basic as they may seem.) Will she or a colleague call you back within two minutes, even at four in the morning—or will you have to wait for the next business day, no matter how urgent the problem?

You may *think* that treating asthma is the most basic of medical skills. But while some physicians can deal with it in their office and request that you come to see them, others will say, "If you're having trouble breathing and you have asthma, I want you to go right to the emergency department."

In the case of heart attack, on the other hand, you should always get to the emergency department as fast as you can. "If people recognize the symptoms of heart attack, they should call the ambulance first," says Dr. Lynn. "Then, if they have the time or the desire, they can call their private doctor after, just to communicate the fact that they think they are having a heart attack and have already called the ambulance. I have seen people who have waited on the phone line for ten minutes while the secretary appropriately says, 'The doctor's busy; can you hold on for a minute?' They sit there with chest pain and the ambulance has not been called. For some, that initial phone call to a personal physician has been lethal."

SIX QUESTIONS YOU MUST ASK YOUR DOCTOR **About Future Emergency Care**

1. If I'm injured or ill, under what circumstances should I come to your office, and when should I go to an emergency department?

2. You know my medical history. Based on my condition, what are the problems or situations that may cause me to require emergency care? How can I recognize these problems and how shall I react when they occur?

3. What key points of my medical history should be written down and carried with me at all times?

4. How can I contact the ambulance in my community most rapidly?

5. Given my situation, which is the best local emergency department for me? For the children? Are there different choices for different problems?

6. If I decide I must leave for the emergency department can you provide me with a procedure for reaching you quickly?

After going over emergencies in general, ask your doctor to review your personal medical history in the context of your individual lifestyle. Situations that may be merely problematic for a svelte and healthy twenty-year-old runner could be quite dangerous for those who are older, overweight, inactive, or suffering from specific syndromes or diseases. If you are a diabetic, epileptic, asthmatic, or hemophiliac; if you are on special medication for any condition; if you've suffered from congestive heart failure, rheumatic heart disease, or rheumatoid arthritis; if you are older than age seventy; if you have gone through premature menopause; if you are pregnant; or if you have had cancer, the emergency guidelines will have to be adjusted especially for you.

If you and your doctor have the time, explore your particular case in detail. What is the most urgent set of circumstances for you? The diabetic experiencing breathlessness might be at risk for cardiac problems, for instance, even at the otherwise unlikely age of thirty-five. A fall to the sidewalk could be particularly serious for the fifty-year-old woman who went through menopause at age thirty-five, even if she has regularly been taking hormone and calcium supplements, since her bones will likely be more fragile than those of other women her age.

If you are pregnant make sure that your doctor explores with you all the signs of a fetus at risk. For instance, she must spell out exactly how many contractions at each stage of pregnancy will necessitate a trip to the Emergency Department.

If you have suffered congestive heart failure have your doctor spell out in as much detail as possible the signs of possible attack that will send you rushing to the ED. If you tend to experience angina (mild chest pain indicative of a heart condition but not a heart attack), find out when the symptoms are severe enough to signal an out-and-out heart attack. What are the signs? How will you know?

While consulting with your doctor it's also a good idea to go over the vital statistics in your own medical history, detail by detail. To function well in an emergency it's often important to know this information thoroughly. While your family doctor is well acquainted with your medical history, emergency department personnel will have only a few minutes, if that, to find out all they need to know to give you the best treatment possible. Any time you have difficulty providing your history, you may delay your treatment and open the door to potentially deadly mistakes: If you're allergic to penicillin, for instance, a dose of it can kill you. If you're a hemophiliac without a sufficient clotting factor, the last thing you'd want to get in case of a heart attack is the anticlotting agent streptokinase, which thins the blood.

In the midst of a medical emergency, you might not think to tell the doctor or nurse all they need to know even if you usually know it cold. Therefore, it's a good idea to prepare. Take a sheet of paper and list the essential points you wish to communicate to personnel in the emergency department. To make sure you've listed everything of relevance, go over the list with your family doctor. Remember to include allergies, chronic ailments, medications, and operations, as well as a rundown of your family history. If your father succumbed to heart disease at age forty-five, that is worth mentioning. If your mother and sisters were diagnosed with cervical cancer, mention that too. If you, yourself, suffer a particular illness, find out if any specialized document will aid in your care. For example, a cardiac patient might do well to carry a copy of his last electrocardiogram. Ideally, the electrocardiogram can be reduced, printed on a credit-card-size card, and laminated.

To make sure your personal medical history is complete, review the following box. If possible, write out a history, using the seven bulleted points as guideposts, and take it when you go to the ED. If possible, carry it with you at all times. Your parents may have told you never to wear dirty underwear or socks with holes in them, because you never know when you'll visit the doctor. Well, don't get caught without your medical

CHARTING YOUR MEDICAL PAST

Make sure to note any major medical problems relating to your heart, your respiratory system and your kidneys. If you have diabetes, lupus, or any other serious, underlying condition, make a note of it. Include any past operations or procedures, even minor ones.

· Preexisting Conditions: Record all your current or recurring medical problems.

· Medications: Record all medications you take regularly. Don't forget drugs that you purchase over the counter at the drugstore including aspirin or anti-inflammatory medications. Be sure to mention birth-control pills and other forms of hormone therapy. Note how often you take each medication and be honest about use of alcohol and drugs. You wouldn't want to be medicated in the emergency department, only to learn the substance reacts badly—or perhaps even lethally—with something you have already taken. Sharing information honestly may save your life.

· Allergies: Make a note of your allergies. This is more important than it seems. Many major infections are treated with penicillin and its derivatives, which can be lethal to those who are allergic to those drugs. And if you are allergic to the anesthetic used to numb the gums in the dentist's office you may also be allergic to lidocaine, the drug of choice for those receiving garden-variety stitches as well as for many patients with cardiac dysrhythmia (a disturbance in the rhythm of the heart).

· Your Doctors: Make a note of your personal physicians and any specialists treating you, including addresses and phone numbers. List the hospitals you've been treated at most recently. These hospitals will be home to your permanent records, and access to those records may greatly facilitate rapid treatment.

· Trips to the Operating Room: Record all operations with a date and place where they were done as well as the best medical description of the procedure you had done (ask your doctor to make certain you don't leave any part out).

- Immunization History: For most people this means jotting down the date of your last tetanus shot. If you've sustained a serious cut or wound you will need a tetanus shot, provided you haven't had one in the last five or ten years. (If the wound is less serious, you can go as long as ten years between shots.) If you are traveling abroad you may need to carry other immunization data as well. Speak to your personal doctor about specific requirements.

- Family Baggage: Jot down any unusual health problems affecting your immediate family—parents, siblings, and grandparents. With genetics a high-risk factor for many forms of disease, this information could be crucial. If you are good at keeping current notes, you might record any communicable diseases suffered by a close family member in the last couple of months.

history list either. Regularly review it. And update it yearly, on your birthday.

Once you've compiled the list above, carry it in your wallet at all times, supplemented by a list of your emergency contacts. This contact sheet, illustrated on the next page, will help the hospital reach your doctor, your closest family members and even your insurance company should you be incapable of verbal communication. If you have been hospitalized in the past, include that information as well. Then, even if the emergency department cannot reach your personal doctor, vital records can be accessed quickly. By including the location of your living will, your wishes can be invoked as soon as possible.

Cut on dotted line

✚ EMERGENCY CONTACT CARD

FOR: _____
                          (name)
MY DOCTOR IS: _____

_____
           (name, address and phone number)
In case of emergency, please contact: _____

_____
              (name and phone number)
_____
              (name and phone number)

I was last hospitalized at: _____
                                        (name of hospital)
                                  date: _____
_____
        (location or address)
My Insurance Carrier is: _____

Policy Number: _____

My Medications: _____

_____

_____

My Allergies: _____

Illnesses I have had: _____

_____

Injuries I have had: _____

_____

Operations I have had: _____

_____

You can find a copy of my living will at: _____

_____
              (location)
_____

37

Keep these lists with your driver's license and your medical insurance cards for easy access by ED personnel. Remember, they're using every second to save your life!

At home, in a desk drawer or other area easy to access, store any X rays, EKGs, or CAT scans that may have a bearing on your past and future health. If you have prepared a living will specifying the type of treatment you would like to receive (or should not receive) should you be unconscious or incompetent, keep that handy as well. Ideally, your close friends and relatives will know where this important information is kept. (For complete instructions, see Chapter 13.)

For those who want to organize medical information in a more official way, an alternative is a medical information card or, preferably, the Medic Alert information bracelet so well known to paramedics around the country and the world. As explained below, the bracelet details all your medical conditions and, as a bonus, enables emergency department physicians to obtain still more information by calling in to a computer data bank that stores many details, including your blood type and your last electrocardiogram. A word to the wise: Experts warn that you must be wary of cheap drugstore imitations, which do not include customized information and cannot provide access to more specific information by phone.

THE INFORMATION SAFETY NET

For special medical problems such as diabetes, epilepsy and food allergies, symptoms might become so severe that communication is impossible. In such instances, medical personnel cannot access important information necessary for your immediate care in the ED. To address this problem, a number of safety insurance services and devices can now be used. Here's a rundown.

The Medic Alert Bracelet

The respected magazine *Men's Health* has called this medical identification bracelet one of the best safety investments around, and probably the cheapest "health insurance." At a cost of thirty-five dollars, these civilian dog tags are a foolproof way to let health professionals know about your medical condition in an emergency. Personalized with information about blood type, contact lenses, implants, food and drug allergies, required medications, and medical conditions such as abnormal EKG, pacemaker, memory impairment, stroke and asthma, the bracelet is also engraved with a twenty-four-hour hotline number that emergency personnel can call for your full medical history, family doctor's phone number, and other data. Call the nonprofit Medic Alert Foundation at (800) 863-3421 or (800) ID/ALERT (432-5378) to order. The bracelet is highly recommended by paramedics, the American College of Emergency Physicians, the Emergency Nurses Association, and others. Application forms can be found in most pharmacies and medical offices.

Vial of Life

Those who use this service receive a small plastic container, or "vial," that holds basic medical information and includes signed releases that authorize medical treatment. The vial is placed in your refrigerator, and a sticker on the refrigerator door alerts emergency personnel that the vial is inside. The vial is offered free of charge in many communities throughout the United States and can be obtained through your local office of the American Red Cross, senior citizen center, hospital, or fire station. Of course, this is only effective if the emergency occurs at home and paramedics recognize the sign on the refrigerator.

Telephone Security System

In this setup, a small console in your home has a *help* button that you can push in the event of an emergency. It also includes a remote *help* button that can be worn on your wrist or around your neck. When you touch the *help* button, a signal is sent to a central station monitored twenty-four hours a day. In response to your *help* signal, the headquarters' staff person will call you for further information; if you cannot be reached, the service will contact your friend or relative; if no one can be reached, an ambulance will be dispatched. This service is generally available through the same companies that provide central station monitoring of burglar and fire alarms in the home. The cost is about twenty to twenty-five dollars a month, plus an installation fee of anywhere from thirty-five to two hundred dollars.

Telephone Buddy

Some communities provide this "reassurance program," in which you receive a telephone call at a specific time each day to see how you are doing.

Community Programs

In some areas, communities have organized programs where mail carriers, gas/electric meter readers and other businesspeople (newspaper delivery, laundry, etc.) look for signs of trouble each time they visit your home. These signs include mail or newspapers piling up at the door or in the mailbox; lighted or unlighted rooms and or failure to answer the doorbell.

Cellular Security

Just a few years ago, most people toting cellular phones did so for business. But these days, as the price of the technology continues to fall, more and more people are buying cellular phones for fast access to emergency care. Especially for those who suffer from serious medical problems, carrying a cellular phone to summon paramedics can provide a means of instant communication not otherwise possible.

Planning Your Trip to the Emergency Department

After you've determined your doctor's capabilities, mastered your personal medical history, and prepared your paperwork, you must plan your route to the ED. If you have a problem that's less critical, for example a cut that needs stitches, or an injured wrist you want to check out for fracture, you might ask a friend to drive you there, take public transportation, call a taxi, or even walk.

We do not recommend that you drive yourself to the ED in most cases. Any injury or illness serious enough to take you to the emergency department could seriously hamper the quality of your driving. Think about it: When you initially become ill or injured, it's difficult to tell how your problem is going to progress. You often have no idea how you're going to feel ten minutes later. For instance, you become somewhat short of breath and anxious, and you think, *I'd better get to the emergency department.* But are you going to be able to breathe at all in fifteen minutes? And if you're unable to breathe in the middle of the freeway, what will you do? Besides, imagine being injured and hunting for a parking spot or circling through the hospital garage while you're in urgent need of care. If you're the patient, you'd better have someone else take responsibility for the car; that person can park at the front door for a minute and get you into the waiting room. Then, once you've been whisked off into the system, the driver can take off for a few minutes to park the car.

Whatever your transportation plan, do make sure that you know how to get to the hospital from your home, your office, or any place you frequently spend time. Be prepared to provide directions to the driver. (The form on page 57 should help.)

It's also a good idea to establish "emergency networks" with friends and neighbors. Long before an emergency occurs, you should line up at least two people available to get you to the hospital in a pinch. If you have children, find someone you can count on to watch them while you get yourself or someone you're helping to the hospital. Talk to your neighbors, your friends, your sister-in-law who lives around the corner; ask them in advance if they would be willing to come in case of a sudden emergency. Put their numbers on the wall, next to your phone. Even though you may call these people every day, when you're in the midst of an emergency, you may draw a blank, or you may be so ill that you'll need to ask someone to make the calls for you.

We also suggest that you stash some "mad money" in the cookie jar; in other words, in the event of a medical emergency and a trip to the hospital, you will definitely need some cash, certainly enough for a few phone calls, and possibly some food from the vending machine or some taxi money to return home.

Calling the Ambulance

If you're truly ill you will want to call an ambulance instead of showing up with a friend. To make sure you have ready access to an ambulance, investigate the appropriate phone number beforehand and place it next to the phone. As noted earlier, dialing 911 now works in most areas; however, many rural and suburban communities still require you to direct-dial the ambulance dispatcher. Often you can reach the dispatcher by dialing O for operator and asking for help. If you're unfamiliar with the procedure in your area, consult your family doctor, the emergency departments of your choice, or the front pages of your local telephone book before your emergency occurs. Knowing the exact procedure often saves precious minutes and may spell the difference between life and death.

One way to get information on ambulance service in your area, suggests Dr. Lynn, is simply by pulling out your local phone book. Look at the very front of the White Pages; along with the number for an ambulance, you will find listings for reporting gas leaks, child abuse, sex crimes, fire, for reaching the poison control center, the police, and more. If you turn to the ambulance section of the Yellow Pages, you're likely to see many commercial ambulance services and a few air ambulances as well. But your best bet is depending upon those listed in the front of the White Pages in your community.

Don't be confused by the number of choices. Many regions, especially heavily populated ones, do have more than one ambulance service: commercial services may seem to offer more options, but in fact, most do not have the response time, level of training and equipment offered by the official designated Emergency Medical Service for your area, usually linked through 911 lines to the fire and police departments. While in some localities 911 Emergency Medical Services have been contracted out to one or more privately owned ambulance companies, in other areas private ambulance companies are designed strictly to transport patients, not rescue them. A patient in a wheelchair must go to the doctor; a private ambulance is summoned to take her there and then back home. An elderly man with the flu must travel from his nursing home to the hospital; a private ambulance takes him, because he is just too weak to walk to the car. If your illness is not very serious, but you'd prefer medical transportation to the doctor's office, or if you're not in a rush yet want to get to the hospital of your choice, then one of the commercial ambulance services listed in the Yellow Pages might be for you.

But if you have a true emergency, the official designated service, with its well-trained paramedics, regulation equipment and rapid dispatch system is almost always best. The response time of the officially designated ambulance service, generally strictly monitored, is often far better than that of commercial services. The ambulance dispatched by 911 is often just roving the streets near your house waiting for a call. They are familiar with all the emergency departments and have been cued in on which facilities are overcrowded, which specialize in cardiac care, and which have social workers to deal with domestic violence or abuse.

If you need an ambulance, you *cannot* get one by calling the local hospital or ED. Most emergency departments do not dispatch ambulances, and even those that do must first patch your call through to central dispatching, usually at 911. Therefore, you'll waste no time if you just call 911—or the designated central number for your area.

There is just one type of dire emergency in which the call to the ambulance should be preceded by another: accidental or intentional ingestion of poison. If you or someone you're with has ingested a toxic substance, you might need an immediate antidote, something to counteract the poison at once; you might not have time for a trip to the hospital. In fact, even if the paramedics show up at your door, *they* might have to call the poison control center to find out what to do. So if poisoning is the problem, call the poison control center first, and the ambulance second. The telephone number of the poison control center should also appear at the front of the White Pages of the phone book. If not, get the number from the telephone operator or your local ED. (The list on page 57 will help you organize all your emergency numbers in one spot.) At St. Luke's–Roosevelt Hospitals' EDs, we call top New York City Regional Poison Control Center at 212-P-O-I-S-O-N-S or your local poison center.

It's also important to know when calling 911 or your local ambulance is inappropriate. Remember that 911 is usually a central dispatch system for police, fire, disaster, and rescue vehicles and should be used only to report crimes in progress, fires, floods, life-threatening situations, and major hazards. Do not use the number to report loud parties, broken car alarms, or other annoyances. Under no circumstance should you ever call 911 to request directions, phone numbers, or the weather.

Summoning an ambulance service in hopes it will get you in and out of the hospital emergency department faster is unrealistic. If you legitimately need emergency medical care, the fastest way to receive it is by calling the ambulance. But if you're just trying to beat the wait, coming in by ambulance will not help.

"People think that because they called an ambulance they won't have to sit around the waiting room for a long time," says Gary Pollino, a longtime paramedic and now a paramedic supervisor at St. Luke's–Roosevelt Hospital Center. "They think that even though they have just a cold, if they come in by ambulance, on a stretcher, someone will see them right away. Well, that fancy taxi ride they just requested will cost about three hundred and fifty dollars just for the ambulance, and another three hundred and fifty in the ED. And if their complaint is minor, the nurse will ask them to stand up and sit out in the waiting room, and they'll wait anyway."

Presenting Your Problem on the Phone

Whether you're calling the poison control center or ambulance dispatcher, your telephone style can make a great difference in the outcome of the case. Perhaps you've seen the dramatic scenarios on the popular television show *Rescue 911,* in which six-year-olds regularly call the Emergency Medical Service (EMS) via 911, alerting dispatchers to a parental seizure, heart attack, or accidental poisoning, ultimately saving the day. Stories in the press bear out the truth behind these dramatizations on TV.

In Glendale, California, a first-grader watched his mother dive into the pool. Instead of swimming around, however, she just floated there, facedown. Afflicted with the rare disease of myasthenia gravis, which caused periods of temporary paralysis, she was completely unconscious. The boy "doggie-paddled" to his mother, pulled her to the shallow end of the pool, then climbed out and dialed 911. From her hospital bed later that day the mother declared, "My son knows that if something goes wrong to call the police. If it wasn't for him, I wouldn't be here now."

In Green Bay, Wisconsin, another fan of *Rescue 911,* age five, awakened to find his father unconscious. Knowing his father was a diabetic, the kindergartner explained his action this way: "I woke up, and I felt his forehead, and I called Rescue Nine One One." Telephone dispatchers walked the child through lifesaving procedures for his dad, telling him to put one of his hands on his father's forehead and the other under his neck to tip his head and open his airway. The boy was just checking his dad's breathing and pulse, under 911 direction, when the ambulance arrived and whisked the man to the hospital. If the child had not followed directions so exactly, medical workers later said, the father would not have survived.

And in Prince Georges County, Maryland, a mother was able to bring her drowned, lifeless baby back to life after calling 911 and receiving instruction in the science of cardiopulmonary resuscitation (CPR) during a three-minute conversation. "When that baby cried," the dispatcher recalls, "it was the sweetest sound I ever heard."

These success stories, say experts in emergency medicine, might have ended tragically had the caller been unable to communicate the problem or follow directions over the phone. With that in mind, it's important for you to think about and cultivate your emergency telephone manner long before an emergency occurs.

For some crackerjack advice you might turn to paramedic supervisor Gary Pollino. The first step, advises Pollino, is to make sure the ambulance knows how to reach you. While most 911 systems now tape your call and flash your phone number and address on a computer screen in what has come to be known as "enhanced 911," many smaller systems or ambulance services are not yet equipped to do so. What's more, technology isn't perfect (clear to anyone who's ever lost a day of work when a computer hard drive went down). Do make sure that the dispatcher has heard your full phone number and address, and always include information on pertinent cross streets or nearby highways.

To be on the safe side, Pollino adds, be sure to post your phone number and address on each and every telephone in your house. Then, no matter who's around to handle the emergency, this vital information can be accessed at once.

Emphasizing the importance of this posting, Pollino recalls a case in the suburban neighborhood in which he used to work as a paramedic. A baby was choking and the baby-sitter, unable to help the child herself, correctly called the ambulance. However, when asked for the address, she gave her own. "Fortunately," Pollino says, "the baby-sitter's house was just up the street, so when the ambulance showed up at the curb, the girl's mother was able to tell us where to go."

After you've established your location it's important to tell the dispatcher about the patient's problem as precisely as you can. "Different situations require different medical equipment," Pollino explains. "We don't want paramedics to go into the house or building and have to come right back out to get totally different equipment. That will waste time, so we want specific information about what's the matter with the patient." Important details to give the dispatcher include the patient's symptoms. Remember to note life-threatening problems, including blockage of airways or profuse bleeding, first. Indicate, if possible, whether the patient's condition is the result of an illness or whether the patient was injured, say in a fall or an assault. Do mention the patient's age—a seven-year-old will require different equipment from a seventy-year-old.

The dispatcher may ask what seems like an endless list of questions: Is the patient sitting up or lying down? Is the patient groggy or alert? Does the patient have allergies? Your natural instinct might be to say, "Just send the ambulance!" and hang up, rushing back to the patient. Don't do that. The dispatcher is asking vital questions that will enable the medic crew to dispense appropriate care; he or she may also give you medical advice over the phone so that you can care for the patient yourself until the paramedics arrive. If your friend's arm has been mangled in a printing press, the dispatcher will tell you how to stem the bleeding. If your elderly father has suffered cardiac arrest and is no longer breathing, the dispatcher will talk you through CPR, allowing your dad to hang on for ten minutes or even more before the ambulance arrives. (CPR can often keep the patient going for longer periods of time, especially in cold weather or after submersion in cold water.) It is definitely in the patient's best interest for you to stay on the line.

This is especially important if you're calling from a phone booth, where the dispatcher will not be able to get back in touch with you. "We had a call a while back," Pollino explains. "The caller told us a lady fell on her head and was bleeding from the nose. Then she hung up. The crew went there with their bandaging bag. True, the lady had a bloody nose. The reason was, she dropped dead and fell flat on her face. She had had a heart attack, went into cardiac arrest, wasn't breathing. The caller forgot to tell us that. The crew rushed back to the ambulance to get all their cardiac arrest equipment to try and bring her back. Minutes, crucial minutes, were lost."

Identifying Areas of the Body

When calling Emergency Medical Services to report an emergency it's important that you correctly identify parts of the body. You can plan for this in advance with this artist's rendering identifying areas of the body as designated by emergency personnel and the American Red Cross.

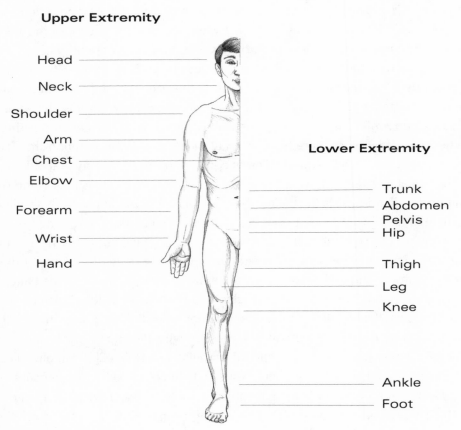

Be Accessible

After you've summoned the ambulance, you must make sure you can be found. "Long before you have an emergency, make sure your address is clearly posted on your house," says Pollino. "You don't know how frustrating it is for paramedics to drive up and down a block unable to find a house because the doorpost numbers aren't there: 'OK, that's number twenty-four, and that's number twenty-eight, so that must be number twenty-six.' Then sometimes we just go knocking on doors." If it's nighttime, make sure your address is well lit, and the houselights are turned up bright. If possible, put a flashing light in the driveway to signal your location.

In cities like New York, a lot of time is wasted because EMS crews cannot get into the locked doors of apartment buildings; because buzzers that are supposed to give them entry from upstairs do not work; because elevators are tied up; and because apartment numbers are not accurately listed on the mailbox or building directory. In extreme emergencies ranging from diabetic seizure to heart attack, these wasted minutes might be lethal. If there are two people available to look after the injured party, we suggest you have one wait in front of your building or house to guide the EMS from the street to the patient. If you live in a building with more than one elevator, commandeer one so it is in the lobby and available when the paramedics arrive. Then they can go right up without waiting at all.

Meanwhile, if possible, have someone in the house or apartment clear the entry-way so it's not blocked by furniture or other objects. If your car is in the driveway, back it out so the ambulance can have easier access to the house. Every time you do something to save the paramedics even ten seconds, you give a critically ill patient an extra chance at life.

Pollino also advises that you lock up any pets, especially dogs, before the paramedics arrive. "Pets tend to be very protective of their masters," he explains. "If somebody is down and not breathing, and they have a pit bull or German shepherd standing over them not letting the ambulance crew in, we can't do anything to save their life. We have to wait for the police to call an emergency service unit that carries tranquilizer darts to sedate the animal before we can do our job." Sometimes, Pollino notes, that means a ten- or fifteen-minute wait. If the person isn't breathing in the first place, by the time the police arrive, it's too late.

EMERGENCY 911 **Tips That Can Save Your Life**

Talk to the dispatcher. If you are having a crisis, you want to get the proper help as soon as possible. For that to happen, you must communicate the problem. Tell the dispatcher the age and sex of the patient and any significant medical history, especially past problems that may be relevant to the present situation.

Know your address. When someone calls 911, the address of the caller may appear automatically on a monitor. However, there is a chance that the address will not show up, and sometimes the location of the problem is not the location of the caller. You cannot be helped if you cannot be found.

Don't hang up the phone. To help you the dispatcher needs as much information as possible. Incomplete calls or change-of-mind hang-up calls mean the dispatcher must call you back for additional information. Precious time should not be wasted when a few seconds can mean the difference between life and death. (Even if you no longer need help, let the dispatcher know everything's OK.)

Speak clearly and calmly. For instance, communicate your address, floor, and room number as individual integers (four, six, Peach Street) and again as whole numbers (forty-six Peach Street). Overpronounce to achieve clarity. The sooner you clarify the nature of the emergency and your exact location, the sooner appropriate help will arrive.

On the Job

Sometimes you're not at home when a medical emergency strikes, but rather, on the job. Though you may not realize it, being in an office surrounded by people can sometimes be isolating; after all, people aren't there to socialize, they're there to work.

Take the recent case of Jack Miller, a computer specialist who suffered a heart attack at his terminal. In the midst of all his coworkers, he was too weak to shout; hidden in his cubicle, he could not be seen. When Miller first felt the chest pain, he later related to the New York *Daily News,* he called his doctor but was put on hold. Soon he was gasping for air. "I was going, and nobody would have noticed," Miller explained. But before he passed out, he had a flash: He could type an SOS and send it out over E-mail. After all, everyone in the office was on-line: HELP. FEEL SICK. I NEED AID, Miller, a fifty-six-year-old employee of Witco Corp. in Woodcliff Lake, New Jersey, managed to type. "I could barely tap out the words," he said. "My chest had this strange coldness, and I just couldn't breathe." But within seconds, dozens of coworkers at the chemical company were darting through the maze of cubicles to help Miller. Some administered CPR, others summoned the EMS. "For me, 'E-mail' means 'emergency mail,'" concludes Miller now alive and well at age fifty-six.

In fact, Jack Miller is more than a little lucky to be alive. Unless your office has an emergency communication network and a preestablished response protocol, it may not be the best place to take ill.

Preparing the office for emergency response is the concern of Richard Marsella, Director of St. Luke's–Roosevelt Hospital's Fast Care^{SM}, a private emergency ambulance service contracted to a number of major facilities and corporations, including Lincoln Center, Time Warner, the Marriott-Marquis Hotel, Paine Webber, CBS, Carnegie Hall, the ocean liner QE2, Viacom, and Radio City Music Hall. In addition to providing ambulance service for these organizations, Marsella explains, Fast Care^{SM} consults with companies so their response to medical emergencies can be as well-organized, as efficient, and effective as possible.

As a first step, Marsella explains, Fast Care^{SM} helps corporate staffs recognize medical emergencies and trains interested employees in first aid and CPR. "We make it clear that all participants are involved on a voluntary basis. Once trained, their job description is not going to change. And people are told that on any given day they may decide to be a good Samaritan, or they may decline to provide hands-on aid."

The voluntary nature of citizen response is vital to the recruitment process, Marsella explains. "It's also necessary so companies can avoid liability that would result if they tried to compel employees to provide first aid. Those trained as first responders must also receive education about blood-borne diseases like AIDS and hepatitis, and training in the use of universal precautions, especially protective barriers like latex gloves and pocket resuscitation masks."

Fast Care^{SM} also helps to establish in-office emergency networks so that problems can be dealt with correctly and expeditiously. The networks, Marsella found, vary from one corporate culture or style to the next. For instance, he notes, "In one law firm we worked with, when people fell ill they would notify their receptionist, Rosa, who had been the company's 'mother figure' for the past twenty years." Other companies relied on in-house nurses, security guards, or even the people in the personnel office. Some places had no policy or procedure for handling medical incidents at all.

If the company has no set procedure, Fast Care[SM] helps to establish one, Marsella explains. If there is a policy, Fast Care[SM] helps to streamline it, then makes certain it is institutionalized—that is, more or less set in stone. "We recommend that each of our clients has a formal, written policy and procedure for managing illness and injury," Marsella says. "Then we train key personnel—those who will be responsible decision makers or coordinators should a medical emergency occur." If security guards are in charge, for instance, they are taught when to call an ambulance, when to alert colleagues trained in first aid or CPR, and when to suspect the individual might just need some lunch. Workers, in turn, are taught to call security the moment a medical problem occurs. If "Rosa in reception" is the conduit, she will be given a protocol for summoning help from both inside and outside the organization, says Marsella. "People are taught that if an employee is having a heart attack or difficulty breathing, they must call the ambulance before they call the person's spouse or private physician. The in-office notification system also ensures that someone is sent to meet the ambulance crew, that someone holds the elevator, and that someone stays with the patient at all times. Someone (usually a friend) should also accompany the patient to the hospital. Fast Care[SM] companies are taught to include *all* employees in the emergency medical network. In-house telephone directories, orientation materials for all new employees, interoffice memos, and postings at water coolers or in kitchenettes are all methods that can be used to ensure that everyone becomes familiar with the emergency medical notification procedure. "Every single employee learns that if a colleague complains of feeling ill, they are not to keep it under their hat." They must follow the established procedure and contact the individual responsible for summoning first responders and professional outside help.

Fast Care[SM] tenets can be put to work in your place of business. At least try to make sure that some people on site have training in first aid and cardiopulmonary resuscitation. Designate one or two people to serve as liaison between the ill or injured person and "responders," from colleagues trained in CPR to the fire department to EMS. Without a plan of action, valuable minutes might be lost. Unprepared employees may be hesitant to act, or they may react quickly and inappropriately. A Fast Care–type system of notification and response can make a difference, and may even prevent a worker's disability or save a life. If this won't work in your company, then make sure everyone has all the appropriate phone numbers affixed to their telephones or posted by their desks.

Marsella advises avoiding a common mistake made in the workplace when illness or injury strikes. "Often, when visiting companies, I'll find that they have what's called a 'quiet room,'" Marsella explains. "It's usually a pleasant little room with a couch, perhaps a medicine cabinet with some aspirin and gauze pads. The person taking me around will proudly say, 'See? When people feel ill, we bring them here, where they can rest quietly.' That's a dangerous thing to do. I like to give the example of the truck driver who told his boss he felt dizzy and nauseated. The boss said, 'Just wait in the cab of the truck, and when your relief gets here, we'll figure out what to do.' When the next shift arrived, the guy was dead." Don't leave a sick worker to sit alone in a quiet room, a ladies' room, a lounge. Report the illness to a designated person, be it "Rosa," the security guard, or someone else. The in-house number must *always* be answered by that person or a surrogate throughout the workday. If that person deems it necessary, call the paramedics. If it's a mistake and the person does not really require a trip to the ED, the paramedics can always give advice and leave. For optimum safety—and protection against liability—places of business, including theaters, hotels, and other public facilities must stipulate a specific method of reporting serious illness or injury to avoid delay in obtaining emergency medical service. This type of policy is a critical part of any organization's risk management program, and constitutes a commitment of responsibility to employees, patrons, and guests.

Choosing the Right Emergency Department

After you've summoned the ambulance or gone to the car with a helpful friend, you're ready to make your way to the hospital. But where should you go? If you've called a public ambulance, you may not have a choice. Paramedics in New York, for instance, are supposed to take you to the closest facility, unless there's a clear-cut reason not to. If a limb has been detached, they may take you to the nearest place capable of microsurgery. If the victim is a child, they will go to the nearest pediatric emergency facility. After all, if you're critically ill, it behooves the ambulance to get you to the closest *appropriate* medical facility as quickly as it can. Of course, sometimes, if the injury is not life-threatening, paramedics will honor a specific request.

If you're allowed to make a request, or if you're arriving on your own, how should you decide? The answer will vary depending on your condition and what's available in your area. The first step is to acquaint yourself with the various emergency departments in your area before a problem occurs. To choose the right emergency department you must investigate the staff credentials and available specialties of all the hospitals in your area in advance.

To start your investigation, ask your personal physician. Where does he or she have admitting privileges? Where does your doctor suggest you go for each of a number of problems, including general illness, heart attack, stroke, broken bones, and psychiatric distress? Where should you take the children? Where should you go in the event of a serious injury?

After getting information from your doctor, do research the situation yourself. If you have friends who are doctors, nurses, or paramedics, ask them. You may also ask neighbors who have had experience in various emergency departments.

In many instances, it's best to go to the facility where your private doctor has admitting privileges. If your doctor knows you're on the way in, she can often call ahead to grease the wheels to facilitate your care. She can consult with the attending emergency physician to help you receive appropriate care. If need be, she can come in and, along with the emergency staff, take a look at you.

But in cases of extreme emergency, a different hospital might be best. In general, the best emergency departments are directed by physicians trained and board certified in emergency medicine. These board-certified doctors should be in the emergency department around the clock to supervise your treatment every step of the way. Just as there are doctors who are trained and board certified in surgery, psychiatry, or pediatrics, there are physicians who are specially trained and board certified in emergency medicine. After four years of medical school, they complete three or four years of residency-training programs in emergency medicine. Under the supervision of fully trained emergency physicians, these emergency medicine residents learn the thought process, the medical skills, and the basic facts that will allow them to practice emergency medicine. After this residency is completed, emergency physicians are qualified to take a certifying examination—one day of written tests, and, one year later, an all-day oral test. Once the doctor passes these exams, he or she will be certified by a recognized board of emergency medicine. Not all physicians working in all emergency departments are "residency trained" or "board certified." Each is a sign of skill and knowledge in emergency medicine; they are valuable markers of quality in an emergency physician. A good emergency department will be staffed by highly qualified emergency physicians. To determine whether an emergency department is top-notch, do ask what percentage of physicians are board certified in emergency medicine. (In a large metropolitan ED, look for at least one, but preferably two or more, of these certified emergency doctors present in the department at any given time. Those with such expertise should be available to you twenty-four hours a day.)

Do not be fooled by a hospital's credentials. Even some highly regarded teaching hospitals may have residents and interns working in the ED with little supervision. Others, particularly those with residency programs in emergency medicine, will have topflight, highly regarded, and seasoned emergency physicians in attendance with the residents at all times. When an experienced and qualified emergency physician is there to supervise the operation on site, the level of care should be fine.

Also check out the availability of physician care. Some emergency departments don't have physicians present twenty-four hours a day. In the wee hours of the morning, you might find a physician assistant or nurse-practitioner running the show. That's fine if you have a cold or sore throat, but if you're having a heart attack, it's probably not the place to go.

You should also find out whether the support staff includes registered nurses and full-time employees or freelancers and temps. The ED nursing staff is absolutely crucial. Often the glue that holds the emergency department together, it's nurses who are right there on the front lines. Those who are experienced can recognize symptoms of heart attack, cardiac arrest, shock, stroke, and dozens of other maladies while less qualified or less experienced counterparts may not. They are there to act as your advocate and guide. A knowledgeable nurse will make sure you get the right treatment— and fast. Indeed, an ED nurse with fifteen years' experience may pick up on a problem long before the on-duty intern physician in training, who's been in the department just a month. He or she can be your lifeline to the care you need.

Investigate the types of specialists associated with local emergency departments. If you have a heart attack, will a cardiologist be called in? Other specialties to look for include pediatrics, psychiatry, obstetrics, neurosurgery, ophthalmology, orthopedics, urology, and plastic surgery. A child with a four-inch slash across his face may avoid the embarrassment of an unsightly scar for life if the stitches are done by a well-qualified emergency physician or a plastic surgeon trained and experienced in suturing.

Find out what specialties a hospital boasts. Is the hospital reknowned for cardiac care, its psychiatric facilities, its pediatric division? If you've broken your hip, where's the best place to go? Perhaps an orthopedic hospital. Similarly, if you've hurt your eye you may want to go to a specialized eye hospital.

There are certain facilities and specialties that are particularly important. Some emergency departments, for instance, have developed special expertise in dealing with heart disease. At St. Luke's–Roosevelt that means a group of doctors and nurses called the MI team (for myocardial infarction, or heart attack) will have treated and stabilized a patient within minutes of the time that he or she arrives at the emergency department.

Also investigate the particular trauma equipment available at your local ED, because technology may vary drastically from one facility to the next. Virtually all hospitals have cardiac units, intensive care units, and operating rooms. However, many lack CAT scans, essential for evaluating head injuries, strokes, and sudden internal bleeding. Long before you are brought to an emergency department with such a life-threatening wound or illness, you must make sure the facility can handle your problem. Otherwise, you may waste precious time.

Make sure you know the location of the trauma center closest to your home. Contrary to popular opinion, the trauma center is not part of the emergency department, but rather, connected to it. The emergency department is the portal to the trauma center, which is a specialized hospital unto itself. Trauma centers must have their own operating rooms, intensive care units, and rehabilitation units, and their own surgeons, doctors, and nurses, enabling them to provide comprehensive care from the moment of entry by ambulance until the moment of discharge. If you've been hit by a truck, if you've been stabbed in the chest, if you've been thrown from a horse and have shattered your spine, a trauma center is, when possible, the place to go.

Though you may not have one in your immediate vicinity, investigate the location of the nearest burn center. Burns, particularly extensive burns, require specialized management. Most major metropolitan areas will have one burn center. In many parts of the country you may be transported two hundred miles by emergency helicopter to get to a burn center. With a serious burn, call 911 or whatever number connects you to your local ambulance and let them do the rest. Nonetheless, it can't hurt to know if you have a burn center down the street.

Parents must determine whether the emergency department is equipped to treat children. Children are not just little adults. They have different diseases that require different medications and radically different treatments from those administered to adults. They require special equipment, including intravenous equipment for smaller veins and breathing tubes for smaller tracheae. Their medicine must be delivered in smaller, precisely measured dosages. Sometimes they require medicine and equipment that is not just smaller, but totally different from that used for adults. Not all EDs have specialized pediatric equipment or a staff capable of recognizing and treating the varied diseases that occur only in children. (See Chapter 7 for details.)

When investigating hospitals, it's also important to look beyond the emergency department. Does the hospital have an intensive care unit or a cardiac care unit? If you're pregnant, you may be interested in a hospital that has not just a delivery room, but also a specialized neonatal intensive care unit, in case your baby is born prematurely or with some other problem.

Assess what you need and locate it in advance by talking with your family doctor and by calling various emergency departments, list of questions in hand. Speak with an emergency physician or head nurse to assess the facility and take notes that you can readily refer to should an emergency arise.

Emergency Medical Service workers who drive an ambulance through one of New York City's outer boroughs confess that when elderly people break a hip they may, if possible, be driven to a hospital specializing in orthopedics in an adjacent borough. "Some emergency rooms will not handle some problems as expertly," one paramedic confides, "and if we feel the patient can take the longer ride, we'll take him to the facility where he's likely to do best."

Some Final Advice

If possible, before you leave for the hospital, call and alert your personal physician. Remember to take important phone numbers and papers, including ID cards, insurance papers, and a list of your medications and medical history. Don't forget to take some cash.

For a quick reminder, before leaving the house for the emergency department, try to collect the items referred to on the list below, which you may post on your wall.

Emergency Checklist

❏ ID cards

❏ Insurance papers

❏ Previously prepared summary of medical history and medications

❏ Money for phone calls and transportation

❏ Emergency numbers

If the situation allows, gather the materials quickly, perhaps while waiting for medics to arrive. Even better, have copies all put together in an easily located single envelope; grab and follow the ambulance.

To access emergency care as quickly as possible, fill out the following form, remove from this book, and post by the phone.

Emergency Phone List

Ambulance Service
name
phone
Emergency Departments in My Area

Closest Emergency Department
hospital name
phone
address
travel directions (emergency entrance)

Emergency Department Where My Doctor Has Admitting Privileges
hospital name
phone
address
travel directions (emergency entrance)

Cardiac Care Emergency Department
hospital name
phone
address
travel directions (emergency entrance)

Pediatric Emergency Department
hospital name
phone
address
travel directions (emergency entrance)

Trauma Center Emergency Department
hospital name
phone
address
travel directions (emergency entrance)

Burn Center Emergency Department
hospital name
phone
address
travel directions (emergency entrance)

Psychiatric Care Emergency Department
hospital name
phone
address
travel directions (emergency entrance)

Personal Physicians for Every Family Member

Family Member	MD	Day Phone	Answering Service

Pharmacies
(the closest)
Name
Address
(open 24 hours)
Name
Address

Poison Control Center

Child Abuse Hotline

Crime Victims Hotline

Sexual Abuse Hotline

Fire

Police

Gas Leaks

Personal Contacts in Case of Emergency
name
address

phone

Chapter 3

The Backyard Medic: Everyperson's Guide to Basic First Aid

I t was September 1990 when seventeen-year-old John Soper, a high school junior, suffered cardiac arrest. Things could have been worse: He had his attack during a break in the second inning of an Orioles-Mariners baseball game at Baltimore's Memorial Stadium. A groundskeeper at the stadium, Soper collapsed in center field not far from coworker Pat Santarone, who, luckily, was skilled in cardiopulmonary resuscitation (CPR). Rushing to young Soper's side, Santarone felt for a pulse. Finding none, he started administering rescue breathing and chest compressions, the CPR two-step. And he wasn't alone. Trauma and emergency physicians out for a day at the game rushed from the stands to help too. Among the three physicians ultimately involved in the lifesaving procedures were a cardiac trauma specialist and one of the Orioles' team doctors. Rescuers thought they had lost Soper twice, but eventually they brought him back.

For Soper, collapsing in the middle of a ball field, next to his colleague who knew CPR, in plain sight of experts was fantastic luck indeed. According to recent statistics, at least a quarter-million Americans a year, one every two minutes on average, collapse when their hearts suddenly stop or short-circuit into chaotic rhythm—the condition known as cardiac arrest. If the victim is lucky, there's someone nearby who can immediately call for help and then start CPR to get blood circulating until the paramedics arrive.

The Chain of Survival

When it comes to cardiac arrest, the ultimate enemy is time. If the pulse is not restarted in minutes, blood and oxygen will halt their life-giving journey to the brain and damage will be irreversible. Thus, victims must quickly enter what the American Heart Association calls the "chain of survival." First there must be an immediate call to the emergency medical service (EMS)—911. Then, within four minutes a concerned bystander must begin administering CPR. Paramedics must arrive within eight to ten minutes equipped with a defibrillator machine that can shock the erratically beating heart back to normal. And finally, the resuscitated patient must be transported to the emergency department. Any break in the links of this survival chain, and death is the likely result.

In many settings, entree to this system is hard to come by. In New York and other crowded urban centers, a sense of anonymity and suspicion, looming high-rise buildings, and the inevitable traffic gridlock, all serve to limit success. The victim may be mistaken for a drug addict or drunk. Potential citizen responders, inundated with news of rampant tuberculosis and AIDS, may fear close contact with a stranger. And professional responders, including police and firefighters, emergency medical technicians, and paramedics, may have trouble navigating the streets, resulting in a survival rate of less than 2 percent. The stats aren't much better in rural areas, where isolation can be profound.

The story is different in suburban Seattle, where victims of a witnessed cardiac arrest recover an impressive 25–30 percent of the time, representing the upper limit of survival. Part of Seattle's success has to do with its infrastructure. Clear roads and low-rise buildings allow paramedics to negotiate the environment, facilitating a speedy response time. The mind-set of this Northwest region is also vital. Still imbued with a small-town sensibility, drivers tend to yield to emergency vehicles immediately. But perhaps most important, large numbers of citizens in Seattle are trained in CPR, thanks to the fire department's superb educational programs. (One local joke has it that Seattle is the worst place in the country to faint in public. More likely than not, you'll find a bystander compressing your chest before you hit the pavement, overjoyed at the opportunity finally to use that training!)

For the rest of us, catching some of this enthusiasm would be a healthy thing. In fact, if the statistics from Seattle are any indication, we could all benefit from training in cardiopulmonary resuscitation and basic first aid. From clearing the airway of a choking victim to stopping loss of blood, the mastery of some vital techniques may enable you to bring those you love back from the brink of death and assist them in times of need.

Your first-aid skills won't go to waste. According to the American Red Cross, United

States citizens suffer almost two million disabling injuries in the workplace each year. Each year injury results in some two million hospitalizations and more than one hundred forty thousand deaths. Accident is the leading cause of death for people under age forty-five. But sudden illness is a killer as well—cardiovascular disease kills about a million Americans a year, while one hundred fifty thousand succumb to stroke.

The First Link: The Citizen Responder

In most of these instances the outcome can be improved when a Good Samaritan—a layperson trained in first aid or CPR—jumps in to help. As the first and often the most important link in the chain of survival, this "citizen responder" can activate the emergency medical service, summoning medical experts and caring for the victim until these experts arrive.

To recognize medical emergencies, refer to this book's first chapter, "State of Siege." But as a citizen responder committed to helping others, you've got to stay attuned to cues from the environment as well. Unusual odors, sights, and sounds can all signal the possibility that a medical emergency is afoot. Screams and moans, the sound of crashing metal, or the smell of smoke are obvious signs of trouble. You must also key into subtler signs: an overturned pot on the kitchen floor; pills spilled across the sink in the bathroom; any strong or unrecognizable odor.

If something seems wrong, do not just rush in like the cavalry. After all, if the victim has been stricken by poison gas, or a downed electric line, you don't want the same fate to befall you. If you sense there's danger from spilled chemicals, oncoming traffic, fire, call for help. Police and firefighters, not ordinary civilians, are the ones who have the training and equipment to deal with such threatening situations. Besides, if you are injured as well, you will be of little service to others.

After you have checked out the possibility of danger, continue to observe. How many victims are there? Remember, the most seriously injured victims are frequently the quietest, because they may be unconscious. Are there any children or babies at the scene?

You've spent a few seconds taking it all in, and now, if you feel it's appropriate, you may provide some help. First, you must determine whether or not the victim is conscious. Is she awake? Possibly moving? Is he moaning or groaning? If the victim is obviously conscious, first simply elicit information. Can the person tell you what happened? Does he have any illness or medical condition that has a bearing in any way on this situation?

If the victim seems unconscious, make an effort to verify. To do so, take both hands and, gently pushing against the shoulders, shout: "Are you OK? Are you OK?" If there's no response, assume she's unconscious. At that point, if at all possible, make sure an ambulance is called at once. If you're the only one around, shout for help in hopes that a passerby can call an ambulance while you stay with the victim. If there's no assistance available, and if the victim is older than age eight, you should leave to call an ambulance yourself before doing anything else. For a victim under age eight, stay in place through the sequence of steps that follow. In this case, your rescue breathing and CPR skills may be more important than anything the ambulance can offer. You will eventually need to call for help, but not now.

As soon as the ambulance has been summoned you must check the victim for the trusted ABC's of survival: an open airway, regular breathing, and circulation (or pulse). To start, make sure the victim is lying on his or her back. If the person is crumpled face-down, roll him over as a unit—"log roll" the victim—so that the head and torso move at once. Then place your ear near the victim's mouth and nose and listen for the sound of breathing for about five seconds. At the same time, watch the chest to see if it rises and falls.

Remember, except to roll a patient over to check for breathing, you are not to move an injured party unless you are faced with the rushing waters of the Mississippi overflowing its banks; the smell of poison gas; or an encroaching wall of flame. (You get the point.) Moving an injured person without the proper equipment will, very possibly, make the injury worse. If you must move the injured party, do so as quickly and carefully as you can.

Opening the Airway

If you detect no breathing, perhaps the airway, or trachea, has been obstructed by the tongue and epiglottis, which normally serves to prevent food and drink from "going down the wrong tube." As a person loses consciousness, the muscles, including jaw muscles, relax; since the tongue and epiglottis are connected to the lower jaw, muscle relaxation may actually cause obstruction of the airway.

In many instances, aiding the victim may be as simple as opening the airway with a simple technique known as the "head tilt/chin lift." To execute, place the palm of your hand on the victim's forehead and push back gently. This will cause the head to tilt or rotate back. (For an adult, you may extend the neck firmly; for a child under eight, use gentle pressure; for an infant, be extremely gentle.) Then, hook the fingers of the other hand under the bony part of the lower jaw. Lift up and forward on the chin until the teeth are nearly closed. (Be certain you lift only on the bony part of the jaw, since pressure on the soft area near the throat could further obstruct the airway.)

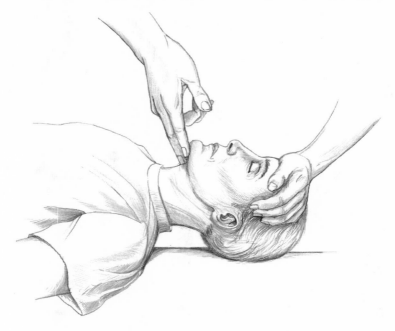

Every Breath You Take

With the airway opened the victim may start breathing on his own. Listen for signs of breathing for about five seconds. If you detect no breathing, you must attempt to restart respiration with the technique known as "rescue breathing."

To execute, pinch the victim's nose shut and make a tight seal around the victim's mouth with your own. The technique is the same for children, but different for infants: Cover the infant's mouth and nose with your mouth. Simultaneously keeping the airway open through the head tilt/chin lift illustrated here, breathe slowly and gently into the victim's mouth until you see the chest rise; the breath should last for about a second and a half. Pause to let the air flow out. Then breathe into the victim's mouth once again. (You can buy a simple face mask in the pharmacy to protect yourself from others' germs. Place the mesh mask between your mouth and that of the victim, and follow through.)

If the chest does not rise and fall you may assume the airway is still obstructed. Repeat the head tilt/chin lift technique and try again. If you still meet with resistance, you may assume the obstruction is a foreign body, like a piece of food.

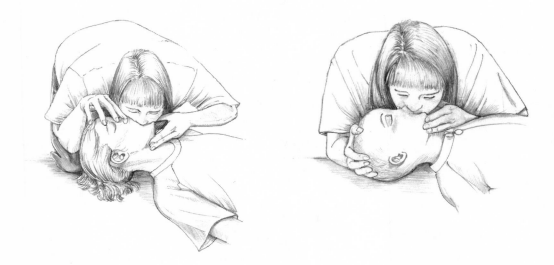

Thank You, Dr. Heimlich

If the airway is blocked by a foreign object, the victim might well be choking to death. Sometimes, choking is obvious: A man eating sirloin at a steak house suddenly starts grabbing his throat with both hands, the universally accepted signal for choking. A toddler playing with a basket of toys suddenly puts one in his mouth and starts gagging. Also be on the lookout for signs that may not be as obvious: the inability to talk or even make a sound, a bluish cast to the skin and lips, loss of consciousness may all be due to choking.

As soon as you realize choking is the culprit, you can utilize the technique developed by Cincinnati physician Harry Heimlich in 1974. The idea for the maneuver struck Dr. Heimlich when he became aware that choking was the sixth leading cause of accidental death in the United States. An expert in the workings of the esophagus and trachea and an inventor of a number of innovative medical techniques, he felt he could arrive at some practical antidote to choking. All that was required was some thought on the problem, a study of the exact mechanics, and a period of experimentation with dogs.

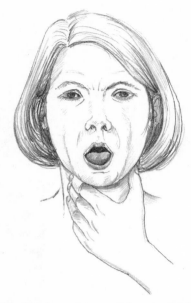

Heimlich eventually submitted a paper on his new technique, which harnessed air already in the lungs to force the offensive object from the body. At first his maneuver was controversial. (So much so, claims Heimlich, that some opposing doctors even accused him of anesthetizing a patient and then forcibly lodging a chunk of meat with a piece of string attached in his trachea in order to illustrate the procedure!) But eventually the technique caught on. Though Heimlich was fond of saying that he himself never had the occasion to perform the maneuver on a living human in a true emergency situation, many others have. With illustrated instructions for the celebrated maneuver posted in nearly every restaurant, the technique is responsible for saving many tens of thousands of lives, including those of Elizabeth Taylor, Ronald Reagan, and Cher.

Performance of the Heimlich maneuver will vary, depending upon the victim's position, state of consciousness, and age. But no matter whose life you think you might be saving, remember one thing: Never, ever practice the techniques described below on another person. Use only a mannequin, ideally during an American Red Cross or American Heart Association course. If the choker is standing, walk behind him and, to steady yourself, place one foot behind him and another alongside. If he is sitting, the back of the chair can provide this essential support. In either case, wrap your arms around the victim's waist. Make a fist, with the thumb side of your fist against the victim's abdomen, just a bit above the navel. Grasp your fist with the other hand and press quickly into the abdomen with an upward thrust. If the object does not come free after

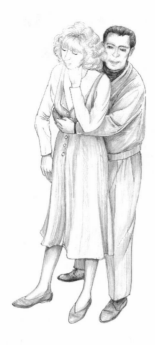
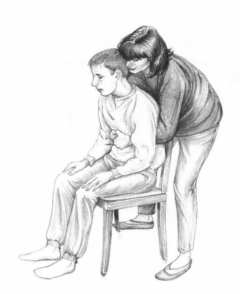

five thrusts, reevaluate the position of your hands and then try again. Continue to thrust and reevaluate, thrust and reevaluate, until the object is dislodged.

For a child or infant obviously choking on food or a toy, you must, of course, modify your efforts. For the child, follow the same procedure specified for adults, but do make sure your thrusts are not overly powerful.

Since such abdominal thrusts can injure an *infant* under about eighteen months of age use another technique instead: Turn the infant over, with head slightly lower than chest, and use your hand to deliver five back thrusts between the shoulder blades. Do modulate these blows so they are powerful enough to dislodge the object, yet not so strong that they injure the baby. Then turn the infant over and deliver five chest thrusts with two fingers of one hand; the fingers should be held in a narrow V, almost as if you are making a victory sign. Visually check the mouth for debris after each cycle, but do not sweep your finger through the oral cavity, since you may then push the foreign body back into the throat.

If the airway has been blocked for too long without relief, victims will lose consciousness. When an infant loses consciousness, alternate each thrusting cycle with two breaths, as described in the rescue-breathing section earlier.

For adults and children, slide the victim to the floor, roll him onto his back, and

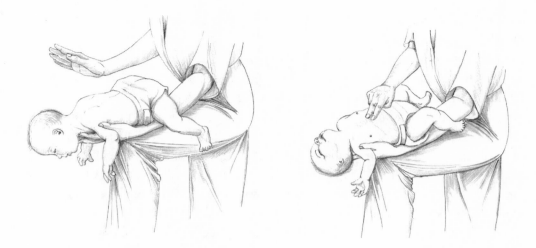

call Emergency Medical Service. Then get back to work. (If you find a victim already uncon-scious, try rescue breathing first. If, during rescue breathing, the victim's chest does not rise with ventilation, you may assume there's an object lodged in the throat. Follow through as outlined, below.) Kneel and straddle the victim's thighs. With one hand directly over the other, place the heel of your hand in the middle of the victim's abdomen, a little above the navel. Be sure your hands are not placed too high; you don't want to break any ribs.

Press quickly into the abdomen and upward toward the head. The force of the thrust should be along the midline of the body, not off to either side. Remember, you are trying to marshal the force of the air inside the lungs to push the object out. Like

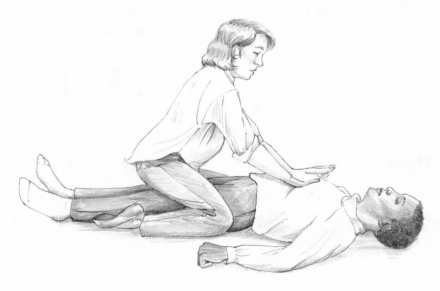

someone pumping a balloon, you may find it effective to perform as many as five thrusts in rapid succession.

After five of these "abdominal thrusts," you are ready to check for the object in the victim's throat or mouth. To do so, grasp the lower jaw, place your thumb on the tongue, and wrap your fingers around the chin. Now lift the jaw to open the mouth and, using your index finger, sweep the mouth for debris. (If you'd prefer, you may don latex gloves, available in any pharmacy, for this task.) Run your finger across the back of the throat and both sides of the mouth and, if necessary, remove dentures.

Hopefully your efforts will be successful; the object will shoot out of the victim's throat and breathing will resume. If the person regains consciousness, you're home free. But this is a best-case scenario. There may be other outcomes as well.

For instance, you may find that despite your best efforts, you are unable to free the object lodged in the victim's throat. In that case, continue with five more abdominal thrusts, followed by rescue breathing, followed by more abdominal thrusts, and so on; as you continue your ministrations, the victim's muscles may relax, allowing the obstruction to come free.

Or, you may find that even though the object has been dislodged and even though the victim can now breathe spontaneously, he does not regain consciousness. In that instance, maintain an open airway using the head tilt/chin lift technique and wait for professional help to arrive.

Sometimes the choking victim will not resume breathing even after the offensive object has popped free. If that's the case, give two breaths using the rescue-breathing technique, then check for a pulse. If you find a pulse, continue rescue breathing, as described above, until the victim can breathe on his own, or until professional help arrives.

If there's no pulse, it's possible that lack of oxygen has thrown the victim into cardiac arrest. In that case, you must move forward with CPR techniques described below.

The Beating Heart

Those of us lucky enough to be alive have a pulse—the beat felt in the arteries with each contraction of the heart. If someone has no pulse, circulation is disrupted because the beating of the heart has ceased. The person is in cardiac arrest; without aggressive intervention, death is guaranteed.

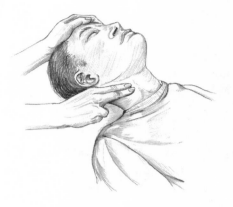
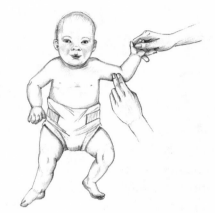

To check for pulse run two fingers along the victim's neck until you find the carotid artery. In infants you must seek out the brachial pulse in the upper arm. You may take up to ten seconds to gently locate a pulse.

If someone is breathing, he also has a pulse, even if you can't detect it. If he isn't breathing and he has no pulse, his heart has stopped.

Once the heart has stopped, seconds count. Without the contractions of the cardiac muscle, oxygen-rich blood cannot be pumped to the brain; and for the brain, oxygen starvation is rapid. If deprived of oxygen for more than four minutes the brain starts an irrevocable slide to destruction. In other words, you have four minutes to start cardiopulmonary resuscitation.

If you find a victim in cardiac arrest, we suggest you have someone else call Emergency Medical Service while you initiate cardiopulmonary resuscitation. (EMS must be told that the victim's pulse has stopped so paramedics will be dispatched with special equipment and medication.) If you're the only one around, start CPR and continue for one minute to get some oxygen to the brain. Then stop to call Emergency Medical Service and resume CPR until help arrives.

You can keep someone going on cardiopulmonary resuscitation for quite a while but not indefinitely, since CPR provides only about one third the normal blood flow to the brain. Most of the time you need medical professionals to step in and bring the rescue to a successful conclusion. A well-stocked ambulance will carry equipment to assist CPR; a defibrillator machine that sends a shock through the chest, causing the heart to beat properly again; medicine to keep the heart going until the patient has reached the hospital; and, most important, skilled and experienced paramedics. While it is important that you start CPR, calling the ambulance could be your most important job.

The Four-Minute Mile: The Road to Rescue by CPR

To become adept at cardiopulmonary resuscitation you should be certified. You can take a course offered by the Red Cross or the American Heart Association. For parents it's possible to take courses that focus on CPR for the very young; you may also consider enrolling your regular baby-sitter. Depending on the level of skill you desire, your course work can span a couple of hours or several weeks. And true skill doesn't stop there. Because perfect execution of the CPR technique requires precise motor coordination and split-second timing, only practice makes perfect. That's why you'll find those best at delivering CPR are lifeguards, nurses, paramedics, and doctors—in other words, those who use the technique all the time. Remember, as with the Heimlich Maneuver, practice only on a mannequin, not another person.

This doesn't mean that in an emergency, when someone's life is at risk, you can't perform CPR yourself. Any CPR, even poorly executed, is better than no CPR, and often even the frantic thrusts of a distraught relative practicing the technique on a wing and a prayer will save the day, providing the brain with enough life-sustaining oxygen until the true experts arrive. To help you through the motions, we provide instructions.

A CPR Primer

To start, make sure the patient is lying flat on the back, on a hard surface like a floor. If the victim is in bed, the soft mattress will limit the success of your efforts. Do move the patient as carefully as possible.

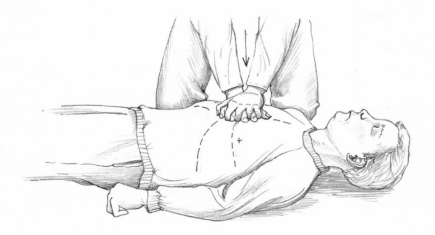

The first step will be the rescue breathing described above: Give two quick breaths and then compress the chest so that blood flows through the body to vital organs, including the brain. Kneel beside the victim, placing yourself halfway between the head and the waist. Lean over the chest and, with one hand, find the notch where the lower part of the breastbone meets the ribs. (To find this "compression landmark" in children, follow much the same procedure you use for adults. In infants, look for the landmark approximately one finger-width below the nipple line.)

Into the soft depression one finger from the bottom of the breastbone place the heel of your hand. Clasp the hand with your other hand.

Keep your shoulders directly over your hands and keep your elbows locked. Then, when you press down, the weight of your upper body will create the force you need to compress the chest. (For a child under age eight, compress with the heel of just one hand. For an infant, use only two fingers.)

Push straight down, allowing the heel of your hand to sink about two inches into the soft breastbone depression in which it rests. Keep it there for about a second and then release the pressure. Keep your hand in contact with the victim's chest, while allowing it to return to its normal position. Give fifteen such compressions in a row.

After you've given fifteen compressions, open the airway with the head tilt/chin lift technique described earlier. Then, using the technique for rescue breathing, deliver two slow breaths. This compression breathing cycle should take about fifteen seconds.

Repeat the cycle three more times and then take about five seconds to check the victim for breathing and pulse.

CPR ILLUSTRATED IN SIX STEPS

Step 1: Find hand position on breastbone.
Step 2: Position shoulders over hand; compress chest 15 times.
Step 3: Give 2 slow breaths.
Step 4: Do 3 more sets of 15 compressions and 2 breaths.
Step 5: Recheck pulse and breathing for about 5 seconds.
Step 6: Do 3 more sets of 15 compressions and 2 breaths.

THE CPR COVENANT

Once you start to administer cardiopulmonary resuscitation, you cannot stop compressing and breathing, compressing and breathing, until the experts arrive.

To do so would be to consign the patient over to brain damage and, probably, death. There are just four accepted reasons for abandoning your mission of medical mercy:

· Another trained person takes over CPR for you.

· EMS personnel arrive and assume care of the victim.

· You are so exhausted you are about to collapse. You just cannot go on.

· The scene becomes unsafe.

By initiating CPR you have assumed a grave responsibility. Try your hardest to bring it to a successful conclusion.

Please cut out the following box and paste it on a piece of cardboard. Carry it with you in your wallet for ready reference.

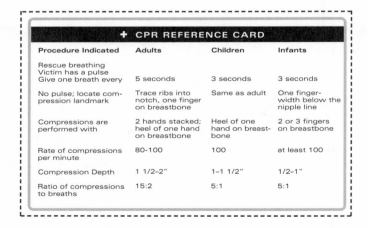

✚ CPR REFERENCE CARD			
Procedure Indicated	**Adults**	**Children**	**Infants**
Rescue breathing Victim has a pulse Give one breath every	5 seconds	3 seconds	3 seconds
No pulse; locate compression landmark	Trace ribs into notch, one finger on breastbone	Same as adult	One finger-width below the nipple line
Compressions are performed with	2 hands stacked; heel of one hand on breastbone	Heel of one hand on breastbone	2 or 3 fingers on breastbone
Rate of compressions per minute	80-100	100	at least 100
Compression Depth	1 1/2–2″	1–1 1/2″	1/2–1″
Ratio of compressions to breaths	15:2	5:1	5:1

ORDINARY PRECAUTIONS, EXTRAORDINARY RISKS

In this age of AIDS, drug-resistant tuberculosis, and a host of other communicable diseases that can pass from person to person through blood, saliva, or (in the case of tuberculosis) even the air, the citizen responder must protect him/herself, especially when aiding strangers. Here are a few guidelines from the American Red Cross:

- Avoid contact with body fluids (blood, saliva, and vomitus) when possible.

- Use barriers such as disposable gloves to cover any cuts, scrapes, and skin conditions you may have. You do not want potentially infected blood entering your body through these channels.

- Carry a pocket mask to place between your mouth and the mouth of the victim when administering CPR.

- Wash your hands with soap and water immediately after providing care.

- Do not eat, drink, or touch your mouth, nose, or eyes when giving first aid.

- Do not touch objects that may be soiled with blood.

- Be prepared by having a first-aid kit handy.

STRANGERS IN THE NIGHT

In New York these days, restaurants and theaters must have pocket masks and latex gloves to facilitate performance of cardiopulmonary resuscitation. These lifesaving supplies may be found in restaurants and theaters in other parts of the country as well.

If you happen to be dining out or attending a play and witness a stranger suffering cardiac arrest, you might feel reluctant to perform CPR. However, if the facility can provide you with basic protective supplies, including mask and gloves, you will be able to intervene, risk-free.

In the eventuality that you must perform CPR on a stranger in one of these locations, request gloves and mask before you begin. Put the mask between your mouth and the victim's so that germ transmission is reduced. Wear the gloves to protect your hands while you sweep the mouth or expose yourself to any bodily fluids.

CAN THE CITIZEN RESPONDER BE SUED?

You see a man collapsed on the street corner. He's definitely unconscious; rushing to his side, you discover he's not even breathing. Certified in cardiopulmonary resuscitation, you know you may be able to help. While someone in the crowd calls the ambulance you get to work. You labor over the victim for some twenty minutes, breathing and pumping, breathing and pumping—in short, keeping his pulse going and ensuring the flow of oxygen to his brain until the paramedics arrive. You later learn your valiant efforts have failed: The patient is pronounced dead at the hospital. Though you put yourself out for a total stranger, his next of kin obviously don't see it that way. A few weeks after the incident, you learn that you are being sued for wrongful death.

Can this nightmare scenario happen to you? It's very, very unlikely, thanks to the Good Samaritan laws enacted in most states—provided you follow a few simple rules. In general, the law states that you will be afforded what's known as "Good Samaritan immunity," as long as you act as a reasonable and prudent person would under the same conditions. In general, the law requests that you use good common sense and a reasonable level of skill not exceeding the limits of your training. According to the American Red Cross, here are a few precautions the reasonable and prudent will take:

· Move a victim only if the victim's life is endangered.

· Ask a conscious victim for permission before giving care.

· Summon emergency help to the scene by calling 911, a local, seven-digit emergency number, or the operator.

· Once you have begun to provide care, do not stop until more highly trained personnel arrive.

If you follow these guidelines, you should easily be able to avoid a lawsuit. Let your conscience be your guide.

Classic First Aid: Dealing with Injuries

Even when the ABC's of survival remain intact, other injuries, illnesses, or emergencies may require immediate intervention. For the qualified citizen responder, knowing how to handle these situations is key. From cuts and bruises to broken bones, from stroke to shock—sudden injury or illness can pose a serious threat to well-being. The heart may be pumping blood, but if a large artery has been cut, the injured party may not have enough blood left to pump for long. Car crashes are, unfortunately, everyday occurrences, and the lives of those involved often depend on how they're treated in the first "golden hour" after injury. That often means having a competent citizen responder on hand. From calling 911, to stemming the flow of blood, the trained citizen responder can offer a lifeline in the minutes before the ambulance arrives. The environment, too, can be an enemy. Extreme cold, for instance, may result in the dangerous condition known as hypothermia, in which body parts, often the extremities, become frozen. For some victims the difference between saving a limb or losing one may be as simple as the skilled citizen responder luckily on hand.

Under the Skin

Your child is running along the sidewalk when he trips and falls, puncturing his shin along the jagged edge of your building's steps.

Your seventy-year-old mother is walking home early one evening when a mugger jumps out of the bushes, grabbing her purse and pushing her to the ground. She walks in bruised and bloody, clutching her wrist.

You're cutting onions with that serrated kitchen knife and, before you know it, you've sliced not just the onion, but your index finger.

You're in the shower when, all of a sudden, the soothing warmth of the water shifts gear; for some unfathomable reason, the cold water just stops running, and you're doused with scorching hot water along your shoulders and back. It takes three seconds before you realize what has happened and jump out of the stall. By then the burn damage feels extreme.

These injuries all have one thing in common: They involve trauma to the body's skin and soft tissue: the skin, fat, and muscle beneath the epidermis, the outer layer of skin. Sometimes these injuries are quite minor; you just clean with soap and water, apply a Band-Aid and wipe away the tears. Other times soft-tissue injuries can be deadly. Cut a critical artery, and you may suffer shock, in which oxygen-rich blood fails to reach the body's organs. Or you can even bleed to death; suffer internal bleeding from a severe bruise, and you may bleed to death within.

SOFT-TISSUE TYPING: **The List of Wounds**

Bruise: In this soft-tissue injury the skin does not break or tear. Instead, blood vessels under the skin break, resulting in swelling and discoloration. Bruises may change from red to dark red to purple, and even green and yellow as time goes on. Do beware: If a bruise is particularly large and painful, it may signify severe internal damage or hemorrhaging.

Scrape or abrasion: A scrape is the wound that results when the top layer of skin is rubbed away. Since dirt and bacteria often get ground into a scrape, it is important to keep such injuries clean. Once the skin is broken, you are at risk for infection.

Cut: A tear in the skin, a cut often results from injury by sharp-edged objects, including scissors or broken glass. Cuts may bleed freely and, if large enough, may bleed severely. Sometimes nerves are damaged as well, reducing the pain of even a critical injury.

Avulsion: An avulsion is a cut in which part of the outer skin or internal tissue is completely cut away. In the most extreme type of avulsion—an amputation— a body part such as a finger or toe is torn off and may require immediate reattachment through the sophisticated technique of microsurgery.

Puncture: When the body is punctured, a sharp object like a knife or a nail pierces the skin, generally creating a single, deep hole. Since a bullet creates the same effect, a gunshot wound is considered a puncture wound as well. Puncture wounds may not always bleed profusely unless they hit a blood vessel directly. However, because such wounds transmit bacteria deep into the body, they often result in infection, including tetanus. If you have a puncture wound you may require a tentanus shot if you have not received one in the last five to ten years.

To treat soft-tissue injuries, make sure you have a first-aid kit like the one described in the box on the next page. Keep one at home and another in the car. As with any medical emergency, check the scene for safety before you leap in. Whatever the victim's problem, if flames are raging or bullets flying, you cannot be effective. Your best bet is leaving to call 911.

THE WELL-STOCKED FIRST-AID KIT

To prepare for an emergency, make sure you have a first-aid kit handy at home, in the car, and at work. You may buy a kit from the Red Cross or your local drug store, or get a box and put one together yourself. The well-stocked first-aid kit should include the following:

gauze pads and rolled gauze of various sizes, especially two and three inches wide

antiseptic ointment and solution

adhesive tape

cold pack

disposable latex gloves

Band-Aids of assorted size and shape

hand cleaner/soap

flashlight with extra set of batteries

scissors

tweezers

Ace bandage

triangular, kerchief-shaped pieces of muslin, available from your pharmacy, to use as a sling

aspirin, Tylenol, or ibuprofen

Poison-control products: The American Red Cross suggests you buy syrup of ipecac, which may be used to induce vomiting, and activated charcoal, which may be used to absorb poisons in the stomach. Do not administer these substances unless instructed to do so by the poison control center. Used incorrectly, they could do more harm than good. However, it is wise to have them on hand.

Keep It Simple

If the scene is safe, you may start to care for the victim, following a few rules of thumb. Perhaps the most important, at least according to respiratory therapist and first-aid instructor Ellen Krasnoff, is the KISS acronym and rule: "Keep It Simple, Stupid!"—something that Krasnoff, with a smile on her face, likes to tell her students. "If there's a simple way to help a victim and one that seems more elaborate," says Krasnoff, "remember, *simple* is almost always best."

In the case of a bruise, use your hand or a dressing in the form of a gauze pad to place direct pressure on the area. This will reduce swelling and help stem bleeding under the skin. You may also reduce swelling by raising the injured area and applying cold.

Don't assume that a bruise can be treated simply. If a victim is in extreme pain, the bruise may signal severe internal bleeding, a broken bone, or damage to a body organ. Call the ambulance and provide reassurance until help arrives.

HOW TO RECOGNIZE **Internal Bleeding**

Signs of internal bleeding include:

a weak and rapid pulse

pale skin

cool or moist skin

altered consciousness, including drowsiness or confusion

any loss of consciousness

The Open Wound

Caring for a small paper cut or scrape is easy enough. Wash, apply some antiseptic ointment or spray, and cover with a Band-Aid.

For a cut that's more serious—longer than an inch, located on the face or some other cosmetically critical area, or wide open, so that underlying tissue is exposed—a trip to the emergency department is a must. These urgent injuries, if left untreated, could result in serious bacterial infection or an unsightly scar for life. To help treat such injuries, cover with a sterile gauze bandage, wrap with roller bandage or simple tape, and hop in the car. Do not wait an hour to see how things go. Your mission is simple: To prevent bacteria from overtaking the wound, rendering stitches impossible and clean, quick healing difficult, you must get to the ED at once. You must get to the hospital within twelve hours—the sooner, the better.

For the citizen responder, the real challenge comes when confronted with a major open wound which is potentially lethal. Often associated with significant tissue damage and severe bleeding, these traumatic injuries can result in serious bacterial infection, shock, or death. To prevent such dire consequences you must act at once.

If a wound seems fairly serious, do not waste time washing it. Doing so could inflict additional damage to tissue. And more important, while you are cleaning the wound, a seriously injured person could go into shock and bleed to death. Instead, remember Ellen Krasnoff's KISS principle: "Keep it simple, stupid!" To start, protect yourself by wearing rubber gloves if at all possible. Then take a sterile gauze bandage from your handy first-aid kit, unwrap, and press firmly against the wound. (If a sterile dressing is unavailable, use any clean cloth.) To slow bleeding further, elevate the wounded area above the level of the heart. Then take your roller bandage and wrap around the dressing until it is entirely covered. (If you cannot find a roller bandage, use anything from a torn sheet to a tie.) Do not make it so tight that you stop circulation. Tie or tape in place.

In many instances this will help the blood to clot and stop the bleeding. If it does not, leave the old dressing alone and place a new one on top. Never remove a dressing from a bleeding wound, because you will destroy any blood clot that has begun to form. Instead, just pack one dressing on top of the next. Open another sterile gauze dressing, place it atop the bleeding area, and apply direct pressure. Try to elevate the injured arm above the level of the heart. Once more wrap with roller bandage.

If profuse bleeding continues you must try a different tack. Locate one of the body's pressure points—spots where major arteries can be pressed against the bone—and apply pressure there. Depressing the pressure point against the bone underneath should prevent blood from surging through the body to the wound, and may stop the victim from going into shock or bleeding to death before the paramedics arrive. Two pressure points—the brachial artery on the underside of the upper arm (see page 81) and the femoral artery inside the upper thigh (see page 81)—will go furthest toward stemming the flow of blood.

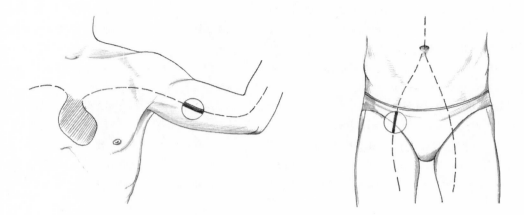

Do not attempt to apply a tourniquet (a bandage twisted tightly around a wound to stem a fatal flow of blood), since experience tells us it most often does more harm than good.

The Deepest Cut

Punctures—caused by penetration of knives, nails, bullets, or anything else that burrows deep—are open wounds as well. They may not bleed as profusely as the conventional variety, but don't be fooled. Someone who has an icepick impaled in his leg is in big trouble whether he seems to be bleeding or not. For the citizen responder dealing with punctures, the first rule is never, ever remove a large object that has pierced through the skin deep into the tissues. On the way out, the object can do more damage, induce more bleeding, and possibly, finish the victim off completely. Instead, using techniques already described out for open wounds, take the sterile dressing and roller bandage and apply around the impaled object so that bleeding is slowed and the object stabilized. Then call the ambulance as soon as possible so the object can be removed surgically, in the hospital, where doctors are skilled at inflicting as little damage as possible and can stop bleeding and repair the injured area at once.

Frozen Miracles

A small boy watching his father power-mow the lawn suddenly runs in front of the moving machine. In an instant, his hand has been severed above the wrist. This victim will need microsurgery to reattach the severed part. But if his caretakers don't know the ropes, getting the severed part to the hospital primed for reattachment can be tricky business indeed.

In case of amputation, the first line of duty for the citizen responder will be stopping profuse bleeding using techniques described for open wounds. After bleeding is controlled, you must find the amputated part, and wrap it in sterile gauze or any clean cloth like a freshly laundered washcloth, cloth, or disposable diaper. Moisten the cloth, place it in a plastic bag, and then put the plastic bag on ice. Never put the severed part directly on ice, and never freeze it; this could damage cells before surgery is performed. Remember to send the severed part to the hospital with the victim.

State of Shock

A few years back, New York paramedics were called to an accident in a subway train. A prankster, riding between the cars, had fallen through to the tracks. Still conscious and wimpering, this young victim was in a bad way: The train, now stopped, bissected his body near the abdomen. "He had been literally cut in half," recalls a paramedic. In fact, though the victim was conscious, aware of all that was happening, he was kept alive only because the pressure of the multi-ton train kept blood from leaving his body. Once workers came to remove the subway car the paramedics knew this young victim would lose all the blood in his body. In seconds, he would go into massive shock and die.

"It happened just as we knew it would," the paramedic recalls. Transit workers moved the train to "free" the victim, releasing him from his life on earth. Says the paramedic, "It was a haunting sight."

Shock in its most extreme form occurs when the circulatory system fails to deliver blood to all parts of the body. And what's frightening is you don't need to be cut in half by a train to go into shock and die. In another recent case, a twenty-one-year-old college student and track athlete was driving on an isolated road late at night when a large deer leaped in front of her vehicle. The ensuing crash left the young woman with two broken legs pinned under the car. A passerby soon called an ambulance, which arrived in about ten minutes. Though the crew went to work immediately, freeing the victim's legs and removing her from the car, she soon lost consciousness and her heart stopped beating en route to the hospital. Despite their best efforts with CPR, paramedics were unable to bring her back to life. The reason: She had lost too much blood and succumbed to the condition called shock.

The injured are in danger of shock whenever blood is prevented from circulating through the body, delivering oxygen to vital organs and cells. If the heart beats irregularly, if blood vessels dilate too widely, if blood loss is extreme, shock may set in.

When all is well, arterial blood vessels work to deliver blood and oxygen to all the body's cells in an equitable fashion so that the brain has oxygen for thinking, the lungs for breathing, and the legs for running. However, when blood is diverted from the body's major organs, for whatever reason, the body tries to compensate. Though you're not conscious of it, the body can direct the flow of blood by constricting some blood vessels and dilating others. Thus, when blood volume falls, the body automatically adjusts by diverting blood to the most vital organs—the brain, the heart, the lungs, and the kidneys, in that order. Slowly, the extremities begin to feel numb as blood rushes to preserve the organs we most need to survive.

However, as blood continues to be shunted from the extremities to the vital organs, cells in the arms and legs begin to suffer. Attempting to compensate, the body may then order blood sent back to the extremities, depriving the vital organs of oxygen instead. The situation is dire. Vital organs now lack oxygen and the heart attempts to compensate by beating faster. If medical help has not arrived, the victim may continue to lose blood and vital organs start malfunctioning. Since the brain lacks oxygen, the victim may become restless, drowsy, or unconscious. Moreover, since the brain inhabits the top of the body's organ hierarchy, blood is ultimately shunted from the kidneys, the lungs, and all other organs to sustain it for as long as possible. As the heart beats faster and faster in an effort to feed the organs, its rhythms may become chaotic—so chaotic that the heart can't pump blood anymore. Without intervention, the outcome is often multiorgan failure, including cardiac arrest and death.

Severe bleeding is particularly dangerous because you don't need to lose that much blood to slide into shock. An average person (weighing one hundred fifty pounds) has ten pints of blood. Losing a single pint—the amount you might give up when donating blood—does not usually cause any symptoms of shock. Just rest and you will regain your equilibrium before long. Lose 20 percent of your blood, or two pints, however, and moderate shock sets in; you may find consciousness drifting in and out, with the victim's affect often combative and restless. Lose 30 percent or more of your blood, or three or more pints, and you have entered the last, most severe stage of shock, characterized by sweating, rapid breathing, and a weak, rapid pulse. If a wound is gushing blood, the victim may go through all three stages of shock quite rapidly, in a matter of minutes. Unless sophisticated medical intervention is delivered at once, the next step could be the last: cardiac arrest.

A child, with far less blood to begin with, can afford to bleed even less before shock sets in. A kindergarten child weighing forty-five pounds, for instance, has just three pints of blood. If that child loses a single pint, he may die. For an infant, loss of even a single ounce of blood can cause shock; total blood volume for that infant is generally just ten ounces.

Shock Therapy

If you happen upon the scene of an accident or injury, guarding against shock will be vital. In accordance with the basic principles of emergency medicine, you must first check a victim for the basic ABC's: airway, breathing, and circulation (or pulse). If any of these basic life requirements are endangered, call 911 and work to treat them first. If you do that, the danger will be severely reduced.

After the ABC's have been accounted for, you may survey the victim again. If you see profuse bleeding, work to stop it, using the techniques outlined previously. While waiting for the ambulance, also make sure the victim stays as comfortable and calm as possible; pain and stress can cause blood vessels to function poorly, accelerating the progression of shock.

Here are some other shock therapy tips as well: If you suspect the potential for shock, lay the patient on his back and elevate his legs about a foot to keep the blood circulating to the body's vital organs. (Avoid this if you suspect any possible injury to the head, neck, back, hips, or legs.) Keep the victim warm if he says he's chilly. Do not give the victim anything to eat or drink, no matter how hungry or thirsty he claims to be; if surgery is required, the stomach should be empty.

Do not attempt to manage shock on your own. You cannot do it. Advanced life support is necessary, so call 911 first.

Burn Clinic

Remember those lazy, hazy days of summer when everyone wore the season's first burn like a badge of honor? These days, we know that sunburn equals skin damage—wrinkles, premature aging, and even skin cancer. Those who test the first rays of summer are instructed to do so with sunblock applied. When burned by the rays of the sun, an electrical appliance, an acidic chemical, or the kitchen stove, salves from butter to aloe are often incorrectly prescribed.

According to first-aid expert Ellen Krasnoff, when it comes to burns, the KISS ("Keep it simple, stupid!") principle applies. For a mild burn on the surface of your body like typical sunburn—on the first layer of skin, or epidermis—chance of infection is almost zero. Yes, the injury is red and painful, but if the skin is intact and there are no blisters, treatment should be minimal.

To treat this first-degree burn, states Krasnoff, keep the injured part under cold water for a few seconds to cool the wound. Do not apply butter, she emphasizes. And that goes for aloe as well. These salves and others may cause infection. First-degree burns will generally heal in five to six days, and will not leave a scar. Aspirin is an excellent treatment if it is safe for you to take aspirin.

Second-degree burns are more problematic. Here, the body develops blisters. And since the surface of the skin is broken, infection may result. In accordance with the KISS principle, do not rub a second-degree burn with butter or aloe. And do not even hold it under water. If, in doing so, you break one of the blisters, infection could result. If possible the burned area should be washed with soap and water and treated with an antibiotic ointment such as Neosporin. Do avoid this, however, if you feel there's a chance the blisters may burst. If blisters are especially severe or extensive, cover the second-degree burn with a sterile gauze pad from your first-aid kit, then secure in place with a roller bandage. The burn should heal in less than a month. But beware: Scarring may occur. Large second-degree burns or those on the face, hands, feet, or genitalia should be seen by a physician.

The real problem comes with the third-degree burn, in which the body is injured through all the layers of the skin. These critical burns may damage not just skin, but also frequently the underlying muscles, fat, and nerves. The third-degree burn will generally appear black or gray, like a piece of meat charred too long on the grill, with white tissue visible underneath. Such burns are actually numb to the touch, since underlying nerves have been destroyed. However, the third-degree burn is always surrounded by painful patches of first- and second-degree burns.

To care for a victim of third-degree burn, have him lie down, unless he's having trouble breathing. As with other types of wounds, raise the burned area above the level of the heart. Since burn victims often feel chilly, make sure the patient stays warm. Cover the burned area with a dry, clean—preferably sterile—dressing. Do not wash the area. Do not apply cold water or ice. Do not remove pieces of cloth that may be sticking to the region. And do not use any kind of ointment, not even an antibiotic like Neosporin. Then call the ambulance and keep the victim as comfortable as possible until paramedics arrive.

Remember, if the injury is bad enough, circulation may be impaired and the victim can go into shock. Thus, when dealing with critical burns, you must take all the precautions outlined in the Shock Therapy section.

For chemical and electrical burns some special instructions apply. For someone who's suffered a chemical burn, flush the area with copious amounts of water, and get rid of exposed clothing. Call for an ambulance at once. Before touching anyone who's suffered an electrical burn, make sure the power has been turned off, and that the victim is no longer in contact with the source of the electricity. If not, *you* can become victim number two. Since electricity sends current through the body, the main problem may not be burned skin but rather two vital functions of survival: breathing and circulation. Check for breathing and pulse and, if necessary, perform rescue breathing or CPR. Since spinal injury is a possibility, do not move the electrical burn victim. And do not attempt to cool the burn or treat with ointment. Keep the patient warm and call for the ambulance at once; electrical injuries can be very serious.

To the Bone: Dealing with Breaks, Sprains, and Strains

The children filling the seats might be gathering for a school party, or, perhaps, a parade. After all, there's plenty of town spirit, with the splashy greens, reds, and yellows of soccer and Little League. But there's a twist. The boy in orange, from the Milky Ways, was playing soccer when he tripped over the ball, landing on his knee. Now, he cannot walk at all. The girl in pink is from the Tigers, a Little League team bent on winning the pennant for their school. She slid to first, only to hear a crack from her wrist as it hit the plate. This "party spot," it turns out, is the waiting room of an emergency department serving suburbia, USA. We are deep in Little League country, with spring sports season in high gear.

Whether you're playing sports or painting your house, it's all too easy to damage your muscles, joints, and bones. Almost all such injuries must be examined by medical professionals. But until you get the victim to the hospital, there's a lot you can do to prevent further damage and reduce pain.

While breaks, sprains, and strains are rarely lethal, they are often quite painful. And if not cared for correctly from the start, some of these injuries can permanently disable a victim. To understand this class of injury, you need some grounding in "anatomy 101."

The adult human skeleton contains more than two hundred bones, structures hard and dense enough to protect internal organs and hold the body up. The spot where any two bones meet is called the joint. Tough bands called ligaments connect two bones to each other at the nexus of the joint, where they may move in relation to each other. Finally, most of the body's six hundred muscles are attached to bones via strong tissues called tendons. The muscles themselves, made of soft tough tissue, can shorten and lengthen, enabling the body to move.

According to the American Red Cross, the four basic types of injuries to muscles, bones, and joints are fractures, dislocations, strains, and sprains. Here are the characteristics of the four:

Fracture: A complete break, a chip, or a crack in the bone. (Yes, a fractured bone and a broken bone are the same thing.) An open fracture is a broken bone that occurs along with a break in the skin. Though relatively rare, open fractures may result in infection. Fractures are life threatening only when breaks are in large bones like the thigh, the hip, or the pelvic area, or when they sever a major artery. In closed fractures (more common) the bone does not pierce the skin.

Dislocation: The condition in which the bone moves away from its normal position in the joint. Often, dislocation results when the ligaments joining bones in the joint area are torn.

Sprain: Characterized by a tearing or stretching of ligaments around the joint. Unlike a dislocation, however, the bone does not move away from its normal position.

Strain: A stretching or tearing of muscles and tendons, often caused when someone lifts something of great weight.

Though it's important for doctors to distinguish between these injuries to deliver appropriate treatment in the hospital, for the citizen responder in the field, specific diagnosis may be impossible and may not be necessary in order to give helpful first aid. No matter what the ultimate injury turns out to be, your job is to call for help, and, in the interim, to keep the injured part from moving, through the creation of a splint. Depending on the body part injured and your access to materials, splints will take different forms.

There are a few specific rules. For instance, only create a splint if you can do so without inflicting further pain. Splint an injury in the exact position in which you find it; under no circumstance should you force an injured area into what you think is the "correct" position. When you make a splint, you must immobilize not just the injured area, but also the joints directly above and below. After you have splinted an injury, raise the area, if possible, and apply ice to keep down the swelling.

Techniques for splinting are depicted in the diagrams.

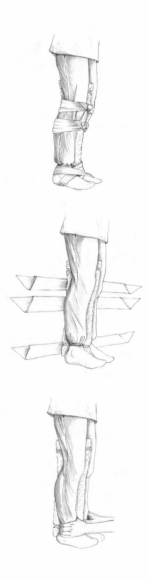

1.   *Anatomic splint:* Splinting one part of the victim's body to another, using the intact part of the body to secure the part that's injured.

a.   Supporting the damaged limb above and below the site of the injury, align it with its healthy counterpart.

b.   Place a pillow, or blanket, between the two aligned limbs and tie with triangular bandages or men's ties.

c.   Tie the bandages securely, fastening the limbs to each other; use the uninjured limb as a splint for the injured one. Do not tie so tightly that you interfere with circulation.

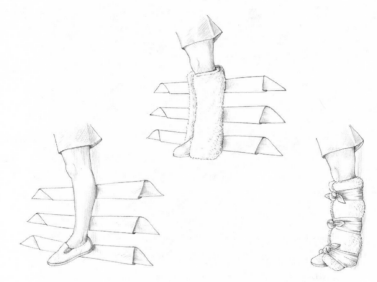

2.   *Soft splint:* Immobilizing an injured ankle or wrist with a soft material.

a.   Place several folded triangular bandages, strips of linen, or even men's ties, underneath the injured area.

b.   Wrap a soft blanket or pillow around the injured area.

c.   Tie the bandages securely, fastening the injured area to the soft material; but do not tie so tightly that you interfere with circulation.

3.   *Rigid splint:* Immobilizing a broken limb with a rigid splint; you may buy the splint in a pharmacy or improvise with something firm, like a magazine.

a.   Use both hands to support the injured limb above and below the site of the injury.

b.   Place the rigid splint under the injured area. Make sure the splint supports not

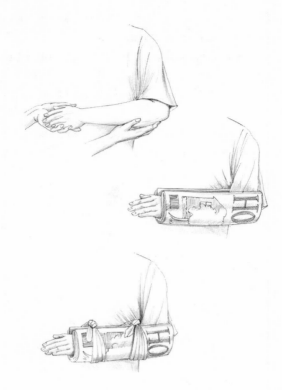

just the injured region, but also the joints above and below it.

c.   Tie several folded triangular bandages, strips of linen, or even men's ties, around the splint and limb above and below the site of injury; do not tie so tightly that you interfere with circulation.

4.   *The sling:* Supporting a broken arm against the body.

a.   Use both hands to support the injured limb above and below the site of the injury.

b.   While supporting the injured arm, place it in the triangular bandage, as shown; tie the bandage around the neck.

c.   Take another triangular bandage, strip of linen, or roller gauze and tie the injured area to the chest, as indicated.

One last point: If you suspect a head, neck, or back injury, you must call an ambulance at once. In these instances, leave the victim lying flat. If the victim has lost con-

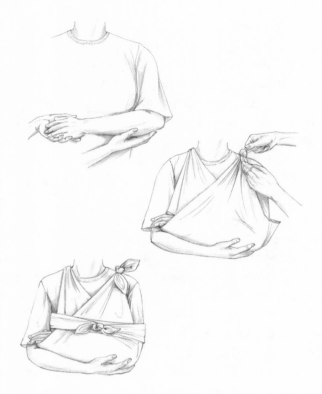

sciousness, maintain an open airway. Do check consciousness and breathing, control bleeding, and keep the victim from becoming hot or chilled. Remember, this class of injury is particularly dangerous, accounting for some two million deaths a year. You should be particularly suspicious of head or spinal injury if the victim falls from a distance greater than his or her own height; if he has been riding in a car; or, if he has been hit by or thrown from a car.

It's Elemental: When Someone Is Damaged by Heat or Cold

In his mystical novel *The Magic Mountain,* Thomas Mann creates a scene in which the hero, Hans Castorp, wanders aimlessly through a snowy realm of cold. First, he suffers loss of sensation, then, altered consciousness. In the end, because he is a literary superhero, he uses sheer force of will to fight death and walk out of the snow.

Despite the poetic imagery and transcendent metaphors, Castorp was the victim of a condition known as hypothermia, in which the entire body cools because it has been so cold for so long that it simply loses the ability to heat itself. Victims of hypothermia slide through a few stages, as did Castorp, from numbness to apathy to loss of consciousness. If help does not arrive, they suffer cardiac arrest and death. You don't have to be the protagonist of a literary masterpiece for this fate to befall you. However, unlike Castorp, mere mortals may need some bona fide medical help to come through the experience alive.

The first stage of cold-related illness, explains first-aid teacher Ellen Krasnoff, is common frost nip, in which the tip of the nose, the ears, or the fingers become red. To treat these areas, just warm them; put on your gloves and pull up that scarf, and you should be fine. "It's like a roast beef you've put in the freezer for a minute," she explains. "When you remove it, the outside may be a little cold, but it hasn't frozen. It will still be OK, as long as you take it out of the cold at once."

In the next stage—superficial frostbite, or second degree—the outside of that roast beef—the outer layer of your skin—has been in long enough to freeze, but the inside is OK. To treat, says Krasnoff, come out of the cold and immerse the frozen part in tepid water no hotter than 105 degrees Fahrenheit. If you do not have a thermometer, simply make sure the water feels the same temperature as your hand, and comfortable to the touch. If it does not, cool it down.

Frostbite is no laughing matter. It results when water in the body freezes. These frozen water crystals can break blood vessels and even nerves. And in its most serious form—deep frostbite, or third degree—underlying tissue freezes with crystals of ice laced throughout. You may recognize deep frostbite if your skin feels numb and cold to the touch or if it looks waxy or discolored. Deep frostbite, notes Krasnoff, is like putting that roast beef in the freezer for the night. When it comes out in the morning, it feels like a rock.

Since your body is not roast beef, treat deep frostbite with respect—especially if you want to get through the episode with fingers and toes (or other injured areas) intact.

As with superficial frostbite, have the victim come out of the cold and warm the injured area with tepid water. Do not rub, since those prickly ice crystals can do irreparable damage. Make sure to use a large container for soaking, and work dilligently to ensure that the injured area does not bang against the sides. Keep the injured area submerged until it looks red and feels warm. Then wrap in a sterile gauze dressing and secure with a roller bandage. If fingers or toes have been injured, place sterile gauze or cotton between the individual digits. Make sure you don't break any blisters. Never try to heat a numb and frozen part of the body in front of a fire or open stove; this may simply add a serious burn injury to serious frostbite. After treating, get the victim to a doctor or your local emergency department as soon as possible.

Even more serious than deep frostbite is hypothermia—the last stop along the treacherous road of cold-related injury before the grim eventuality of death. When the entire body becomes so cold that even shivering stops, internal organs start to chill and the frozen heart starts to beat erratically—a condition known as ventricular fibrillation. If untreated, the heart will ultimately just stop.

Signs of hypothermia include shivering, followed later by the cessation of shivering; slow or irregular pulse; numbness; and changes in consciousness, ranging from a remote, faraway affect and apathy to loss of consciousness.

Note that the thermometer does not have to register below 32 degrees Fahrenheit for hypothermia to result. Those who have spent long periods in wet clothing or cold water may be prey to the condition, as are those with special medical problems rendering the body's self-warming machinery less than efficient. Specifically, look for signs of hypothermia in the elderly and the very young, and in those with diabetes, stroke-related illness and a brain tumor.

Once you recognize hypothermia, seek emergency assistance immediately through a call to Emergency Medical Service. While waiting for medics to arrive, warm the victim gradually. Remove any wet clothing and cover the victim in blankets; if you have hot water bottles, heating pads, or electric blankets, place them over the first layer of warming material you've applied. Give the victim warm liquids to drink. Do not, under any circumstance, warm the victim too quickly by immersing in a tub of warm water; this might initiate erratic heart rhythms, resulting in cardiac arrest.

Since hypothermia is a medical problem of the highest order, you must continue to monitor victims, especially unconscious ones, for the ABC's of survival. Be prepared to perform rescue breathing or CPR. And make sure you call an ambulance as soon as you safely can.

Of course, cold isn't the only way to go. Internal overheating—sometimes known as hyperthermia—can be deadly as well. Like hypothermia, hyperthermia is the last stop on the path of heat-related illness before the body succumbs for good. There are many steps along the way, and if you look out for them, hyperthermia is something you will never have to face.

The first heat emergency to look out for is the painful muscle spasm known as heat cramp. Due in part to loss of fluid and salt from heavy sweating, heat cramps most commonly occur in the muscles of the legs and abdomen. To treat, have the victim rest in a cool or shady area and drink water or a commercial sports drink like Gatorade. Make sure the drink is not cold or icy and that it is consumed slowly—not more than half a glass, or about four ounces, every fifteen minutes. After a while, the victim can stretch his muscles and, very lightly, massage them as well. When the cramp has subsided, activity may be resumed provided the individual continues to drink plenty of fluid.

Heat cramps usually subside, but they may also be a sign of further heat-related illness to come. The next sign of trouble is a condition known as heat exhaustion, which sometimes follows long periods of strenuous activity in high temperatures and/or humidity. Do not treat heat exhaustion lightly. According to the American Red Cross, it is an early indication that the body's temperature-regulating mechanism is becoming overwhelmed. Signs may include moist, pale skin, nausea, dizziness and, of course, exhaustion.

In its earliest stages, heat exhaustion can be treated easily much like heat cramps, with shade, water, and rest. However as the condition progresses, shock may be a risk as well. Fluid is lost through sweating, and, at the same time, blood flow to the skin increases, reducing blood flow to the vital organs. If you think shock is a possibility, get the victim to a doctor or emergency department as soon as you can.

Heatstroke, or hyperthermia, is the most dangerous of the heat-related illnesses. If you ignore the early signs of heat exhaustion, heatstroke could be the unfortunate result. Signs can include fast, shallow breathing; a rapid, weak pulse; confusion or loss of consciousness; and body temperature soaring to 106 degrees Fahrenheit or higher. If help is not immediate, the victim can die.

To treat, do all you would have done for victims of heat cramps and heat exhaustion. Move the person to a shady area, provide water at the rate of no more than one-half cup every fifteen minutes, and stay on the lookout for problems with any of the ABC's of survival. Call an ambulance as soon as you can. And finally, since the victim of heatstroke is often unable to sweat, you may help simulate the process until professional help arrives: Soak towels or sheets in cool water and apply to the skin, then fan the victim to increase the rate of evaporation.

The Poison Patrol

Unfortunately, most of us are exposed to or can access literally thousands of poisons in our normal everyday activities. The scenarios are virtually endless: An elderly man, deeply depressed over the death of his wife, swallows some rubbing alcohol; an infant visiting an aunt's house crawls under the sink and swallows some cleaning fluid; it's winter, and a man warming up his car inside his garage lets the engine run too long, filling the area, and his lungs, with toxic levels of carbon monoxide.

Poisons may be swallowed intentionally or accidentally. They may be inhaled, or they may reach the victim through the skin, as in the case of insecticide poisoning. Whatever the source, toxins are substances which, when introduced to the body in sufficient quantity, cause illness, injury, or death.

According to the Red Cross, between one and two million Americans are poisoned each year, and of that number more than 90 percent of the poisonings occur in the home. Most victims are under age five; of that group, less than 5 percent actually die. In fact, while safety measures in the home and in packaging have reduced poisoning deaths in children over the past thirty years, adult deaths due to poison, mostly suicide and drug-related, have drastically increased.

The most important first step in dealing with toxin-induced illness is recognizing that exposure has occurred. Look for clues at the scene. Ask the victim for information. Search for empty pill or medicine bottles. Look around for open or emptied containers and try to detect any odd smells or fumes. Examine the victim's skin for signs of bites or injections with hypodermic needles.

You must be attuned not only to these man-made substances, but to poisons in the natural environment as well. Make sure your toddler has not ingested part of a plant; come in surface contact with poison ivy, poison sumac, or poison oak; or been bitten or stung by any number of critters, from ticks and insects to marine life and snakes.

Also be on the lookout for one or more of the symptoms of poisoning, including nausea, vomiting, dizziness, diarrhea, difficulty breathing, chest or abdominal pain, alterations in consciousness, including fainting or seizures, pale or bluish skin, and burns or other unusual marks around the mouth or skin.

Having concluded that poison may be the trouble, remove the victim from the poison source, if appropriate. For instance, if someone has succumbed to carbon monoxide poisoning in a garage, turn off the car's engine, open the garage door, and, if you can, carry or drag the individual outside.

Then call your local poison control center at once. Hopefully, the number will be posted visibly right by the phone. At St. Luke's–Roosevelt Hospitals' EDs in New York City, we call the New York City Poison Center at 212-P-O-I-S-O-N-S; you may call it, your local poison center, or your telephone operator. Communicate to the operator as clearly as possible the clues you have gathered and the symptoms you observed. Then

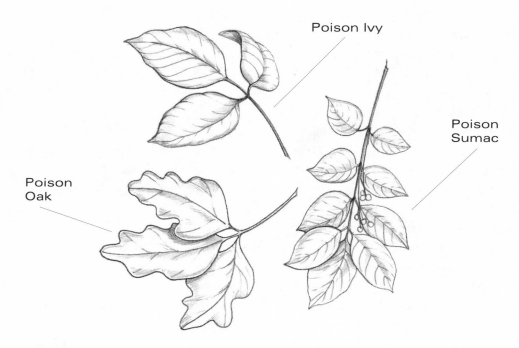

Poison Ivy

Poison
Sumac

Poison
Oak

await instructions. As with talking to an ambulance dispatcher, you must stay on the line to answer all questions. Then follow instructions as quickly and precisely as you can.

For instance, you may be asked to report on the victim's level of consciousness, breathing, or pulse. You may be asked to save some of the vomitus so the possible poison can be analyzed. Then you may be asked to give the victim milk or water, or instructed to induce vomiting. Remember: Do not give the victim any food or water or induce vomiting unless you are instructed to do so by the poison control center or some other medical professional.

If the poison victim is completely unconscious, you may want to call the ambulance before you call the poison control center. Frequently, the ambulance dispatcher will send an emergency crew and then patch your call through to poison control.

Stinging Advice

If someone has been stung by an insect or bitten by an animal that seems rabid or poisonous in any way, get the victim away from harm without endangering yourself. In the case of a venomous snake or a mammal that might be rabid, try to remember where you saw it and what it looked like. Then call your local emergency number, which can, if necessary, dispatch professionals to bring the animal in for testing.

Wash wounds from animal bites to guard against infection. If you suspect the possibility of rabies, help the victim access medical care at once.

For an insect sting, remove the stinger with your nail or a plastic credit card (using tweezers may break the venom sac, releasing more venom). Wash the site, cover with a Band-Aid, and apply ice to reduce swelling.

In the instance of a snake bite, make sure the victim gets medical help within thirty minutes. Even though the vast majority of snake bites are not poisonous, it's always better to err on the side of caution. Until medical professionals enter the scene, wash the wound, immobilize the injured area with a sling, and try to lower it below the level of the heart. If you are in a wilderness area too remote to access medical care within half an hour, make sure you are carrying a snake-bite kit.

Beware of bites from marine mammals such as stingrays, sea anemones, and jellyfish. As a citizen responder, protect your own hands before removing any tentacles or stingers from the victim. Wash off the wound in salt water. If the victim has trouble breathing, or has been stung in the face or neck, call your emergency medical service at once.

Bites and stings can sometimes result in severe and often deadly allergic reactions called anaphylaxis, characterized by hives, itching, and rash as well as wheezing, difficulty breathing, nausea, and dizziness. Sometimes, as respiratory problems due to anaphylaxis progress, the victim's airway is blocked, resulting in death. Once you have recognized the possibility of this severe allergic reaction, you must act by calling the ambulance at once. Help the person into the position that facilitates breathing. When the paramedics arrive, they will give the victim an injection of the drug epinephrine, sometimes called adrenalin, to counteract this deadly allergy attack. (Sometimes, people who know they have a tendency to anaphylaxis carry kits available by prescription; often, they will use an EpiPen—a device shaped like a pen that can inject a measured dose of lifesaving epinephrine. If they have one and tell you they need it, you may help them use it; the directions are written on the kit.)

When Sudden Illness Strikes

A diabetes patient forgets to take her insulin and suffers diabetic coma. Hours after a meal out at a fast-food restaurant, a small child develops severe abdominal pain and bloody diarhhea. A teenager breaks out in huge, beet-red hives. Sudden illness takes many forms. Sometimes, as in the case of the diabetic, it's possible to guess just what's wrong, particularly if the victim is a friend or relative; other times, diagnosis is impossible without sophisticated blood and urine tests or X rays. The victim may be suffering from stroke, heart attack, the violent onslaught of a sudden virus, pneumonia, allergic reaction, or a host of other ills. Symptoms may range from dizziness, nausea, and profuse sweating to loss of consciousness; from debilitating pain to seizure. Whatever the cause, the symptoms you observe require immediate care.

In fact, for the citizen responder, it is possible to treat sudden illness without an actual diagnosis while waiting for expert help to arrive. Treating the symptoms is an important part of initial emergency care. The basics are just like the first-aid protocols: Check the environment to make sure no dangers lurk; then take a few seconds to stand back and examine the scene. Try to get the big picture. Is there any unopened medicine laying around that might signal the victim's problem? Any other clue as to what might have gone wrong?

Next, approach the victim and ask him to tell you what's wrong. Ask about regular medications and chronic problems or allergies. Key into reports of nausea or vomiting, seizures, chest, abdominal or head pain, and blood passed in the urine, bowel movements, or phlegm. Notice changes in skin color and changes in cognition, including dizziness, lightheadedness, confusion, or loss of consciousness. Make sure to check the victim for the ABC's of survival: airway, breathing, and circulation.

Then, if the victim seems desperately ill, call for an ambulance before you administer any care. You must call an ambulance if the victim is losing consciousness or has lost consciousness; if his speech is slurred; if he has trouble breathing; if he passes blood; or, if he appears poisoned.

Finally, you are ready to treat the patient. If rescue breathing or CPR are required, administer these immediately. If not, attempt to comfort the victim. Make sure he's resting. Prevent him from becoming overheated or chilled. If he's conscious, you may provide some food or water.

There are specific rules for individual symptoms:

Dizziness and nausea: If the patient feels faint, position her on her back and raise her feet eight to ten inches. Loosen tight clothing. If the victim has fainted, check the ABC's. If the victim is nauseated, roll her on her side so the airway will remain clear in the event that she vomits. Keep her eyes closed.

Weakness, dizziness or blackout can be associated with diabetes: If the victim is diabetic, illness may result from high blood sugar (too much sugar and too little medication) or low blood sugar (not enough sugar combined with too much medication or too much exercise). These problems stem from the nature of diabetes itself. For all of us, including diabetics, food is broken down into simple sugars. In healthy people, the pancreas produces a hormone, insulin, which then helps the sugars enter the body's cells. In diabetics, the pancreas produces insufficient insulin, and sugar remains in the bloodstream, where it cannot fortify the body as it should. To deal with the problem, diabetics today are fortunate enough to have access to supplemental insulin by injection (and other medicine in pill form), which helps their cells utilize sugar as if the proper hormone had been generated in the pancreas itself.

But if the diabetic takes insulin, then fails to eat, insulin builds up in the blood, and blood sugar falls, resulting in the condition called hypoglycemia, or insulin shock. The condition may also result if the diabetic receives too much insulin, overexercises, burning up all available sugar, or experiences undue emotional stress. Whatever the cause, the outcome is the sudden onset of insulin shock which, if not treated immediately, may mean death.

On the other hand, if the victim has eaten but failed to take insulin, the result can be hyperglycemia, too much sugar in the blood. If the situation is not corrected, the diabetic may slowly slide into a coma over a period of days.

The citizen responder should, if possible, communicate with the victim to learn what's wrong. If the person is conscious, you may simply ask the source of the trouble. If the person seems alert, and if the answer is emphatic, take the person at his or her word. Provide food and drink, as requested, only if the person can talk and swallow with ease.

However, if the victim is unconscious or confused, both hypoglycemia and hyperglycemia must be handled exactly the same way. The reason: Symptoms, ranging from rapid pulse and breathing to drowsiness, dizziness, and eventually, loss of consciousness, are the same in either condition. The difference is that the diabetic experiencing hypoglycemia is in danger of sudden death. This lethal possibility must be addressed with administration of sugar, preferably common table sugar, in granulated form or dissolved in water. If the patient is unconscious, pour the sugar right into the corner of his mouth. If the patient is hypoglycemic—in need of sugar—you will have saved a life. However, if the patient is hyperglycemic—in need of insulin—you won't really do any harm. In either case, call Emergency Medical Service and let paramedics handle the rest.

Seizures: These electrical irregularities in the brain are often due to epilepsy; they may also be caused by high fever in the very young. Seizures range in severity from mild blackouts to severe muscular contractions.

Contrary to common wisdom, you should not hold a seizure victim down or place a spoon in his mouth. This may cause injury to the victim as well as yourself. Instead, your goals are twofold: to monitor the airway and to prevent injury. Make sure the person in seizure has a clear path for breathing, unblocked by vomit or saliva. If you see any saliva, vomitus, or blood in the individual's mouth, turn his head to one side to drain. Also remove dangerous objects and place a pillow or cushion of cloth underneath the victim's head.

You need to call an ambulance only if the seizure lasts more than a minute or the person appears to be injured. You must also seek immediate medical help if there are repeated seizures in a short span of time, or if the victim is pregnant, diabetic, or a juvenile.

Weakness or numbness: When it occurs in the arms, legs, or face, often on one side of the body, this set of symptoms may point to stroke, in which blood clots or other factors disrupt the flow of blood to the brain and may cause permanent damage or even death. To care for a victim of stroke, call an ambulance at once; the sooner the victim is treated, the higher her chances of recovering as much function as possible. In addition, while awaiting the arrival of the ambulance, monitor the stroke patient for the ABC's.

Crushing chest pain or pain radiating down the arm: These and other symptoms of heart attack have been covered extensively in Chapter 1, which deals with recognizing a medical emergency. We suggest you know them well. If you suspect someone is having a heart attack, have the person stop the task at hand and rest. The sitting position may often be preferable since it may ease the task of breathing. Call for an ambulance at once. The sooner the patient enters the emergency medical system, the greater the chances of survival. Until the ambulance arrives, continue to monitor the victim for the ABC's of survival. If the person loses consciousness, stops breathing, and has no pulse, he has gone into cardiac arrest. Administer cardiopulmonary resuscitation until the paramedics arrive.

FIRST-AID MYTHS

A young mother going off to work has hired a nanny for her child. A matronly grandmother, the caretaker seems to bring to her job a lifetime of wisdom. One day, the mother comes home to a typical problem. Playing in the park, the little boy has gotten a splinter from a bench, and the nanny is about to remove it. Before doing so, however, she will sterilize the needle in her own special way: She will run it through her hair, which, on this day, happens to be teased, lacquered and dyed. Appalled, the mother grabs the needle and instructs the nanny in the art of sterilization as taught by her own mother: She holds the needle in the fire of a gas-burning range until the tip has turned coal black. Squirming wildly, the child finally has his splinter removed. A week later, relating the story to her pediatrician, the mother finds her own notion of sterilization-by-fire is less than state of the art, but certainly better than her nanny's. These days, the doctor instructs her, "needles are doused in rubbing alcohol, the best sterilization technique of all."

Just talk with a random sampling of friends and relatives and you'll be amazed at how many medical myths we harbor, how many questionable practices and beliefs we embrace in our homes as science itself marches on. In the following pages, we list the reality behind some of the most prevalent emergency and first-aid myths. Read this carefully. You might be a myth-maker yourself.

The myth: Seizures are rare and, once started, extremely difficult to stop.
The reality: Seizures are far more common than most people understand. They are seen all the time in the emergency department. All seizures stop, most within a minute.

The myth: Place a solid object like a spoon or pencil in the mouth of a seizure victim to prevent him from swallowing or biting his tongue.
The reality: This is an inappropriate practice. The seizure victim will not

swallow his tongue but may, in fact, bite you or swallow the object you place in his mouth. There have even been cases in which the would-be helper has had a finger bitten off. To help the seizure victim, perform the "head tilt/chin lift," described on page 62, so that you establish an airway. You may move the seizure patient if her arms or legs bang against a hard surface like ceramic floors, furniture, or the walls, or if she falls off a bed or chair.

The myth: In children, seizures associated with high fever may be especially dangerous.

The reality: Febrile seizures in children, though frightening, usually last only a few seconds, and are almost never serious. (Of course, any such occurrence should nonetheless be reported to a physician.)

The myth: Put butter on your burns.

The reality: It is best not to put honey, butter, or milk on your burns. The best thing to put on a burn is nothing. Butter on the burn might well make it more painful, especially when the butter must be removed, and harder to evaluate by the emergency department. The application of cold water or ice is acceptable and will relieve pain, but should be done only for small burns and over a short period of time. The reason is that when the skin is burned, it looses the ability to prevent the loss of heat and exposes the body to the potential for hypothermia. Too much cold over too long a period could render the burned area hypothermic, inflicting the same sort of damage as frostbite.

The myth: If a wound is not too severe, you can put off treatment for a couple of days.

The reality: If a wound requires medical attention, it must be treated within the first twelve hours. Otherwise it will be overrun with bacteria, making it difficult or impossible to treat without a high risk of infection or an unsightly scar.

The myth: For a person with diabetes in the midst of an attack, the most deadly substance you can think of is sugar.

The reality: Though most people with diabetes are told to avoid large amounts of sugar, in an emergency sugar will not be harmful, and may well help. If sugar or glucose levels gets too low, the diabetic may suffer brain damage. In fact, most diabetics will carry a candy bar in a pocket to pump up sugar level during the early afternoon. If a diabetes patient is unconscious, take a pack or two of loose sugar and pour it into the mouth. (Don't use a candy bar, since this may cause the patient to choke.)

The myth: In the case of a victim bleeding profusely, the first thing a citizen responder must do is stem the flow of blood by adding pressure at the site of the wound.

The reality: The most sensational symptom may not be the most critical. No matter what symptom you observe in any ill or injured patient, always make sure to check the ABC's of survival—airway, breathing, and circulation—first. Stop the bleeding with pressure afterward.

The myth: For those who have frostbite, the goal is to thaw the frozen limb as quickly as possible, no matter where you are.

The reality: If you thaw a frozen limb in the middle of nowhere, you will convert a numb foot that can walk, perhaps with difficulty, into a painful, immobile extension that can no longer be used. The patient, stuck in the middle of a wilderness, will then be exposed to the possibility of total body hypothermia.

The myth: To stop profuse bleeding, tie a tourniquet around the damaged limb.

The reality: Never attempt to stop bleeding with a tourniquet, because it can do far more harm than good. Use pressure to stop bleeding instead.

The myth: Q-Tips, or cotton swabs, are extremely effective tools for cleaning out the ear.

The reality: Never use Q-Tips (or paper clips) to clean out the ears. Never put anything in your ear that is smaller than your elbow.

The myth: Insect bites should be treated with ammonia.
The reality: Insect bites should be treated with ice and antihistamine.

The myth: It's best to cool an overheated child with rubbing alcohol or just cold water.
The reality: An overheated child should be cooled with tepid water only.

Cold water or rubbing alcohol will induce shivering and may thus actually increase temperature.

The myth: If you can't do perfect cardiopulmonary resuscitation, don't do it at all.

The reality: If the heart has stopped, imperfect CPR is always better than no CPR at all.

The myth: Sipping cognac or other forms of alcohol is a good treatment for hypothermia.

The reality: The bottle of cognac with the picture of a Saint Bernard with a cask hung below her neck may give you that "warm-all-over feeling," but will actually result in more rapid heat loss.

The myth: If you have a black eye, an uncooked steak is the best compress.

The reality: Forget the steak. For the first twenty-four hours, treat the black eye with ice. Then apply some heat.

Chapter 4

A Ride on the Wild Side: The Ambulance Illustrated

The young man—just a teenager—made deliveries around the meat factories of Flushing, Queens. Among other things, the factories were known for their giant ice machines—particularly hazardous because huge blocks of ice had to be toted to the top, then pushed through a grinder. It was this boy's misfortune to slip. Tragically, instead of shredding the ice, the grinder tore up his foot.

By the time the machine was switched off, part of the boy's foot had been virtually pulverized. It was attached to his leg by strips of tissue, nothing more. The paramedic on the case could have simply loaded the boy in an ambulance, in the process further injuring him. "Instead," the paramedic relates, "I climbed to the boy on top of the freezing ice machine, attached an IV line, and cradled him in my arms." The city dispatched one of its emergency service units, adept at negotiating mechanical emergencies, including separating body parts from machines. Against all odds, the shredded foot was salvaged. By now almost as frozen as his patient after the long wait atop the ice, the paramedic rushed the boy to a major Manhattan trauma center known for its groundbreaking microsurgery team. There, true to form, a couple of gifted surgeons reattached the foot.

The place was Manhattan's Riverside Park. It was a pleasant Sunday afternoon, with children playing soccer some twenty yards away. There, St. Luke's–Roosevelt Hospital paramedics were on a mission of mercy indeed. A man was stabbing himself in the stomach, and, witnessing the self-destruction, one paramedic decided that despite the possible danger, he would intervene. "I grabbed the knife," he related some time later. Said his partner, "It was dangerous, and a little bit crazy, but it was heroic." Elaborating further, the hero explained: "It's comparable to the situation in which there's a house burning down; the fire department isn't there, and you hear a child screaming inside. If you don't jump in yourself, the child will die." Added his partner, who ultimately helped as well: "Call it heroism, call it crazy. Once he committed himself to this course, I had to, too."

A sixty-year-old woman, despondent over the death of her husband, has swallowed sleeping pills, then called her daughter across town to say good-bye. Getting through to the local 911 number, the daughter initiates an immediate response. Paramedics arrive but cannot get through the door of the older woman's seventh-floor apartment. But entering a neighboring apartment, they climb over terrace walls above a major highway, through the windows, and finally, into the now-unconscious victim's room. In the end, their death-defying efforts save her life.

These stories do not come from a television show or the pages of a dime-store novel: They come from the mouths of New York paramedics, working some of the toughest beats in the world. Though they might earn far more money through managerial or nursing jobs, these EMS workers have chosen to patrol the city aiding the ill and injured as their lifework. They can bring you out of insulin shock, back from a heart attack, or—sometimes—back from the dead. Well versed in the tools of their trade, they carry oxygen and intravenous fluid, heart and blood pressure monitors, splints and neck collars, regularly performing first aid, cardiopulmonary resuscitation, defibrillation, and more.

According to some, in fact, paramedics are often better equipped to handle medical emergencies on the street or in your home than many physicians. Indeed, when people ask if there's a doctor in the house, they expect that physicians can save lives in an emergency. But often, a better question might be, "Is there a paramedic in the house?" If you are desperately injured or ill, it will be your good fortune to encounter one of these brave and generous souls.

Of course, medics, like folks of other disciplines, come in all stripes. Thus, as you come into contact with EMS workers, you would do well to view them as you would anyone else in the helping professions. Recognize and accept the expertise that's usually available, but DO ask questions when doubts arise.

The goal of this chapter: to teach you to negotiate the ambulance experience. You have already learned to deal with emergency dispatchers via phone. But once the paramedics arrive, you must learn to communicate with them effectively face-to-face, helping them address your critical problems and concerns. If you have special allergies or health problems, you must explain them immediately. If you feel treatment is inappropriate, you must say so. If you wish to change the driver's destination to the hospital of your choice, you must know when it's appropriate to do so—and how.

To advocate for yourself in the ambulance you must understand the ambulance workers, including the highly trained paramedic and the emergency medical technician (EMT), who is often sent out on less dire calls. What is her education and background? What level of stress does he endure? What has she been doing before she was called to your home or office, and what will she do after leaving you to patrol the streets again?

Familiarize yourself with the geography of the ambulance itself. From the splints stored in side cabinets, to the detachable stretcher, to the cylinders of oxygen, the ambulance has a medical layout and modus operandi all its own. Indeed, the treatments provided en route to the hospital, while lifesaving, may seem unfamiliar to anyone who's never taken the "bus." The "big black bag" the paramedic carries and the "little black bag" your doctor once toted are very different. If you know what to expect you'll be more likely to leave things entirely in the hands of the paramedics or EMTs when appropriate, and to advocate for yourself when you should.

The Good Old Days

Most people don't realize that today's sophisticated Emergency Medical Service system, with its computerized network of dispatchers, well-equipped vehicles, EMTs, and highly trained paramedics, evolved only relatively recently. While the 911 Emergency Medical Service has its critics, those of us accessing the ambulance these days have it pretty good. Things weren't always this way.

Dan Mathisen, now director of ambulance services for St. Luke's–Roosevelt Hospital remembers what happened when he broke his leg during a football game back in Pittsburgh at age thirteen. "It was a situation that required an ambulance," Mathisen relates, "but what showed up was a sheriff's car, a station wagon, to be exact. I was tossed in the back and, with no medical care whatsoever, was rushed off to the hospital. I was in great pain."

In the mid-1960s, the art and science of emergency transport was crude. Most ambulances were operated by funeral directors and private firms, many without two-way radio equipment and without attendants who had even a Boy Scout's training in first aid. Each year, tens of thousands of Americans lost their lives as a result of treatment that was inadequate, inept, or simply too late.

From the farmlands of Iowa to the cosmopolitan cities of Boston and San Francisco the experience was much the same. Whether the patient was an indigent mother on welfare or a captain of industry ensconced in a mansion, until reaching the hospital that individual was virtually on his or her own. Often, lack of medical care during these crucial minutes meant irreversible damage or death.

We've all heard the litany of time constraints biology has saddled us with. For the victim of cardiac arrest, four minutes without oxygen and the brain starts to die. For the trauma victim, commence treatment even a little beyond the critical "golden hour" after injury, and chance of survival plummets. When intervention begins in the ambulance, on the other hand—when an intravenous line is started so medicine can be delivered, when CPR is initiated, getting oxygen to the brain—precious seconds, and lives, are saved.

The practice of the 1960s and even the 1970s—carrying the critically injured in vehicles virtually without medication or medical personnel—was shocking, especially in light of all the progress modern medicine had otherwise made. In an age when doctors were performing heart transplants, bypass surgery, and even sophisticated neurosurgery, dumping the desperately ill and injured in the back of a truck like mere cargo was something that had to change.

War-Zone Medicine

Surprisingly, when change finally came, the guiding lights were soldiers sent a world away, to the ravaged, wartorn jungles and rice paddies of Vietnam. While critically ill Americans at home were tossed in the backs of vans and driven, untreated, to the hospital for care, soldiers in Vietnam had the treatment taken to them.

Gus Pappas is now division chief for the community affairs unit of Emergency Medical Service in New York City, and one of the most experienced paramedics in the United States. In 1968, he was part of the Tet Offensive in Vietnam. Trained as a medical corpsman by the navy and assigned to Fleet marine service, Pappas helicoptered into war zones from Khe Sanh to Phu Bai, treading regions where doctors would not go. "In Nam," Pappas explains, "doctors stayed in the 'safe zone.' Members of the medical corps, on the other hand, went into 'MASH' zones on what we called 'medevac runs.' Sometimes we went in with helicopters, sometimes on foot. We were cross-trained in a full gamut of medical skills. We learned to do the initial triage, deciding who needed care first, and who we had to turn our backs on to save the others. We learned to stabilize those with fractures and severed limbs, often giving intravenous infusions to prevent shock. We were even trained in the art of surgery, which was sometimes essential to save a life out in the field. Using our surgical skills, we often removed pungi sticks and grenade fragments and even sutured before transporting the wounded back to base."

Pappas himself was wounded by a hand grenade in June of 1969 and was sent back to the States. Imagine his disappointment when, as an employee of the Health and Hospitals Corporation in New York, he went to work in the old-style emergency room as part of another, less-celebrated corps. "We were the bedpan pushers," Pappas says. Indeed, despite their skills, Pappas and others of his ilk had been demoted to mere errand boys. "We emptied bedpans and assisted the staff in menial tasks," Pappas explains, but without any civilian credentials, he was not allowed to do much more.

Determined to utilize his training, Pappas went back to college, earning a premed degree. He might have gone on to medical school, but a growing awareness merged with the return of Vietnam's medical corps to suggest a new possibility in New York and around the United States. Why not do here what he'd been doing in Nam? Someone was driving the ambulance anyway, right? Why send a glorified driver to the scene when you could train a "medic" in six months to a year, and start critical medical intervention on the spot?

Slowly, the notion of Emergency Medical Service (EMS) systems emerged. To operate properly, its architects insisted, such a system would draw together a variety of elements, including adequately equipped ambulances, specially trained personnel, and a communications network between doctors at the base hospital and technicians in the field.

"Lying in the jungle covered in mud, I would always think about the white picket fence and the kids and the dog in the yard," Pappas relates. "I wanted to start my family soon. So when I had the option of training to be a medic instead of going on to medical school, I decided that was the path for me."

A Corps Is Born

As part of the first generation of emergency medical personnel in New York, Pappas was classified an emergency medical technician (EMT) in 1973. Pursuing his training further, he earned the advanced status of paramedic a year later.

A bold new health care initiative had begun. In New York, for instance, the fledgling Emergency Medical Service received four thousand calls a day. In Chicago, the medical pioneer Dr. David Boyd created an EMS that served as a national model. Other major cities, including Miami, Seattle, Los Angeles, Pittsburgh, and Charlottesville, established impressive EMS systems as well.

Soon paramedics had become national symbols of survival. In 1972, in a tribute to our culture's latest icons, television pioneer Jack Webb, creator of *Dragnet,* launched the popular series *Emergency,* profiling the heroic efforts of paramedics in Los Angeles.

Its importance duly noted on national television, the Emergency Medical Service set out to improve its performance and, every so often, invent itself anew. Fueled by government grants, emergency services—especially in the large urban areas—were soon tied to 911: Call that single number, and, depending on the situation, a dispatcher could hook you up with paramedics, fire department, or police. Some systems even came through with what the experts call a "tiered response": The first responders, emergency medical technicians perhaps (EMTs), got there in minutes and started providing basic care. They would be backed up by paramedics trained in more sophisticated techniques, depending on need.

Pinellas County, Florida, which includes Clearwater and St. Petersburg, is known for its state-of-the art EMS system. Each time the emergency system is tapped, the victim, no matter what the problem, gets help from a fire department rescue truck and an ambulance, each manned by two rescue workers.

And in Tulsa, Oklahoma, a computer knows in an instant the ambulance nearest an emergency; instead of being parked at a station house, each vehicle moves around under guidance of the computer, which calculates when and where accidents and heart attacks are most apt to happen. Radar tracks the ambulance, shown as a magenta blip on a thirty-inch electronic screen, so it can't get lost. Ambulances must respond in eight minutes 90 percent of the time or the private company that runs the service is fined.

Man the Decks

But Emergency Medical Service is more than just an organization. The more you understand about the *people* who care for you, the better you'll be able to communicate your needs when an emergency occurs.

Emergency medical workers come from many backgrounds. Some come to the job with just a high school diploma, others have Ph.D.s. They also come from a wide variety of cultures and nationalities. "It's significant," says Richard Marsella, director of St. Luke's–Roosevelt's Fast Care[SM], "because you're putting them together, elbow-to-elbow, in what I liken to the front of a space capsule. They're in this very confined space in the front of the ambulance for eight hours. They don't need to become the best of friends, but they do need to work effectively in situations often very demanding of cooperation. When paramedics and EMTs work together for a long time, they start to anticipate the other's actions—they develop a rhythm, a sixth sense, that greatly enhances performance."

While each municipality is set up differently, the megasystem functioning in New York, the nation's largest, can be used to portray the range of human roles. We've described some of these individuals before, but here the chain is complete:

Tour commander: In New York and any other sizable EMS system, the tour commander coordinates all operations, from the initial 911 call, to the dispatching of ambulances, to multiple casualty ambulances.

911 operator: When you dial 911, you reach the city's call-receiving station, where the first person you speak with is the 911 operator. After hearing that you want an ambulance, the operator retrieves such basic information as the location of the emergency, the call-back number, and the caller's name. The information, and the call, are then transferred to an EMS call-receiving operator (CRO) via a computer and telephone link.

EMS call-receiving operator: The CRO verifies the information, and then, determines the exact nature of the medical emergency. In many cases, you will receive crucial "prearrival" instructions on what to do for the patient until the ambulance arrives.

Registered nurses: If additional medical information is required, the CRO may transfer the call to a registered nurse, who can provide more elaborate phone help until the ambulance arrives.

Dispatchers: Information is sent, again via computer link, from the call-receiving computer to a local dispatch terminal, where a dispatcher is standing by to send the appropriate ambulance, depending on the medical problem. Dispatchers radio the appropriate ambulance, at the same time sending pertinent information over a mobile computer data terminal.

First responders/first-aiders: These people, who are often the first on the scene of a medical emergency, have completed varying levels of training, from as little as four hours on up to a month or two. They may provide only the most basic care, including control of bleeding and CPR. First responders may include police officers, firefighters, or laypeople. They will have limited equipment, supplies, and knowledge, and are intended to provide immediate care prior to ambulance arrival.

Emergency medical technicians: EMTs are basic life-support personnel trained to assist with childbirth, to splint fractures, control bleeding, stabilize spinal injuries, perform CPR, and treat shock. In addition, they have been equipped and trained in the use of cardiac defibrillation. They also go through a certification process and must be recertified every three years.

Paramedics: Trained in advanced life support, paramedics (often called just medics) assess and treat the seriously injured and ill. In addition to the skills and techniques of the EMT, they have at their disposal medications that stabilize heart rhythms and restore the functions of vital organs; advanced airway devices for opening the breathing passages, a procedure known as intubation; a variety of intravenous fluids used to transport vital fluids and nutrients, including electrolytes, throughout the body; and defibrillators that normalize rapid, uncontrolled heart rhythms.

Paramedics may, depending on local protocol, perform many invasive procedures that can be performed in an emergency department. Instructions for these procedures are often "standing orders" previously authorized by a physician, and do not require that medics contact a doctor on the spot. Sometimes, in more complex or life-threatening situations, when more unusual treatment is required, doctors on call may give medics instructions via radio or telephone-medical directory.

In New York, a paramedic can be certified after twelve hundred hours of training. He or she also goes through a certification, or testing, period, and must be recertified every three years.

Emergency physicians: Doctors are hooked up with the EMS system twenty-four hours a day to help paramedics make decisions before initiating some of the more complex medical procedures, including initiation of medication.

Depending on your situation, you can expect an ambulance to respond with a team of EMTs or a team of paramedics. If you have a broken wrist, expect a team of EMTs to show up at your door. If you're having a heart attack, an asthma attack, or have been in a car accident, paramedics will be sent, though EMTs may show up first as part of the "tiered response," so that help arrives as soon as possible.

Take It to the Streets: A Day in the Life

Despite rumors to the contrary, working the ambulance is not usually one long dirge, not a series of grizzly traumas and deaths, one after the next. For a couple of St. Luke's–Roosevelt Hospital paramedics, the four-to-midnight shift one rainy day and night went like this:

First stop, around four o'clock in the afternoon, was a doctor's office, where the patient complained of heart problems, high blood pressure, and a condition the paramedics termed prostatic hypertrophy—the constant desire to urinate, frustrated because the prostrate is enlarged, preventing the urine from coming out.

The sixtyish patient, grateful to be getting help, explained that he'd been a salesman at Macy's for thirty-one years. During the ride, he showed a paramedic pictures of his daughter.

"You have a number of serious medical problems," the medic advised. "If you treat them, you'll be OK. If you don't, you may die. If they want to admit you to the hospital, don't fight it. Just stay."

After drop-off at the hospital, the paramedic team cruised the streets. They stopped for coffee and a snack, and, while sitting in the ambulance, read the newspaper and talked. At six o'clock, they were summoned again: Farther uptown, the dispatcher said, a man lay unconscious on the street. The ambulance arrived within minutes; only problem was, the victim was no longer there.

More cruising, more talking, more coffee, until 7:55 P.M., when the dispatcher called again: A man had collapsed on the Broadway uptown local subway train. Taking their stretcher underground, the paramedics finally found the patient. A well-dressed man, complete with briefcase, suit, and tie, was surrounded by police. He didn't seem to know his name, the date, or the location—something the paramedics call "disoriented times three" (for this patient, time, place, and identity are all unknowns).

Again, the medics made an assessment: This was a seizure patient, they determined, one who had *not* taken his medication. The paramedics put him on the stretcher and, despite his pleas not to go, took him to the hospital. If the patient is "disoriented times three," they explained, and if police are present to confirm, they don't need his permission to take him in. They do what they feel is in the patient's best interests.

Again the paramedics started cruising—and cruising and cruising—until ten o'clock, when they were summoned to Harlem, to a tiny tenement apartment crowded with tattered furniture and guarded by a giant but gentle dog. An old man, already diagnosed with thoracic cancer, could hardly breathe. "The tumors in his chest have probably metastisized," one paramedic guessed before providing oxygen, seating him on an upright stretcher and taking him to the ED.

That's the way a typical shift goes: short, high-stress periods on call punctuated by longer periods of downtime. On this particular day, there is no carnage—no burned or beaten children, no brutal murders, car crashes, or rapes—though, the paramedics insist, they have seen it all. Even during this quiet tour it's all work, of course, make no mistake. Even while chatting, while drinking coffee, the paramedics are girding themselves, gathering emotional resources for the moment they are called on again.

The stress of the job is real. According to experts, EMTs and medics are far more prone than most other workers to bouts of depression, drug abuse, and suicide. Psychologist George Everly, Ph.D., of Union Memorial Hospital in Baltimore, an expert on critical-incident stress who has studied EMS workers, explains, "The unusual shifts, long hours, and dramatic fluctuations in endocrine levels of EMS crews create extraordinary stress. The work generally consists of hours of boredom, punctuated by moments of sheer terror," he says. "You'll be sleeping, all of a sudden have a massive adrenaline surge, then go back to sleep again."

In recent years the stress has been exacerbated because medics fear for their own safety during work. "I've had people throw rocks, bottles, and eggs at me while on the scene of fires and medical runs," says a paramedic from Baltimore.

"Hunting for an address in the middle of the night with no real idea of the situation is a constant stressor," adds a 911 dispatcher and emergency medical technician from California. "I've had a patient carrying a concealed handgun, and have even walked in on a murder with the shooter, the victim, and the hysterical wife of the victim still in the house."

A paramedic from Washington says, "Here in the District of Columbia, we have a very violent society. People here know how the game is played. Let me give you an example. Your friend has been shot, but you don't want the cops because you have been engaged in what is not exactly a legal activity. You want your friend to get help, but you want to be gone by the time the cops get there. So you dial 911, but instead of reporting the truth—that there has been a shooting—you tell the operator your friend is having a heart attack. The police don't respond on heart attacks. Fire trucks and medic units do."

For fellow rescue workers, the medic from Washington gives this advice: "All I can say is listen to that little voice inside you. When the voice says 'Get out,' do it! If you roll in on a scene that is going bad, put the patient in your truck and get out! After you are clear, then work the patient. Do they teach you this in school? No. But the instructors don't have to worry about a situation like this sitting in a classroom, do they?"

Despite the adrenaline, EMS workers often deal with the relatively mundane. As St. Luke's–Roosevelt Hospital's Dan Mathisen points out, "Most people have a skewed view of what it is EMS people do, because all they've seen is Johnny and Roy and Squad 51 on *Emergency,* or William Shatner and *Rescue 911.* People don't realize that most of the calls are not life-and-death; as much as anything, we're there to provide what we call psychological first aid—calming somebody down and helping them understand what just happened to them. The majority of those we care for are disoriented—whether they've fallen and broken a leg or have been in a car crash, they've never been in this situation before, and they need to know it's OK."

Medicine on Wheels

When the EMTs or paramedics finally arrive at *your* house or office, what can you expect? Except in instances of dire emergency, the procedure will go as follows.

Before you are put in the ambulance, EMS personnel will conduct a physical exam and get your medical history so they can determine as accurately as possible what the problem might be. Since paramedics generally work in teams of two (as do EMTs), expect one partner to do the hands-on assessment while the other jots down information, including the details of your medical history and your complaint.

As part of the physical assessment, Emergency Medical Service workers will try to determine whether you are oriented as to identity, time, and place—whether you know who you are, where you are, and the time—or whether you are conscious at all. They will examine wounds and injuries, assess the color of your skin and take vital signs, including respiration rate, blood pressure and pulse. Expect some pinching, touching, and poking, and expect someone to listen to your chest and lungs.

Many patients become impatient answering a lot of questions, but as a rule such history is critically important to correct diagnosis. As with the 911 dispatcher you spoke to earlier (see Chapter 2), it is in your own best interest to communicate as clearly and calmly as you can. Communicate the name and affiliation of your personal physician, any medication you may be taking, any prior illnesses and any allergies you may have.

Do not assume that just because this information was given to the dispatcher it has been relayed to paramedics on the scene as well.

At this point, if the responders are emergency medical technicians, they may decide to summon paramedics, who can deliver a higher level of care. If paramedics are second on the scene, chances are they will repeat some of the physical exam and questioning. They may also hook up a portable electrocardiogram to check the heart and start an IV to keep a vein open for delivery of drugs later, if necessary. Medications may also be injected into the skin, delivered as oral or nasal mist through a nebulizing machine, or channeled through a tube inserted in the trachea (known as an endo-tracheal tube).

Whether your final responder is an emergency medical technician or a para-medic, your condition will determine the care. Sometimes, paramedics will just calm you down, lift you onto a stretcher, and take you to the hospital. Other times, they will start treatment in your home or office or in the ambulance itself. If you have trouble with your ABC's—airway, breathing, or circulation—they will address those problems first.

According to Plan

Whatever techniques are applied, they will always be drawn from the paramedic's set of rules. Indeed, paramedics and EMTs are bound to follow very specific protocols as outlined in an accepted tome of guidelines called *The Standard of Care*. To make the split-second decisions emergency medicine requires, they rely, without question, on this medical "cookbook" linking a set of protocols to presenting signs and symp-toms. While dermatologists or neurologists may have the time to research and consider the best course of treatment, paramedics must do the job *now*—and according to plan.

For patients with acute asthma, for instance, paramedics will first ensure an open airway and administer oxygen. Then they will establish an IV lifeline and, if needed, administer medication, including epinephrine, inhaled Proventil mist, and other bron-chodilators as well.

In case of acute myocardial infarction, or congestive heart failure, medics will administer oxygen; sit the patient up with legs dangling; set up an intravenous lifeline; monitor the heart with electrocardiogram; and then deliver one or more of a number of possible medications, including nitroglycerin, furosemide, or morphine sulfate.

For patients in cardiac arrest, medics may "camp out" at the scene, running a "code"—or cardiopulmonary resuscitation—without attempting to move the patient at all. This makes sense. If the patient is going to be resuscitated, it's going to happen in the first few minutes after the arrest. Why waste valuable time carrying Grandma down six flights of stairs when paramedics can bring the power of emergency department drugs and techniques to her?

It is, of course, impossible to go over the details of each and every malady and the related protocols, equipment, and drug therapies here. But to familiarize yourself with some of the medicines, equipment, and lesser-known techniques of the ambulance corps, refer to the summary below.

"PARAMAGIC"

Emergency medical technicians and paramedics may use these tools and techniques to see you through.

Suctioning: When the mouth or throat fills with vomit, blood, or secretions, a suctioning device helps remove the material. To help paramedics remove blood or vomitus from the airway, most ambulances have a fixed suction, powered by the ambulance engine, and a portable suction that can be taken to the patient.

Laryngoscopy: The technique by which paramedics look directly into the larynx, with a laryngoscope, to remove foreign bodies obstructing the airways of choking victims or to insert an endotracheal tube.

Endotracheal intubation: The technique by which a tube is passed directly into the trachea through either the mouth or nose, enabling paramedics to open the airway or, when necessary, deliver medicine directly to the lungs.

Cricothyrotomy: The surgical opening of the skin and tissues in the neck to create an airway.

Oxygenation: When impaired heart or lungs or compromised circulation limits delivery of oxygen to the body's cells and vital organs paramedics can make up the deficit through oxygenation. To oxygenate, medics use oxygen contained in an oxygen cylinder aboard the ambulance and in a portable cylinder brought to the patient's side. Oxygen passes from the cylinder, often through a humidifier, before delivery to the patient. Your Emergency Medical Service team may deliver oxygen through a number of conduits, including nasal cannulas (soft rubber tubes placed in the nostrils) or a plastic face mask.

Ventilation with bag-valve-mask: Instead of mouth-to-mouth resuscitation outlined in the first aid chapter, EMTs and paramedics generally use this device, consisting of a face mask, a valve, and a bag that is squeezed to pump oxygen into the lungs. The bag-valve-mask may pump regular air or tap a supply of pure oxygen.

The oral airway: A curved plastic device that fits over the back of the tongue, helping deeply unconscious people breathe without interference.

The nasal airway: A soft rubber device inserted through the nose, allowing the passage of air from the nose to the lower airway.

Intravenous (IV) therapy: Paramedics insert intravenous lines to replace fluids in those patients who have lost blood, and to deliver vital medications fast. If the IV is used to replace fluid, paramedics typically use a regular saline solution. Drugs delivered intravenously may include lidocaine to control the heart's rhythm or morphine for heart failure.

Tourniquet: Though you yourself should never use a tourniquet as part of your first-aid strategy, EMS workers may, on very rare occasions, apply one to save a life. In general, a tourniquet is a wide, flat material tied around a limb to stop an otherwise fatal flow of blood.

Spinal immobilization: To stabilize the neck, usually before removing the patient from a car crash or the scene of other traumatic accidents, paramedics apply a cervical collar. They then place a short backboard behind the head and neck and finally, to stabilize still further, put a neckroll under the neck. Stabilized with neckroll, short backboard, and cervical collar, the patient may then be strapped to a long backboard, or whole body splint, to be carried away from the accident scene.

Splinting injured extremities: From rigid splints to inflatable air splints, EMS workers will carry a range of devices to stabilize breaks, sprains, or dislocations until the patient arrives at the hospital.

Monitoring the heart: In the event of extreme high blood pressure or cardiac emergencies, including dysrhythmias or cardiac arrest, paramedics will monitor

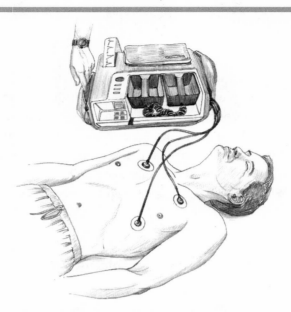

the heart with an electrocardiogram, or EKG. First, monitoring electrodes are applied directly to the chest, arms and legs. Once the electrodes are hooked up, the monitor is turned on and trained paramedics may then get a better idea of what is happening.

Defibrillation: Once the individual muscle fibers of the human heart are out of synch, once the heart stops beating in a single, coordinated rhythm, danger of cardiac arrest is grave. To halt such fibrillation, restoring the heartbeat to normal and sometimes, in case of cardiac arrest, bringing victims back from the dead, paramedics use a machine called a defibrillator. After the machine is turned on, the paddles attached are lubricated. When applied to the chest, these electrically charged paddles send a jolt of electricity to the heart, momentarily paralyzing all its component muscles. When the muscles regain their function, they will often start beating in unison, restoring the heartbeat to normal.

THE AMBULANCE APOTHECARY

Paramedics are generally certified to use specific drugs. Following protocols established in advance, paramedics may administer these drugs orally, or sublingually, by injection, through inhalation via a mask, by intravenous lifeline, or down the breathing tube. Paramedics keep these pharmaceuticals in a drug box, and are advised to double-check the dosage with literature on hand before each and every administration. Those pharmaceuticals found in the ambulance are listed below. Some brand names are given in parenthesis following generic or chemical name.

Activated charcoal USP: Used in some cases of poisoning or overdose to absorb harmful compounds.

Albuterol (Proventil, Ventolin): For fast relief of asthma, bronchitis, or emphysema, to dilate the breathing tubes.

Aminophylline: Relieves constriction of the brochial tubes in cases of asthma.

Amyl nitrite (Vaporole): To treat cyanide poisoning.

Atropine sulfate: Used to accelerate the heart or treat some cases of poisoning.

Bretylium tosylate: Sometimes used to replace or aid defibrillation of the heart and to restore heart rhythm.

Dextrose, 50 percent: Used in cases of low blood sugar and coma to restore blood-sugar level.

Diazepam (Valium): This muscle relaxant may be used to suppress brain seizures or relieve severe anxiety.

Diphenhydramine hydrochloride (Benadryl): Used in the treatment of severe allergic reactions.

Dopamine: Helps restore blood pressure and promote urine flow in cases of shock.

Epinephrine (Adrenalin): Used to enhance defibrillation in cases of cardiac arrest, and to treat life-threatening allergic reactions as well as acute attacks of asthma.

Epinephrine, racemic: Used in children to treat upper airway problems, especially croup.

Furosemide (Lasix): This potent diuretic is used to control fluid overload during congestive heart failure.

Lidocaine (Xylocaine): Used in certain instances to prevent ventricular fibrillation of the heart muscle after electrical defibrillation.

Magnesium sulfate: Used, under particular circumstances, to treat heart failure, asthma, and eclampsia.

Morphine sulfate: Used to treat pulmonary edema associated with congestive heart failure, and to relieve pain associated with heart attack, burns, and other conditions.

Naloxone (Narcan): Used to treat narcotic overdose and coma of unknown origin.

Nitrous oxide, "laughing gas" (Nitronox): Relief from pain in instances of heart attack, trauma, burns, and other conditions, including labor.

Oxygen: Reverses the damaging impact of oxygen loss on the brain, heart, and other vital organs. Used in instances of cardiac or respiratory arrest, chest pain, shock, coma, chest trauma, drowning, pulmonary edema, inhalation of toxins, acute asthma, stroke and head injury, and critical injury.

Sodium bicarbonate: By neutralizing excess acid, this drug helps return blood and body fluids to normal in instances of poisoning, shock, barbiturate overdose, electrocution, asthma, and trauma, as well as during prolonged CPR.

Syrup of ipecac: Used to induce vomiting, thus emptying the stomach of ingested poisons or drugs in a conscious patient.

Terbutaline sulfate (Brethine): Used in some cases of asthma or other lung disease.

Thiamine (Vitamin B1): Used in cases of chronic alcholism or other instances of malnutrition as well as prior to administration of 50 percent dextrose in those suffering coma.

Verapamil (Calan, Isoptin): Used in some cases of cardiac arhythmia.

How to Advocate for Yourself in the Ambulance

Emergency medical technicians and paramedics have been trained to deal with a wide range of problems. They must prove themselves capable through continuing-education courses and rigorous recertification tests taken every three years. When a new technique is accepted, as a matter of course it becomes part of the armamentarium used by the Emergency Medical Service across the land. EMS workers are under constant scrutiny: It takes only one big mistake to have that certificate taken away. Most emergency workers on the job have proven themselves worthy of the responsibility they bear. And EMS workers go out in pairs. If someone is new on the job, that rookie will be assigned to a veteran who has handled the beat for years.

These safeguards ensure that most EMS personnel who come your way will be highly competent. However, even when paramedics are highly qualified, they are not psychic. They cannot know or guess every detail of your condition, and in a high-stress situation such as a multiple car accident with many victims, EMTs or paramedics may not ask.

In short, there may be situations aboard the ambulance where you find it necessary to advocate for yourself or for someone you're helping who is injured or ill. But when is it really appropriate to intervene on your own behalf, and when will a dispute with EMS simply put a life at risk? Which issues are really important, and which are of little consequence in terms of the patient's ultimate health? If you must intervene, how should you approach paramedics so that they take your concerns seriously—without taking offense?

To answer these questions we have polled EMTs and paramedics across the country. Their answers have helped us create a powerful guide for ambulance patients everywhere.

The point paramedics make first is that patient intervention can hinder appropriate care. Advocating for rights, for instance, didn't work out for one pregnant Queens, New York, woman whose family called EMS after she went into labor and started to bleed. Paramedics wanted to take the woman to a hospital just a mile from her house. The woman's family requested she go to her physician's designated hospital four miles away. Argument over the destination continued for twenty minutes before EMS supervisors resolved the argument—in the family's favor. By that time, though, the fetus had been lethally compromised. The baby, suffering from a rare anomaly in which normally enclosed umbilical veins were exposed, bled to death during the labor.

Paramedics in this case were accused of serious wrongdoing. Critics charge that they allowed the pregnant woman to walk to the car herself, and failed to examine her on the spot. In addition, the woman's own hospital, although farther than the paramedics' choice, was still within the ten-minute travel time allowed—and they, as well as the woman's family, had argued on and on.

But whether or not one takes issue with the paramedics, we contend that, given the life-threatening nature of the woman's condition, it would have been in her own best interest to stop arguing (even if she felt she was right) and get to the closest emergency department. After examining the facts of the case, St. Luke's–Roosevelt Hospital's Dr. Lynn states, "The problem afflicting this child was extremely rare, and there's no way paramedics could have picked up on it in the field. In this case, rapid transit was clearly necessary and five minutes might have made a difference. This woman would have been much better off going to the closer hospital. Even though her physician was associated with the second hospital, he wasn't there when she arrived, he didn't perform the surgery, so the fact that she had a relationship with him didn't benefit a soul."

Adds Dr. Lynn, "The policy of going to the closest hospital serves to protect the community as well. While this patient was arguing, she was not only jeopardizing her own fetus, but also, other people waiting for the ambulance, who were not going to get care because the ambulance was delayed."

The bottom line is this: If you or a loved one are seriously ill or injured, and if there's any chance that condition may lead to permanent debility or death, don't waste more than a few precious seconds negotiating with paramedics about destination. Instead, just *ask* to go to the hospital of your choice, explaining your reasons as clearly as you can. And do make the request reasonable. One New Jersey paramedic points out that patients on his run have demanded hospitals in New York City, two and a half hours away, Philadelphia, three and a half hours away, and even Connecticut, five hours away. Obviously, those requests could not be honored and tended to antagonize the paramedics involved. After you've made your request, accept the team's decision with equanimity. Even if you feel they are wrong and you're right, go with the program. They always have your best interest at heart!

When someone is bleeding to death, even a minute or two can save a life. For the person in cardiac arrest, two minutes can mean the difference between an intact or permanently damaged brain. For the devastated mother in Queens, taking on EMS meant a serious, perhaps deadly, delay. You've heard of the "golden hour, " but EMS workers have another, favorite term: The "platinum ten minutes." The meaning is obvious. For the seriously injured or ill, rescue work done as close to the time of injury as possible is key. Moreover, since the trauma patient needs to get to an operating room within sixty minutes from the event, and since ten, twenty, or even thirty minutes have been lost between the time of the trauma, the call to EMS, the dispatch, and the response of the rescuers, it's to your benefit to minimize any wasted time on the scene. Ideally, you should be assessed, treated, and loaded into the ambulance en route to the hospital in ten minutes or less.

Arguing with paramedics over destination will not only waste time but also jeopardize the quality of your care. Medics often know things you don't. They know which hospitals are overcrowded on any given day; which hospital has that inexperienced new resident in charge; and which place just happens to be blessed with the board-certified emergency expert who can restart the heart and remove five bullets with aplomb. They also know the location of the burn center, the trauma center, and other modes of specialized care.

Just think about it: If you've been admitted to your second- or third-choice hospital for emergency care, you can still be transferred later to the hospital of choice for surgery up the road or a long-term stay.

On the other hand, paramedics point out, sometimes patient intervention can help save a life. One paramedic from Michigan concedes, "There are times when the patient is right and we are wrong." Specifically, the Michigan paramedic recalls "a simple run" involving "a heart patient in critical need to reach the hospital fast. Air was the way to go," explains the paramedic, because speed was of the essence. But the patient, who had a moral fear of planes, refused to fly. "I do not have wings," she told the EMS crew. "If God wanted me to fly, you would be seeing feathers instead of hair."

"Due to her extreme fear of flight," the paramedic explains, "we almost lost her. When we agreed to drive, her vital signs bounced back." En route, the ambulance crew honored other requests as well. "We agreed to no lights and no siren, because she hated the thought of all that fuss. We used a lot of oxygen, IVs, and monitoring, and she did fine." Adds the paramedic: "We later learned she almost died on a chopper with a previous crew because of her fear of flight."

Of course, unless you are declared insane, incompetent, or "disoriented times three," you have the legal right to determine what care you receive, or whether you get any care at all. If you explicitly refuse a procedure the paramedic deems necessary, that procedure may be performed only if the paramedic can establish what lawyers call "implied consent," a legal principle by which society seeks to protect those who cannot protect themselves. For example, in most jurisdictions the EMT or paramedic in charge has "implied consent" to treat minor patients until a parent or guardian can be found, despite the objections of the child. Similarly, people under the influence of alcohol or drugs may not be able to give valid consent, paving the way for the EMT or paramedic to have the last word. (Such patients might later be able to validly refuse treatment when they sober up.)

In most instances, however, the demands of the patient prevail. One paramedic who is also a lawyer states: "The notion that every person has the right to self-determination over his or her body has a long and strong background in this country." Adds another paramedic, "As long as they're a conscious, competent adult, we can't force them to go to the hospital—that's kidnapping—or to accept treatment—that's assault. We had a seventy-five-year-old lady, conscious and 'oriented times three,' with fluid in her lungs. We tried eight ways till Sunday to convince her to go to the hospital, but she wouldn't budge. Finally, she signed an RMA/AMA [Refused Medical Attention/Against Medical Advice]. We advised the family to call us again if she passed out."

In short, unless you are underage, under the influence, or insane, you have the right to refuse treatment. But if health, not debate, is your agenda, you will approach EMS personnel in a psychologically savvy way. Before you argue with a medic over treatment, ask him as politely as possible to do things your way, or to explain what he's doing and why. The best emergency medical technicians and paramedics espouse communication as a goal. For veterans of the street, dialogue is key. Every so often, however, you may have to help the process along.

Ask your questions in a firm, polite manner: "Do I really need to have my clothes cut off and destroyed? Can I show you a way to remove them without inflicting any damage?" is one way of phrasing things. And another approach: "Why do you feel oxygen is necessary? Couldn't I do without it?" Make your point—respectfully.

Do alert EMTs or paramedics whenever your condition changes in any way. "People must understand that if their symptoms change or progress, get better or worse, they need to tell the ambulance staff," says Dr. Stephan Lynn. "Even if the staff doesn't ask, the patient has an obligation to inform, though most patients don't. They are so overwhelmed by the circumstances it doesn't occur to them."

If you have been cordial, EMS workers are more likely to accommodate your requests if they possibly can. If they can't, you will find that, in the overwhelming majority of cases, their actions are ultimately for your benefit.

Because medicine "in the street" is so different from conventional medicine, patients may sometimes feel treatment is at odds with prior understanding of an illness or injury. For example, a patient with chronic asthma or emphysema may have been told by a primary-care physician never to take more than two liters of oxygen per minute. In an emergency situation, however, high concentrations of oxygen are crucial to survival, and if there are any side effects, well, the paramedics are there.

If, after listening to the explanation, you want to reject a treatment, it is in your own best interest to explain why. Perhaps you have an allergy you failed to mention? Perhaps there's a past illness or injury of which the paramedic is unaware? After all, if you've failed to communicate crucial information, the initial diagnosis and possible course of treatment are called into question.

As the patient and end-user, carefully consider the treatments, including their benefits and detriments. Don't be shy about asking whatever questions you have. After all, a well-informed patient will most often make the appropriate personal decision.

After discussing the treatment, if you still believe it is wrong, you may request that the EMT or paramedic call into base. There, a doctor in charge may decide your view is correct (or incorrect), sometimes even verbally altering instructions set forth in the protocols.

You can reject a treatment, but may not demand that paramedics perform novel procedures outside the purview of their training. Emergency medical technicians and paramedics must follow instructions set forth in their standard book of protocols; to veer from the path is to invite trouble, including the patient's death, lawsuits, and the loss of a job.

Last Rights

Perhaps the most distressing situation for patients advocating for their rights emerges in the case of the terminally ill. An old woman, suffering from advanced abdominal cancer, is in constant debilitating pain. She has begged her family to let her go peacefully, keeping her off dehumanizing life-support machines when her time comes. But one day, weeks before the expected end, she clutches at her chest, sensing the sharp stab of a heart attack. Her family, unsure what to do, dials 911.

That's when the woman's worst nightmare comes to pass: Paramedics rush into the house, using all the tools at their disposal. She has gone into cardiac arrest, so CPR and defibrillation are brought to bear. Now, at the hospital, hooked up to a respirator, she is told she will pull through this one—but she has been deprived of the chance to go quickly, as she wished, burdening no one and ending her pain.

In this case, a trip to the "eternal care unit," not the intensive care unit, was what the patient wanted. But for those in similar situations, *without the proper documentation,* neither the patient nor the family will be able to intervene. If the patient wants *no* intervention, it is probably best *not* to call the Emergency Medical Service.

To advocate for the dying after calling 911, it is necessary for the patient to have in his or her possession a valid, properly documented DNR, or "Do Not Resuscitate" order, which, in essence, instructs paramedics to lay off. When such individuals suffer cardiac arrest or stroke, they will be able to go quickly and peacefully without losing their dignity shackled to life-support machines, or burdening family and friends. If your elderly dying relative has suffered cardiac arrest and wants to go peacefully, do not—remember, *do not*—call EMS unless you have a DNR order. Once the system is activated, medics are legally bound to carry through. (See Chapter 13 on death and dying.)

If you don't have a DNR order, and wish to summon nonemergency transport for a relative or dear friend who rejects lifesaving techniques, call a private ambulance company.

A Word to the Wise

We end this chapter with a word of advice. If you are very ill, if you have chest pain, or respiratory distress, if you think you may be suffering severe allergic reaction—in other words, if there's any chance you may jeopardize your health if you do not receive medical care within thirty minutes—don't waste even a second by trucking over to the emergency department on your own. Call an ambulance. The emergency medical technicians or paramedics will be able to stabilize you; they can prevent or treat shock; keep oxygen flowing to your brain and other vital organs; open your airway; and reverse the effects of sudden, deadly allergy. If your medical situation is an emergency in the truest sense of the word, your chances of recovery are greater by leaps and bounds if you summon your local EMS.

VIEW FROM THE BUS: **A Dictionary of Ambulance Slang**

Emergency medical technicians and paramedics spend so much time together in the "bus" and on the street, they have developed a language all their own. Some of the terms, gathered from EMTs and paramedics around the country, may seem somewhat flip. But EMS workers insist these "inside terms" help them deal with tragedy and ventilate stress on a job that is "much harder than 99.9 percent of the public realizes." So that you can tune into "EMSspeak" while riding the ambulance or speaking with paramedics on the scene, we provide the lexicon, below. We have resisted the temptation to put these terms in alphabetical order, and instead, have grouped them by meaning. For some insight into EMS culture, read on.

walky talky: A patient who can ambulate and converse.

frequent flyer: An individual who constantly calls for an ambulance.

lock and load: Putting the patient on a stretcher and getting him in the ambulance, fast.

Paramagic: When a paramedic makes a really great save.

WADAO: Weak and dizzy all over.

doc-in-the-box: A little urgent care center.

MAGGOT: Medically able to get other transportation.

ECU: A patient admitted to the ECU, or eternal care unit, has died.

ICE: Impending cosmic event.

roamin' in the gloamin': Walking through the woods looking for a lost person.

Singer technique: Rapid and repeated plunging of the IV needle attempting to find a vein. Considered bush league.

bus, taxi, truck: All terms for the ambulance.

WWI: Walking while intoxicated.

PHD: Personal hygiene deficit.

nose hose: The tube used in nasal intubation, employed to open the airway.

eating plastic: Describes a person who's been intubated through the mouth.

Edison medicine: Term used to describe application of defibrillator for cardiac arrest.

peanut butter ball or phenobasketball: Phenobarbital.

coma cocktail: Narcan, D50, and Mazecon (an antidote to Valium).

CHAOS: Chief has arrived on the scene.

white wave: Anything more than one supervisor on the scene.

lead overdose: Death by shooting.

gravity storm: What causes a person to slip or fall.

family plan: When twelve family members pile in the ambulance for the two-block ride to the hospital.

Allstateitis: Syndrome exhibited by the patient complaining of neck and back pain after an accident, just to collect a settlement from the other driver's insurance company.

The Rule of Threes

EMS personnel throughout the country have taken to positing rules in threes. These rules vary, but we present a few favorite versions here:

From Dallas and Boston:
1. All bleeding eventually stops.
2. All patients eventually die.
3. If you drop the baby, pick it up.

From New York:
1. It is three in the morning; . . .
2. there are more than three flights of stairs; . . .
3. he weighs more than three hundred pounds; . . . *he walks!*

From Miami:
1. Patch the holes.
2. Blow the air.
3. Drive the bus.

Chapter 5

From Triage to Treatment: What to Expect in the Emergency Department

T he end-state AIDS patient, his immune system so compromised his blood can no longer clot, bleeds from all his facial orifices: nose, mouth, eyes. Donning double latex gloves and face-eye masks, Dr. Maurice Wright, assistant director of the St. Luke's ED, an emergency medical resident, and nurse, stand packing the patient with hundreds of tiny gauze strips in hopes the bleeding will stop. "We just want to make him more comfortable," says Wright, acknowledging the patient's chance of survival is slim to none. "He'll never leave here," Wright explains. Still, Wright works on until, with a series of wracking coughs, the patient spits up a large bloody bolus of tissue. "You don't want to know what that is," Wright tells a visitor. "His diseased, necrotic lungs. I guess we've lost this battle," Wright adds.

Maybe so, but that doesn't stop him from fighting. He dives back into the room to finish the job and, eventually, with great effort, the team stops the bleeding. The patient's mother, a bent, worried, gray-haired woman is summoned, and the two are sent "upstairs."

The scene, one of despair for the afflicted, delivers a message of hope as well. The doctor who fights so fiercely on behalf of a dying man is an emergency physician—a gifted one; and for those who pass his way, it's comforting to know how hard he'll work to diagnose an illness, fashion a treatment, and save a life.

Tall and slim, age thirty-five, Wright says he learned his sense of discipline in a strict Jamaican boys' school where caning was the rule. Today he leads a team of emergency physicians and nurses at St. Luke's Hospital, the uptown site of the St. Luke's–Roosevelt Hospital Center in Manhattan. This inner-city sanctum just across the street from Columbia University and the world-famous Cathedral Church of St. John the Divine is crowded. On a busy day, the patients' stretchers may touch metal to metal, and extend out of established stations into the hall. Just look around and you'll find the elderly grandmother with chest pain; the truck driver with a virus so debilitating he must call in sick at work; the teenager who has been stabbed in the arm or the gut.

Fortunately for these patients, Dr. Wright—in a testament to what must be amazing powers of recall—stores every last detail about every one of them in his brain. The cool, calm eye of a medical storm, he walks through the emergency department like Norman Schwarzkopf in the Gulf. And as he makes his rounds, his instructions are medically incisive, and to the point. "Get that woman started on a thrombolytic [blood thinner]," he instructs one nurse. "Get that man cleaned up," he tells an aid after viewing a patient so ill he has not shaved or showered in what is likely a week. Viewing a woman with chest pain, he shouts out, "Anyone have some nitro in their pocket?" No one does, but a nurse rushes to the drug cabinet to follow through. No detail, apparently, is too small: "Change that bedsheet," Wright tells one attendant. Going over the charts, he notices one aspect of a patient's care has not been duly noted, and, annoyed that the record is incomplete, summons an assistant to set it straight.

On this day, Dr. Wright, heroic though he is, is less than pleased by the demanding attitude of another patient—a woman whose stretcher is right outside the room where he works on the man with AIDS. Oblivious to the uproar, she keeps calling Wright and others on the staff to her side. Admitted to the St. Luke's emergency department with a series of vague symptoms—her shoulder hurts, her stomach hurts, her head hurts—the woman is given a thorough exam and battery of tests. "I have spent well over an hour on this patient," explains Wright, who has scrutinized every test result and ordered still more tests throughout the day. Calling for the woman's records, he determines that she is a psychiatric patient who has missed her clinic appointments and failed to take her medication. Apparently, nothing physical is wrong. "For this woman, this was an emergency," he said, "but it's a drain on a system with limited doctors and so many people who are truly, urgently ill."

The ED staff will spend the next few hours attending to three asthmatics, who must breathe Proventil through nebulizer masks; a victim of drug overdose; an elderly gentleman who's just suffered a heart attack; a young man with a viral infection so severe that his intestines have been damaged and must be restored; a man whose hand has been gashed, requiring specialists from surgery; a case of food poisoning; and more.

"The first thing you need for a top ED is great nurses," Dr. Wright says, "and we have them here. You need a sense of camaraderie, and a sense of humor."

Maurice Wright isn't kidding. The nurses, interns, and residents, who all call him

Maurice, tease him mercilessly about his wife, his kids, and his house in the 'burbs. (His wife, like one of those favorite off-camera characters on a TV show, is often mentioned but never seen.) They also solicit his opinion on everything from a vacationing resident's love life to Broadway shows. After ten grueling hours of work, Dr. Wright's parting comment as he flies out the door is, "Call my wife and tell her I'm so exhausted she needs to get me to the ED."

His wife might take him some sixty blocks downtown to the ED at Roosevelt Hospital—St. Luke's sister institution and a harbinger of the future, where the high-tech science of emergency medicine reigns supreme. Located on 59th Street, near Central Park West and the Plaza Hotel, this ultramodern emergency department, state-of-the-art for the late 1990s, is housed in a new building its architects have dubbed "the hospital for the twenty-first century." Boasting everything from soothing lights and designer colors—peaches, violets, aquamarines—to the latest and greatest emergency equipment medicine has yet devised, the Roosevelt ED is a monument to its craft. For all who can read the writing on the wall—writ large in the form of cardiac arrest clocks, nebulizers, and oxygen ducts built in alongside electric and phone outlets—the message is clear: In a society hooked on speed and efficiency, the age of the emergency department is here.

At the Roosevelt ED, the psychiatric division contains a "quiet room," with floor-to-ceiling tiles in soft, rubberized gray linoleum. The ED obstetrics room, where babies are born, contains ultrasonic heart monitors and specially heated bassinets. The trauma room, a well-stocked surgical theater, has powerful overhead X-ray equipment that can be positioned to work from virtually anywhere, and spotlights that can be moved, remotely, so that already-powerful beams converge. Especially impressive are the computerized monitors located at every patient station. Like the sensors in a nerve network, these intelligent nodes track heart rate, blood pressure, temperature, and oxygen saturation, electronically reporting the stats to the nurses' station and sounding an alarm when things go awry.

Even the layout is innovative. Hospital architects, with a special knowledge of medicine, have created a visual space that brings problems into rapid view. The emergency department's outer chamber, for instance, is walled on one side by plate-glass windows and doors. Clearly visible from the street, its presence advertised by a large red sign, it is a clarion call for the ill and injured. As patients walk in, they are visible to the triage nurse, who faces the entry and can see everything in the wide-open room. The inner chamber, meanwhile, contains a centrally located nurses' station from which all patients are visible—even those in quarantine. Isolated patients, once closed off behind solid doors and walls, are now placed in well-ventilated rooms with clear Plexiglas sliding doors that provide the needed protection, without shielding them from view.

But in the end, the care at Roosevelt, as at St. Luke's, has less to do with the surroundings than with the devoted, highly skilled staff: Dr. Stephan Lynn, director of emergency medicine for the St. Luke's–Roosevelt Hospital Center, sets casts, applies dressings, and sutures wounds like a medical Michelangelo, and also diagnoses an amazing range of diseases, from common to rare. His philosophy is profoundly egalitarian, as it must be if he is to head both sites of this huge metropolitan ED: "My job is to listen to the patients," says Dr. Lynn, who knows this is the first rule of diagnosis. "They're feeling the pain. They're feeling the anxiety. They know their past history, their social circumstances, their surroundings, and their resources. They are probably best able, at least initially, to judge what needs to be done."

And Lynn is not alone: The cast of characters at Roosevelt includes Dr. Gregg Husk, director of the hospital center's new emergency medicine residency program, who can often be seen huddled with students, discussing the merits of treatment for a given case, the more complex the better for teaching the art and science of emergency medicine, and Suzanne Pavel, a nurse who spends much of her day coordinating continuing education for the Roosevelt emergency department nursing staff.

Spending time in the emergency departments at Roosevelt and St. Luke's is more exciting, and far more draining, than watching an hour of *ER* on television. First of all, while the patients on TV are creations, those on the floors of these functioning EDs are soberingly, frighteningly real. An emaciated woman with AIDS, a former prostitute, frets about how she will break the news of her illness to her estranged son—before her "witch of a mother" gets to poison his mind yet again. Five teenagers hurtle at a hundred miles an hour down the West Side Highway, in one last hurrah before a friend goes off to jail on drug charges. Predictably, if tragically, the car bounces off a curb, flies through the air, and ricochets off some trees. When relatives gather to mourn the dead—there are three victims—it is in the outer waiting room of the emergency department at St. Luke's.

In the real emergency department, when doctors and nurses converse they talk a technical language all their own; nothing need be "dummied down," after all, for the lay audience of television. Once you understand what's going on, however, you realize that these dedicated professionals have mastered not just some clever story lines and a few standard techniques, but rather a wide range of sophisticated skills and high-tech strategies across the spectrum of medical disciplines, from cardiology to neurology to orthopedics to radiology and more. Indeed, while the docs on television are mostly residents, physicians in real-world big-city EDs like Roosevelt and St. Luke's are usually board certified in emergency medicine. Highly trained professionals with many years of experience, they have chosen emergency medicine as a lifelong career. The reason for that choice is clear: They love to solve mysteries, and thrive on the intensity of the situation, where their special ability to hyperfocus is pushed to the max. At a pace that is sometimes dizzying—what one paramedic has called "Wham, bam, save your life, mam!"—they respond to literally hundreds of novel and swiftly evolving problems every day in their theater-in-the-round, the ED.

Nurse Suzanne Pavel explains that for her, novelty is what makes the job so rewarding. "To work in the emergency department, you really have to be a generalist," Pavel says. "You're dealing with life from birth to death; babies are delivered here, and at the same time, you have the ninety-five-year-old person who experiences death here. We see every patient population, the whole gamut of ages, cultures, and economic groups. It's completely multicultural; it's the soup-to-nuts of society. You see the homeless and, because Roosevelt is right in midtown Manhattan, the VIPs. It's also exciting because you're taking care of people when they're coming in—they still have their street clothes on; before they're diagnosed, you really don't have any idea what's going on with them, and it's your job to solve the puzzle, to find out."

It's no wonder, given the complexity of the modern emergency department, that patients and visitors may sometimes find it hard to know what's going on. At Roosevelt and St. Luke's, patients may witness high-tech medical alchemy performed by dozens of medical and support personnel: doctors, nurses, aids, social workers, paramedics, emergency medical technicians, residents, interns, medical students, specialists in radiology, neurology, surgery, and more.

In the pages that follow, we will clarify the terrain. Consider the rest of this chapter, in part, a walking tour of the ED. We will orient you as to time and place, summing up how a patient advances through the system from triage to waiting room to the inner sanctum, where treatment begins. Once we have helped you understand this medical stage, we will review actors, scenery, and props: the variety of staff you will encounter, the range of diagnostic techniques, the medicines, the treatments, and the tools.

Finally, because the ED, like any complex environment, is easiest to negotiate when you are prepared, we will suggest some useful patient strategies: How can you best present your case to the triage nurse? How can you make sure the doctor understands your true problem? How can you advocate for your patient rights in myriad effective ways? For the answers, read on.

Triage: Portal to the Emergency Department

In Vietnam, medics had a system for deciding who would be treated first and who, due to lack of resources, might be left to die. Called *triage,* the french word for sorting and sifting, the system first came into being in the nineteenth century, during the Napoleonic Wars. Simply and brutally, it involved literally choosing who would receive the limited medical resources first. Since those in the military were primarily concerned with getting soldiers back into battle, they often treated the least injured first: In that way, there would be more soldiers available to wage the war, though sometimes, due to this difficult choice, the most severely injured died before treatment could be dispensed.

Those who go to an emergency department, either by ambulance or on foot, will find a triage system in place, though in reverse. In a hospital, after all, the goal is not to win a war, but to save lives. So the triage nurse, who generally sits behind a desk near the entrance, sorts out the sickest patients—those having heart attacks, those in shock, those bleeding to death—and rushes them in to be treated first. It's comforting to know that emergency departments take the term *emergency* seriously: If your life is at risk or if you are in excruciating pain, the triage nurse will recognize it and send you through before filling out a chart or, possibly, even taking your name.

THE TRIAGE TOP TEN

If the triage nurse believes you have one of these ten conditions, you will be sent through to the inner emergency department at once.

shock

obstruction to the airway

cardiac arrest

heart attack

chest injury

crushing injury

amputation

open fracture

hemorrhage

major burn

In addition, if you have any of the following urgent conditions, the triage nurse will try to arrange for you to see a doctor as soon as possible.

fractured hip

severe laceration

asthma

difficult or labored respiration

In all but the most dire instances, the triage nurse will sit you down for a brief intake interview in which she can use her significant medical acumen to assess what's going on. During this brief assessment, the triage nurse will measure vital signs, including temperature, pulse, respiration, and blood pressure and will inquire about medications regularly taken, and why. He will ask you about allergies to medications.

Perhaps most important, the triage nurse will ask you to describe your major problem: What is it that has brought you to the emergency department in the first place? Within the context of this question, the nurse will try to find out exactly what is going on.

In a nutshell, questions such as the following should help the triage nurse *quantify* your problem: Can you rate the severity of your pain from one to ten? How long have you had your symptoms? Have you coughed up a teaspoon of blood or a bowl of blood? And, in the case of vaginal bleeding, how many vaginal pads have you gone through within the last six hours?

Not only will your answers alert the triage nurse as to the severity of your problem, they will also define the type of care you probably need. Since not all rooms in the emergency department have the same type of equipment, it's important for the triage nurse to determine where you belong. Do you require a room with a cardiac monitor? Are you going to need to see the orthopedist and have an X ray taken? Do you need sutures? Do you need the facilities available only in the OB/GYN room, or psychiatry?

When speaking with the triage nurse, says Dr. Lynn, you must be specific, forceful, and direct. "If you come in and say, 'I don't know, it hurts a little bit. I'm not really sure. I've been bleeding for a while,'" he notes, "the nurse is going to get the sense that it's not horribly serious. But if you come in and say, 'I've had severe pain for the last six hours, and I've bled two quarts of blood,' the nurse will know you have a true emergency, and will bring you right in to be seen."

If the nurse decides you are urgently ill, she will, providing doctors are not busy with even more urgent problems, send you on through to the inner ED at once. On the other hand, if you are deemed to be less critical, you will be asked to take a seat with the registrar, who will record your name, address, phone number, next of kin, and form of insurance or payment—though these will not determine if and when you get care. Instead, in accordance with the rules of triage, you will be asked to take a seat in the outer waiting room, where your medical need, and that factor alone, will determine when you are called.

Finally, in busy EDs like St. Luke's and Roosevelt, those with minor problems such as ear infections, small cuts and bruises, or common viral or bacterial infections will often be sent to a "fast track" area. There, doctors trained in emergency medicine and functioning in an atmosphere reminiscent of the classic family doctor's office will dispense treatment on a first-come, first-served basis. Even if you have a serious problem like a sprain and break, a wound no longer bleeding but requiring sutures, or a high fever, on a very busy day you may have to wait a while.

Observe the triage nurse for an hour at any major hospital and you'll hear an enormous spectrum of complaints: patients with chest pain and shortness of breath, indicating heart attack; those who seem disoriented, indicating possible stroke; end-stage AIDS patients bleeding to death; those with insomina, depression, knife or gunshot wounds, broken bones, sore throat and fever. Sometimes, the injuries have occurred just minutes before, as in a soccer game right near the hospital grounds. Other times the problems have been around for a while. "I've had this rash for the last six months," said one Roosevelt patient who finally decided she definitely needed care. "I've had a headache for two years," said a man. Think of any health problem you've every heard of, and, at some point or another, it will be present at the emergency department.

Patients, of course, are as diverse as the health problems they report. Some sit quietly, state their case, and do as the triage nurse asks of them, from offering an arm for a blood-pressure reading to waiting their turn. Others get swiftly angry; in discomfort, and unfamiliar with the system in place, they deem it intolerable when asked to wait.

For those without life-threatening problems, waiting in the emergency department is often to be expected. It is part of the system, part of what enables the ED to direct all the resources necessary to save a life whenever a life is at stake. If your life were hovering in the balance—and next time it might be—you wouldn't want your ED allocating crucial resources to treat the man with a broken ankle or the woman with a gash on her leg while you silently slipped away.

The next time you go through triage, remember that your complaint will be judged in the context of all of the other patients who are waiting for space, equipment, staff, and service. And although your complaint may be legitimately urgent, on any given occasion there may be one or two people whose problems are even more urgent.

BEHIND THE NUMBERS: **Understanding Your Vital Signs**

"Blood pressure is 140 over 90. Pulse is 78. Oxygen saturation is 98 percent." The triage nurse duly notes these measurements on your medical record, saying them aloud to you as he writes. But what does it all mean? The emergency department is confusing enough without having to interpret a series of numbers—digits, it turns out, that provide crucial information about your health. While normal vital signs vary with the individual, below is a general guide to the numbers for your general understanding.

Pulse rate: Should be between 50 and 100. Anything lower than 50 is too slow, and, in general, anything higher than 100 is too fast for healthy adults. (People who are in very good physical health, particularly athletes, frequently have low pulse rates, but usually not lower than 50.) Children can have far higher pulse rates: A newborn baby can have a pulse rate of 140 to 160, and a young child can have a pulse rate ranging from 100 to 120. Hospitals usually measure pulse with a cardiac machine, but nurses can also clasp their fingers against your wrist and count the beats.

Blood pressure: This physiological measurement has two numbers: an upper, called systolic; and a lower, called diastolic. In general, diastolic blood pressure is the more crucial measurement. Blood pressure is usually considered elevated when the lower number is greater than 90. In most cases, the systolic blood pressure will be less than 140, though in senior citizens it may normally reach 160. If you are thirty-five years old and hear the nurse say your blood pressure is 140 over 90, you may assume you are at the borderline of hypertension. The lower limits of normal blood pressures are harder to determine, but usually, a patient with a blood pressure lower than about 90 over 60 is considered to have low blood pressure. An exception can be seen in some particularly small, thin people, who will normally have blood pressures lower than 90 over 60. Very low blood pressure is sometimes associated with shock. Blood pressure is measured with soft blood pressure cuffs that circle around your arm with Velcro. The cuffs are pumped with air and then deflated until the nurse hears a "pop," indicative of the blood pressure. At Roosevelt Hospital, a monitor automatically blows up and deflates blood pressure cuffs and then takes the measurements.

Oxygen saturation: A healthy patient breathing normally will have blood with an oxygen saturation of between 96 to 98 percent. Anything less than 90 percent is considered significantly abnormal. The blood does not have enough oxygen, showing problems with either breathing or circulation. Oxygen saturation is measured with a device that focuses a red light on the fingernail; the machine detects changes in nail color: a redder shade indicates more oxygen.

Temperature: Normal temperature is defined as 98.6 degrees Fahrenheit (for those hospitals that measure in centigrade, that equals 37 degrees). Doctors generally consider temperatures of 96–100.4 degrees Fahrenheit to be normal; thus, a person can have a temperature between 96 and 100 degrees Fahrenheit, and still be healthy. But when temperature rises above or falls below these levels, it is abnormal and may indicate an infection or some other medical problem. The upper limits of temperature are generally 106 or 107 degrees, though in very rare cases, including instances of hyperthermia, even higher temperatures have been recorded. Temperatures below 95 degrees Fahrenheit may indicate shock, severe infection, or hypothermia. Temperatures below 90 degrees Fahrenheit indicate severe illness, though the numbers may fall to 75–80 degrees Fahrenheit before a person will succumb.

In the emergency department, temperature is generally measured with an electronic thermometer covered with a new plastic sheath for each patient. It requires just a few seconds, not the usual three minutes, for hospital thermometers to register a precise, digital reading. Newer techniques actually measure temperature by placing a device in your ear. This technique is usually simpler than taking temperature by mouth.

Advocating for Yourself in Triage

Emergency department professionals consider triage a high-level skill. "They don't let you do triage until you've been working in the ED for at least a year," explains one nurse who worked at Roosevelt for twenty-five years. With good reason: Recognizing the true emergency and differentiating it from urgent problems that must be treated in twelve to twenty-four hours is a complex task indeed.

The task is so complex that occasionally it's possible for the triage nurse to miss a crucial clue. That's why, as the patient, you can be your own best advocate during triage intake. The more articulate you are about your problem, the more likely it is the nurse will accurately assess what's wrong.

For instance, if you go in with a bleeding finger, you will be sent to the outer waiting room. If you fail to mention that in addition to the finger injury your chest hurts, you feel dizzy, and you're sweating, your nurse might miss the fact that a myocardial infarction—a heart attack—is underway, too. Indeed, it might have been the dizziness caused by the cardiac distress that caused you to injure your finger in the first place.

When describing your complaint to the triage nurse, don't leave out anything, as insignificant as it may seem, and even if you believe it is totally unrelated to the problem at hand. If you have been taking over-the-counter or prescription medicine; if you have a headache, stomachache, or any pain whatsoever; if anything strikes you as unusual, do make sure you mention it to the triage nurse. Strain to recall anything that may be relevant, and do not eliminate any potential clue.

"The ED is an extremely difficult, demanding, and stressful environment not just for the patient, but also for the physicians and nurses," explains Dr. Lynn. And unless the patient is able to articulate his or her concerns or problems, they simply may not get dealt with in the appropriate way.

"As doctors and nurses, it's our job to see patients as expeditiously as is possible, based on our assessment of the urgency of their medical complaint," Lynn adds. "Given that fact, it's clear that all patients must advocate for themselves in the ED. They need to make certain that they clearly articulate their complaints and concerns, and when things don't seem to be going appropriately, they need to ask."

How to accomplish this crucial feat? "You need to speak forcefully," says Lynn. "You need to make certain that your points are made, and that you make them frequently, but not, ideally, loudly and belligerently. In most circumstances, undue aggression hurts more than helps."

Are there any symptoms the triage nurse will look for when deciding to send a patient right through? It makes sense that, like all experts in medical emergency, the triage nurse will be most concerned about threats to the ABC's: the airway, breathing, and circulation. That means choking, asthma attacks, heart attacks, profuse bleeding, and shock. What the triage nurse looks for when scouting out such emergencies, however, are accurate descriptions of the symptoms, not a diagnosis seized upon by the patient in hopes of seeing a doctor soon. If you're too emphatic about a particular diagnosis without describing the related symptoms, if you complain desperately about problems that are truly minor, you may be perceived as the boy who cried wolf.

For instance, don't walk up to the triage nurse and announce, "I'm having a heart attack." If you're *truly* having a heart attack, you'd do better to report the symptoms: "I know I have high blood pressure, and I have this pressure pain in my chest that's been bothering me for the last half hour."

A more complete, even more convincing, description would sound like this: "I have pain in my midchest, behind my breastbone, that feels like somebody's standing on my chest. It's been there for thirty minutes. It started when I was walking up the stairs. It got better when I stopped walking. I've had minor pains like this before that the doctor has called angina. Sometimes, the pain goes to my left arm; sometimes, the pain takes my breath away. The pain has been getting progressively worse over the last half hour, and there's nothing I can do to make it go away."

Along the same lines, do not walk up to the triage nurse and say, "I broke my leg." You will score more points—and obtain a more accurate assessment and better level of treatment—if you state, simply, "I tripped on the sidewalk and I have excruciating pain below my knee."

If your child has the dreaded, much publicized "hamburger disease," the one associated with the *E. coli* bug found in undercooked chopped meat, this description might help the nurse assess what's going on: "My child's been sick for the last two days. It started out like the flu. He felt tired and didn't want to go to school, and didn't feel like eating. Then he had aches and pains all over, and complained of a stomachache. He's had diarrhea. Initially, the stools were a little loose, but today, he's gone to the bathroom every hour or so, and it just looks like dark water coming out. Every once in a while, there's some blood mixed in, and he's been getting sleepier and sleepier. By the way, he ate a burger at a fast-food place three days ago, though I don't know if that's related to his problem now."

As for the proverbial broken ankle: "When I tried to get up, my ankle hurt. It got black and blue and, since I can't put any pressure on the ankle, I can't walk."

In the emergency department, most presentations are of pain. Therefore, before you ever get to the triage nurse, you might rehearse describing your pain as accurately as you can. If something hurts, remember to report exactly where it hurts. Explain how the injury occurred. Describe the severity of the pain. For instance, if you were to grade your pain from one to ten, where ten is the worst and one is the least pain that you've ever experienced, how bad would this pain be? If you can, describe the essential quality of the pain: Is it a pressure pain? Like a toothache? A burning sensation? Like a knife? Where does the pain go? Does it stay in one position, or radiate to different parts of your body? How long has it been there? Is it getting better or worse? Are there specific things—such as pressure, heat, cold, or medication—that make it better or worse?

In short, as an advocate for yourself in triage, your best weapon is your ability to describe your problem as precisely as you can. If you are polite to the triage nurse, moreover, you will find he or she can be a helpful advocate, as well.

There are other ways to advocate for yourself in triage. Report to the triage nurse any time your condition changes or worsens. Report chest pain as soon as you feel it; you will then get sent back to the inner ED immediately. Mention special requests to the triage nurse in advance. For instance, if you have a deep cut on your face and wish to have it sutured by a plastic surgeon on call instead of the attending physician, that is something that can sometimes be negotiated in advance. If your personal doctor is at a hospital across town and you wish to be transferred as soon as possible, mention that as well. And remind the triage nurse you are there and still waiting, every half hour or so.

Through the Looking Glass: What to Expect in the Inner Emergency Department

If the triage nurse finds that you are critically ill, she will escort you through the "portal" to the ED's inner sanctum and place you in an appropriate room, where doctors and nurses will converge to bring you back from the brink.

If your problem is deemed less urgent, you will be called inside when space and staff are available. Either way, your care will be turned over to an emergency department nurse, who may start an intravenous line, draw blood, put you on the cardiac monitor, or do whatever else is necessary to prepare you for evaluation. Sometimes the nurse will get assistance from other technical personnel: IV technicians specializing in establishing intravenous lines; EKG technicians who perform cardiograms; and respiratory therapists who specialize in cardiopulmonary resuscitation and a host of respiratory ills. Do expect some amount of undressing so that medical personnel can access the body part in question. If your injury is particularly serious, emergency workers may even need to cut away some of your clothes so they can administer treatment quickly, without causing you undue pain. One recent patient at Roosevelt, for instance, came in complaining of what seemed like a broken leg after a particularly brutal fall. Nurses and doctors cut away virtually all his clothes to check him for other breaks—and perhaps more important—head and spinal injuries and internal hemorrhaging. Fortunately, almost miraculously, no major injuries beyond the one broken leg were found.

Once you have gone through the appropriate "prepping," a doctor will assess you and make the diagnosis so that treatment can begin. A summary of presenting problems and treatments appears later, in Chapter 6. But whatever your issue, be prepared to enter the unknown. In the event of a life-threatening problem, doctors practicing the rapidly changing field of emergency medicine will pull out all the stops, tapping high-tech equipment, new (and better) medications, and a host of innovative techniques.

To get an idea of the sophisticated rescue efforts in the modern emergency department, all you need do is follow what happens to the person who stumbles in with chest pain. At the St. Luke's and Roosevelt sites—and at most other facilities labeled "heart stations"—diagnosis of cardiac problems in triage triggers a series of events resembling a clocked relay race. The "runners" in this case are doctors and nurses on St. Luke's–Roosevelt's MI (myocardial infarction) team. An MI is, of course, a heart attack (myocardial infarction).

To maintain its heart-station status, Roosevelt must not only meet certain standards, but must also beat the clock. "Once you've been seen in triage," says nurse and MI team runner Suzanne Pavel, "if you have any cardiac symptoms, not just chest pain but also dizziness or nausea, we're going to have you hooked up to a cardiac monitor in ten minutes or less. Actually, we strive for five minutes as our goal, and a lot of the time, we have people hooked up in three."

Within five to ten minutes, upon completion of the EKG and blood tests, insertion of an IV line, and delivery of supplemental oxygen through a nasal tube, the situation is reviewed by one of the attending emergency physicians, an MI team runner who may either say, "Oh, man, normal as can be!" or, "God! Look at the elevations! We have an evolving MI!"

At this point, with no seconds to spare, the patient will be assessed for thrombolytics—streptokinase or tissue plasminogen activator (tpa)—which break up the blood clots that may be blocking arteries, preventing the heart from working as it should. In some cases the patient is disqualified. If there is any condition that makes the patient prone to bleeding—hemophilia, ulcers, a history of aneurysm, a recent stroke, recent injury, or major surgery—thrombolytics could make things worse. But if the MI team feels all systems are go, the thrombolytic medicine will be pumped into the body, drop by drop, through the preestablished IV. The goal is to get these thrombolytics into the body within thirty minutes of the time the patient has walked into the ED. After these "big clot-busters" have been administered, the MI team maintains the steady state of thinned blood with the anticoagulant Heparin also pumped in drop by drop through a portal in the IV.

The MI team stands by with other treatments as well. For those who develop trouble with bleeding, fresh-frozen plasma, or blood, is pumped in to replace it. If blood pressure goes up, nitroglycerine is provided. A defibrillator is handy, just in case the heartbeat becomes irregular or cardiac arrest occurs. Lidocaine can be pumped in through the IV to prevent further fibrillation of the heart muscle after electrical defibrillation has occurred.

Most emergency departments will buttress their arsenal of medical technology with a system of personal support. At the St. Luke's ED, for instance, one nurturing presence is social worker Jorge Rey. Known for the pot of aromatic drip coffee he brews in a staff lounge near his office—available to all staff and even patients or family members —Rey spends his time haunting the ED, almost invisibly, the proverbial fly on the wall. But the second a patient or family member becomes distraught, the second someone needs help coping with stress—nurses, doctors, or administrators only need beckon, and Rey is there.

Rey is there to find a helper for the elderly man abandoned by a home-care worker who wants a couple of days off; for the young, retarded woman found naked in the park and in need of placement; for the mother whose son has, tragically, just died. He is there with his list of support groups, therapists, and city services for the abused and for the alcoholic. When a young man with cerebral palsy was abandoned at the St. Luke's ED by hostile relatives, Rey took him personally, by cab, to a temporary placement home. He also called the man's relatives down south, and implored them to take him in. (They did.) When a sick old woman arrived from a dingy single-room-occupancy hotel, Rey called the city and had someone go in and clean the filthy room she was simply too frail and tired to clean herself. When a patient in the outer waiting room grew so distraught he started yelling, Rey rubbed his shoulder and brought him lunch. "After he ate," says Rey, "he felt so much better, all his anger just left."

BLUEPRINT FOR EMERGENCY

Anyone entering a large metropolitan emergency department for the first time can feel more than a little disoriented by all the energy, motion, and commotion. There are dozens of sick and injured patients clamoring for care, and dozens of health-care workers providing it, using all manner of strange medical terms, foreign tools, and elaborate techniques. When you add in the life-or-death nature of the scene, it's to be expected that for the uninitiated, the confusion quotient will be high. Sometimes, there's nothing like floor plans to clarify confusion over space.

YOU WERE WONDERING?

Whether your emergency room is in an urban or rural area, some general rules apply across the board. Summarized here are the most frequent questions asked by patients who utilize emergency departments.

WILL THERE BE A WAIT?

Most patients are initially evaluated by a triage nurse, who determines which individuals have the most serious problems. Since the primary responsibility of the emergency room is to care for those who are critically ill or injured, you may be asked to wait.

WHO WILL TAKE CARE OF ME?

The answer, of course, depends on the emergency department. The best-equipped facilities are run, night and day, by physicians who are specialists in emergency medicine. At these top facilities, often in teaching hospitals, you may find psychiatrists and pediatricians on staff as well. And specialists of all types, from orthopedists and ophthamologists to heart surgeons, will be available on-call in the hospital, just minutes away when they are needed. Watching or sometimes assisting in treatment, you may find residents in emergency medicine or general medicine.

In more remote locations or smaller facilities, you may find emergency departments run by residents or physician-assistants. All emergency rooms, of course, have nurses who, ideally, have received special training in emergency nursing.

In many larger hospitals, you might find other staff members as well. These include social workers, there to assist with information about community services and resources, and to offer counseling and support. You might also find patient representatives, who provide a direct link to the hospital administration and can help you solve a wide range of problems.

IN GENERAL, WHAT MEDICAL FACILITIES ARE AVAILABLE IN THE ED?

The largest, best-equipped emergency departments often contain a separate trauma room for the gravely injured; a cardiac room for those who have suffered heart attacks; a psychiatric area; a pediatric area; an obstetrics and gynecology area; and X-ray facilities. If your emergency department is part of a major medical center, the hospital should also provide you with access to many sophisticated imaging technologies for diagnosing soft-tissue injury, from CAT scans (computerized axial tomography), a highly detailed X ray, to MRI (magnetic resonance imaging).

Operating rooms and critical-care units will be available, should you need them, as well.

Because emergency departments have become so busy recently, some hospitals have also set up "fast-track" areas to run in tandem with the primary emergency facility. If you come in with a cold, a cough, or a minor scrape, you may be lucky enough to be referred to qualified professionals who can treat you expediently, without the long wait.

WHAT ABOUT FAMILY AND FRIENDS?

The emergency department may not be the appropriate place for numerous friends and relatives to gather 'round. One friend or relative is all you need to accompany you into the treatment area—and then, only when the doctor or nurse deems it appropriate. The reason is obvious: In a crowded space, where stretchers often line the hall and staff needs space to rush back and forth with drugs and equipment, extra people add unacceptable levels of congestion.

WHAT ABOUT FOLLOW-UP CARE?

When you need additional medical attention after you leave the emergency department, you may return to your regular physician. If you have none, the emergency department staff will refer you to a doctor or clinic where you can receive additional care.

WHAT ABOUT COSTS?

Most emergency room visits cost at least several hundred dollars just to walk in the door. Laboratory tests, X rays, medication, and special procedures may cost more. Most insurance coverage will pay the basic cost of emergency care as well as the fee charged by the emergency physician. If you have requested a specialist such as a plastic surgeon or a dermatologist, that person will charge you separately. And even the hospital radiologist, who reviews your X ray to confirm the diagnosis rendered by the attending emergency physician, may send you a separate bill. In most emergency departments you do not pay at the time of your visit, but receive a bill. If you cannot afford to pay, the emergency department staff will still treat you and bill you later. No one is turned away.

WHAT IF I AM ADMITTED TO THE HOSPITAL?

If you are to be admitted, the emergency department physician and nurse will discuss the reasons with you carefully. Then you will wait for a bed. Sometimes, you will be transferred up to a room immediately; however, sometimes you will be faced with a wait.

Cast of Characters: Staff at a Glance

It's important for any patient in the emergency department to understand which staff member performs which function. Who's the medical director—the board-certified physician—in charge of the ED? Who's the resident, the medical student, the nurse, the social worker, the aide? This knowledge is crucial for any emergency department patient who hopes to be informed and thus capable of watching out for his or her personal best interest throughout.

For instance, should you require an intravenous line, you'd do well to have it inserted by the intern or nurse. At this particular task, these staff members should be adept. But if you're receiving stitches on your face, you may want to insist that the emergency medicine specialist—or a specialist in plastic surgery—be the one to suture. Need a bed? Feel your care has been inadequate? To advocate for yourself, you must learn to proceed, tactfully, of course, up the chain of medical command.

To help you out, we provide a list of health care workers normally found in the emergency department.

Doctors: For emergency physicians, the primary goal is rapidly assessing the problem presented in the *chief* complaint, appropriate treatment, and disposition ranging from discharge to admission to the hospital. The doctors you will encounter may include:

ED director: At large metropolitan hospitals, this physician is likely to be board certified in emergency medicine, and is responsible for medical care and staff around the clock, whether he or she is physically present or not. If there is confusion as to how to proceed, the director may be called upon to make the final decision. In the chain of command, this individual is the highest you can go. Very large emergency departments—like the dual-site department at St. Luke's–Roosevelt—may have associate and assistant medical directors, who are also generally physicians trained and board certified in emergency medicine. Emergency department directors supervise all staff, including attending physicians, ED administrators, and the head nurse.

Attending physicians: Board certified in emergency medicine, surgery, or internal medicine (or psychiatry in the psychiatric emergency department and pediatrics in the pediatric ED), these experienced doctors provide direct patient care, control the flow of patients through the ED, serve as liaison to nursing, administration, and EMS, and supervise medical students, interns, and residents. In general, the attending physician is the person responsible for individual patient care.

House staff: In large teaching hospitals, medical students as well as residents and interns from such departments as emergency medicine, medicine, surgery, and pediatrics may rotate through the emergency department on a twenty-four-hour basis. These students and doctors, still in training, are supervised by full-fledged attending physicians. If you feel a resident's call may not be on target, do not hesitate to request medical attention from the attending physician, one step up the chain of command.

Nurses: Responsible for delivering quality care to all patients. They do so by assessing the patient and administering appropriate treatment, ordered in consultation with a physician. Like doctors, nurses function through a chain of command. In general, the clinical nursing coordinator or head nurse is responsible for the nursing department whether physically on the premises or not. A charge nurse, who reports to the clinical coordinator, is in charge during each eight-hour shift. Emergency department nurses report to the charge nurse on each shift.

Nurses aides or orderlies: They assist the nurse and physician with patient care and prepare the patient or the patient's room for needed evaluations.

EMS personnel: Emergency Medical Service staff who bring patients into the emergency department often assist the in-house staff during the transition stage, under the supervision of an attending physician or charge nurse. The emergency medical technician's emergency department duties may include patient transport, splinting, wound management, and opening of the airway. The paramedic may assist with these duties as well as intubation, starting intravenous lines, defibrillation, and other advanced life-support techniques.

Administrators: The administrative staff of the ED is generally responsible for overall operation of the area, including all clerical functions from processing insurance, to accepting payment, to implementing policies of the department. The administrative staff develops budgets, orders and maintains supplies, performs quality assurance audits, and handles patient complaints.

Patient support staff: These personnel may include a patient representative, who intercedes between patients and staff to guarantee that the patient's interests and needs are attended to. The patient rep may try to get the patient a bed; may ask the nurse why treatment is taking so long; may communicate with or bring a relative or friend into the ED; or may simply bring a cup of coffee or sandwich. Support staff may also include social workers, who work to refer patients in need of a variety of social services. The social worker may refer an AIDS patient to a support group; a battered woman to a shelter; an unexpectedly ill or injured senior to a home health aide; or a retarded, abandoned teen to a residential home. For patients who are distressed, social workers and patient representatives are there to talk.

WE'VE COME A LONG WAY, BABY

Emergency medicine wasn't always the high-tech specialty it has become today. Eleanor Mulligan, former head nurse and Roosevelt employee for some twenty-five years, remembers it way back when.

In the good old days, Mulligan recalls, the Roosevelt ER—for emergency room—was an intimate place with a few staff members who knew each other well. "In 1960," Mulligan explains, "we had four nurses who staffed the ER round the clock. People were brought from in-house for meal relief. By 1968, we had ten nurses with staggered shifts for coverage twenty-four hours a day. Of those ten, we'd have maybe three people on day shift, three people on evening shift, and one or two people through the night."

"Back then," Mulligan explains, "those who worked in the emergency department were required to have no special skills beyond the training afforded most doctors and nurses of the day. A nurse was a nurse was a nurse, and they just put you wherever they needed you. Now, we've got to go through extensive training and orientation, but back then, they just handed you the keys and told you to begin."

As for the doctors, they were generally residents going through the paces of training. "Back then, we didn't have attending physicians especially trained in emergency medicine," says Mulligan. "Instead, we had residents there as part of their rotation at all times. Generally, there was a surgical and a medical resident on every shift."

Though physicians in the emergency departments of the 1960s were still in training, Mulligan says the ones she worked with at Roosevelt "were very sharp. I would have put my family in their hands," she states. "They were capable of delivering state-of-the-art emergency care of the day. And there was always an attending physician in-house, in the hospital itself, who could be called, and who oversaw what they did." (This ER of the 1960s is what you see on *ER*, the TV show.)

In a sense, the emergency room—like life itself—was simpler back then. "Mostly," Mulligan explains, "we had true emergencies coming in on the ambulance." The staff treated those with the most serious problems first: If someone was having a heart attack, if someone had been shot, everyone mobilized to help them survive. Of course, treatment was simpler because medicine was less evolved. For instance, there were no thrombolytics, or blood thinners, for patients with blood clots or heart attacks." And unlike today, back in the 1960s, minor problems like sore throats and splinters were rarely ever seen.

Indeed, at Roosevelt and other topflight metropolitan emergency departments, the halcyon days of the straightforward, intimate ER Mulligan remembers with so much affection are gone: The dual-site ED of St. Luke's–Roosevelt, for instance, includes about twenty-five full-time and seventy per-diem attending physicians who rotate through both sites to provide staff for the twenty-four-hour-a-day, seven-day-a-week schedule. Specialists on call around the clock include doctors from the in-house departments of gynecology, neurology, dermatology, surgery, pediatrics, plastic surgery, orthopedics, anesthesiology, urology, cardiology, and more. The dual-site nursing staff consists of eighty-eight nurses, including sixteen nursing aides. Administration includes thirty-six employees who work round the clock addressing patient needs, resolving conflicts, reviewing records and paperwork, and sending bills.

As always, time and science march on. But for what it's worth, loss of intimacy is a small price to pay for the lifesaving advances in technology and medical science that can save our lives today.

How to Advocate for Yourself in the Emergency Department

The major metropolitan emergency department is a complex environment with multiple levels of staff attending to many patients suffering a wide range of injuries and ills. In well-oiled settings like those at St. Luke's and Roosevelt, where attending physicians are certified in emergency medicine and nurses go through months of training and orientation, it's hard to imagine patients slipping through the cracks. Talk to enough people visiting EDs around the country, though, and some unsettling stories emerge.

One woman we know broke her foot and rushed by car to a small emergency department in suburban New York. After examining the X ray, the attending physician on duty told her she had no break at all. He gave her an Ace bandage and sent her home to ice her foot. In this case, no harm was done: The excruciating pain caused the woman to stay off her foot through the next day, when a staff radiologist reviewing emergency department X rays for the hospital discovered the woman's fifth metatarsal in her foot had been fractured. She was able to make an appointment with an orthopedist in her area for the appropriate care.

Another person tells the story of being stabbed by a maniac on a street in Queens. Emergency department personnel—in this case, the resident—discharged this woman quickly, though her husband sensed something gravely amiss. When the patient's husband insisted the attending physician have a look, too, it was found the woman was still bleeding profusely, internally. Her hemorrhage discovered, the woman was rushed into surgery. In the end, thanks to appropriate patient advocacy, an astute physician in charge, and heroic surgery, her life was saved.

As these stories suggest, it's important for the patient to advocate for him or herself in the ED. As in triage, expressing your problem clearly, calmly, quickly, and accurately is the way to obtain the highest quality of care. "Unless patients are able and willing to speak for themselves, they're not always going to be well served," states Stephan Lynn. "There are so many things going on in the emergency department that the patient who doesn't communicate forcefully and effectively will probably not be as well received, and may not end up getting the rapid or appropriate service needed."

One rule of thumb, for instance, is stating the problem in your own words, as opposed to waiting for the doctor or nurse to try and figure out what it is. "When I ask about the problem," says Lynn, "some patients turn to me and say, 'You're the doctor; you tell me what's wrong.' That doesn't always cut it. It can work, of course. I can ask all the right questions, but it takes a lot of time, and sometimes, given the nature of the ED, I don't always have the time to spare. I'm much better able to help the patient who can articulate the problem himself."

Other general advice includes reporting a change in your condition as soon as it occurs; asking questions so that you know what is being done to you each and every step of the way; determining which staff member, at which level, is performing what procedure; requesting that medical students or doctors-in-training refrain from performing any particularly complex procedures (remember, the intern might be better at establishing an intravenous line than the ED director, since he does it all the time); and insisting you receive the treatment you believe you need, even if it means going up the chain of medical command.

For instance, at one Massachusetts emergency department not long ago, a boy prone to "nursemaid's elbow"—in which the elbow joint becomes dislocated—was brought in so the doctor could twist his elbow back in place. The doctor on the case, a resident, gave a twist and sent the child packing, insisting he'd done the job. However, the mother, who had been through this problem with this particular child many times before, realized the joint was still displaced. After going out to her car, she thought the better of it and marched back to the ED. As politely as she could, she informed the resident she did not believe the joint had been restored, and requested that a more experienced physician come to her aid. The attending physician came out, repaired the child's elbow in seconds, and this time, mother and child gladly went on their way.

Indeed, knowing when and how to move up the chain of command in the emergency department is an art in itself. According to Adrienne Shiloff, patient representative at the Roosevelt emergency department for many years, whatever the problem, the first person to consult is the nurse assigned to your case. Whether you need an extra pillow, want some pain medication, would like to talk with the doctor, or want to get a bed upstairs, your nurse is the individual likely to help you most. If the nurse assigned to your case is unable to help, for whatever reason, ask to speak with the charge nurse or nursing supervisor. If you have already been assigned a doctor, you may speak to her.

If your problem is very serious—you've received inadequate treatment, for instance, or feel your condition has been incorrectly diagnosed—ask to speak with the attending physician or emergency department director in charge. These professionals can reevaluate your condition, perhaps picking up clues others have missed. Do not be afraid to ask a nursing supervisor to intervene if you feel a doctor has rendered treatment that is inadequate or incomplete. Often the head nurse can go over *everyone's* head to the ED director. If she agrees with your assessment, as a trained patient advocate, she is likely to do just that.

If your concerns remain, suggests Shiloff, or if your requests for care are ignored, ask to speak with the patient representative kept on staff by many large emergency departments to field complaints, or with a representative from the hospital's administration department. People from administration, Shiloff notes, can sometimes perform miracles. "Much of the time, complaints to the patient representative involve waiting time. We can explain the reason for the wait, and can also check to see whether something can be done. Sometimes it's as simple as digging out the patient's chart, which has somehow become buried under a blizzard of unrelated paperwork, causing the case to be passed over time and again." And, adds Shiloff, "there's nothing like a call from administration to help find out why your room isn't ready or your lab results have not been returned. They can sometimes help facilitate the process if, in fact, that bed is lying empty, say, but the room must still be cleaned."

Shiloff and other experts from Roosevelt point out that if your dissatisfaction involves the waiting time, often little can be done. Fact of the matter is, you have gone to the ED, where triage reigns. If other patients' problems are more urgent, they must be seen first. However, in cases where you are dissatisfied with the quality of care itself, Shiloff says, the patient representative can request that the doctor reexamine you; can facilitate consultation from the ED director; or can aid in obtaining input from a specialist on call.

Without a patient rep, of course, you must negotiate this difficult terrain on your own. If your requests have been met with nothing but frustration, says Shiloff, and if there's no patient rep on the ED floor, your best bet is to ask for the phone. Though there may not be a phone in your particular cubicle, virtually all emergency departments have phones that can be moved. If the phone cannot be moved, request that your stretcher be moved to the phone. Place a call to hospital administration and ask for help with your problem. "Night or day," says Shiloff, "someone from administration should be available to field your call."

This last-straw strategy should work just about anywhere, even in the remote, small-town outposts of emergency medicine, where board-certified experts may be rare. It's a situation most of us dread. In the middle of a trip through some lovely little town in Anywhere, USA, you or someone you're with suddenly takes ill. But instead of tapping the high-tech centers of emergency medicine available in your city, you are suddenly rushed to what paramedics driving the ambulance call "The Doc in a Box"—the local emergency room, staffed by a lone, relatively untrained practitioner whose experience with dire medical problems is slim. Though many doctors staffing these smaller emergency rooms are immensely skilled, if you happen to hit one you feel is not, where do you turn? "You can still call administration on the phone," Shiloff informs us. "There are *always* other doctors in the hospital, in departments from cardiology to OB/GYN. If you request another physician, one can be sent down."

Dr. Lynn suggests you might use that phone to contact your personal doctor. "Your private physician is one of your best advocates in the ED," says Lynn, "whether he is associated with the hospital that houses that particular emergency department or not."

Your own doctor can be counted on to know you medically. And he or she has the appropriate authority and status, enough personal clout to request that you get specific, often special, care. If your private doctor has particular requests as to the nature of your care, physicians in the ED will, if at all possible, generally comply.

Even if you're traveling and your private physician is hundreds of miles away, a call to the ED can help smooth the way. "When talking to doctors in another city, " states Dr. Lynn, "your private physician brings his or her authority to the table in negotiating your cause. Even if that doctor has not seen your injury—and even if the problem is in an area of specialty other than your doctor's—he or she is familiar with your past and knows how you respond, knows what type of support system you have at home, and what type of person you are. Thus, in some instances, your private doctor may be better able to suggest a treatment plan than the doctor on the scene."

Remember, as you deal with emergency personnel and administrators, try at all costs not to lose your cool. Don't insult anyone, don't yell at anyone, don't get belligerent or cast blame. "I cannot emphasize enough the importance of tact," Shiloff says. "If you want someone's help, it's best not to make them feel you are on the attack."

In one masterful stroke of self-advocacy at Roosevelt, for instance, a patient in terrific pain after breaking his leg was being X-rayed. The X-ray technician, adjusting the patient's leg for the machine, inflicted unbearable levels of discomfort. "You are hurting me too much," the man said calmly, gritting his teeth to stay as pleasant yet assertive as he could. "I would like the director of the department to position my leg." Though miffed, the technician summoned Dr. Lynn, who, with his golden touch, was able to manipulate the injured limb for the X ray while inflicting no extra pain.

To get such results, there's often a special way of phrasing things, of presenting your position, so you seem reasonable, serious, and correct:

"I have been through episodes like this many times before, and I feel I can say with some certainty that the treatment has not fully alleviated the problem. If you feel you cannot do anything more for me, I would like to request that someone else deal with this."

"I feel strongly that something is still the matter here. Can you please ask the director of the department to see me and join in the dialogue on this case?"

"I understand that this is a teaching hospital and that doctors need training and experience. However I would like an attending physician to perform this procedure."

"I know you have my best interest at heart, but I'm not comfortable. Can I get someone else to look at me?"

"Excuse me, I've been waiting a very long time. I understand that you must treat the sickest patients first, but I wonder if it's possible just to check and make sure my chart has not been misplaced?"

Dr. Lynn suggests that patients or family members can sometimes advocate effectively by asking pointed or pertinent questions.

"I don't understand why I need this medication. Can you please explain it?"
"Can you please explain why you're not admitting my friend?"
"Why have you decided not to take an X ray?"

The answers might satisfy your doubt. And if they do not, it will lead to dialogue in which you can advocate in the best interest for yourself, your friend, your parent, your child, or your spouse.

By phrasing requests and doubts politely, you will probably see results. If you pair this tact and assertiveness with the realization that whether you are a prince or a pauper, homeless or the president of IBM, you must wait your fair turn—you should be effective at protecting your own best interests in the emergency department.

One issue you may question quite naturally is participation in drug research studies, sometimes conducted in emergency departments around the country, especially in teaching hospitals. In general, if a nurse or doctor asks you whether you would be willing to be part of a study as to the efficacy of medicine A as opposed to medicine B, it may be in your best interest to be cautious. While no competent doctor would ever intentionally jeopardize your life for an extra data point in a research report, the additional seconds required to carry through with research protocols may be meaningful. You also have the right to refuse to be photographed and videotaped, and you may ask that attending physicians not gather large groups of medical students, interns, or residents around your bedside to teach about some rare—or quite ordinary—disease, unless these people will be part of your care.

Finally, Shiloff suggests that you advocate for yourself in the emergency department even as you're being discharged. "Often," she notes, "the doctor will examine you, walk away, and return for a final consult. The period between is a good time to think about any questions you might have." Get a piece of paper from the nurse and write all your questions down. It's a good idea to number them. Ask the doctor to address these questions one at a time, and to repeat or further explain anything you don't understand. After all, you're sick or injured, and no one should expect you to process every detail the first time around. Do make sure you know what to do for your problem at home. Ask for written instructions if you feel you may not remember all the details.

If you are being discharged before all your test results are in, make certain you know where and when to call for the final reports. If you are told to schedule a follow-up visit with a particular clinic or physician, be sure to clarify how and when you should schedule the appointment.

It's the Law

As a patient, your rights in the emergency department are spelled out not just by moral imperative, but also by federal, state, and local law. In New York, for instance, the Medical Emergency Services Reform Act of 1983 protects your right to care at the ED regardless of your ability to pay. If Emergency Medical Service designates a hospital as a receiving station, that hospital *MUST* comply with EMS requirements. It must, for instance, agree to care for all patients regardless of ability to pay, and without discrimination based on sex, race, religion, age, or national origin.

Finally, patients at the emergency department (or anywhere else in the hospital) can turn to a Patients' Bill of Rights. While the particulars may vary from state to state, we present New York State's version, hanging in the waiting rooms at Roosevelt and St. Luke's emergency departments.

PATIENTS' BILL OF RIGHTS

As a patient in a hospital in New York State, you have the right, consistent with law, to:

1. Understand and use these rights. If for any reason you do not understand or you need help, the hospital must provide assistance, including an interpreter.

2. Receive treatment without discrimination as to race, color, religion, sex, national origin, or source of payment.

3. Receive considerate and respectful care in a clean and safe environment free of unnecessary restraints.

4. Receive emergency care if you need it.

5. Be informed of the name and position of the doctor who will be in charge of your care in the hospital.

6. Know the names, positions, and functions of any hospital staff involved in your care and refuse their treatment, examination, or observation.

7. A no-smoking room.

8. Receive complete information about your diagnosis, treatment, and prognosis.

9. Receive all the information that you need to give informed consent for any proposed procedure or treatment. This information shall include the possible risks and benefits of the procedure or treatment.

10. Receive all the information you need to give informed consent for an order not to resuscitate. You also have the right to designate an individual to give this consent for you if you are too ill to do so. If you would like additional information, please ask for a copy of the pamphlet "Do Not Resuscitate Orders: A Guide for Patients and Families."

11. Refuse treatment and be told what effect this may have on your health.

12. Refuse to take part in research. In deciding whether or not to participate, you have the right to a full explanation.

13. Privacy while in the hospital and confidentiality of all information and records regarding your care.

14. Participate in all decisions about your treatment and discharge from the hospital. The hospital must provide you with a written discharge plan and written description of how you can appeal your discharge.

15. Review your medical record without charge and obtain a copy of your medical record for which the hospital can charge a reasonable fee. You cannot be denied a copy solely because you cannot afford to pay.

16. Receive an itemized bill and explanation of all charges.

17. Complain without fear of reprisals about the care and services you are receiving and to have the hospital respond to you and if you request it, a written response. If you are not satisfied with the hospital's response, you can complain to the New York State Health Department. The hospital must provide you with the Health Department telephone number.

When to Request a Specialist

It shouldn't have been that shocking when one six-year-old, only in kindergarten and already diagnosed by psychologists as hyperactive, ran into the wall. The tragedy was that his head hit the corner, which sliced right through him like a knife. When the blood stopped gushing quite so profusely, the deep trajectory of the cut was agonizingly clear: It traveled like a gully down the center of the boy's forehead, from the top of his hairline to the space between his brows.

The frantic parents rushed their child to the emergency department of a suburban hospital with one attending physician, an internist moonlighting to supplement his day job. They were sitting in the waiting room, sick with worry, when the husband of another patient inquired as to who would do the stitches. Concerned only with having their child's head closed, the parents were waiting for the attending physician, who would do the suturing. No one on the hospital staff, after all, had suggested anything else. But the gentleman across the room did: "It's your child, it's his face!" he expounded. "Get a plastic surgeon to do the stitching."

When approached about that possibility, the emergency department nurse said the hospital did indeed have a plastic surgeon on call. Though it was late in the evening, it took this specialist just thirty minutes to get to the hospital. Utilizing a special, internal stitch that would not leave railroad tracks across the child's head, the plastic surgeon told them they had done the right thing.

Most of the time, a specialist is not needed. If you have sprained or broken your leg, for instance, the ED doctors are probably capable of setting it. Nonetheless, if you require an orthopedist the hospital will be there to meet that need.

But remember, doctors who are board certified in emergency medicine are specialists, too. When it comes to saving your life, *they* are the experts. Of course, you'd want a cardiologist to manage your heart condition over the long term, but if you've gone into cardiac arrest, there's no one like the ED doc to bring you back from the brink. Only a neurosurgeon should remove that bullet from your brain, but if your vitals are dropping because you're slipping into shock, count on the emergency medicine specialist to stabilize you adequately so that surgery can begin.

Some specialists on call in the typical emergency department include:

anesthesiologist (gives general and local anesthesia)

radiologist (performs and reads X rays and other imaging technologies)

cardiologist (heart doctor)

dermatologist (skin doctor)

hand surgeon (repairs the hand)

neurosurgeon (specializes in surgery of the brain and spinal cord)

obstetrician/gynecologist (expert in delivering babies and caring for woman's reproductive system)

oral surgeon (dentist with surgery training)

orthopedist (bone doctor)

plastic surgeon (expert in cosmetic and reconstructive surgery)

urologist (expert in the urinary tract)

pulmonologist (lung doctor)

gastroenterologist (expert in the digestive and intestinal systems) otolaryngologist (ear, nose, and throat specialist)

intensivist or critical-care physician (expert in critical care)

In general, if you want a specialist, request one. If the request is appropriate, the emergency department will, as a rule, comply. But remember that emergency medicine specialists are trained to handle most problems that come to the ED competently and completely.

Patient Dismissed: Leaving the Emergency Department

After you have been observed, diagnosed, and treated, it will be time to leave the ED. For those who arrive with minor cuts or abrasions, the process will be simple. The doctor will apply a dressing and give you a sheet of instructions for follow-up care at home, then will sign your discharge papers and wish you well.

Sometimes, however, the ED is just a doorway to other parts of the hospital. Depending on your situation and your condition, you might be sent to an intensive care unit or a cardiac intensive care unit for specialized round-the-clock care; the operating room for surgery; a trauma center; or a bed in the hospital.

Sometimes, you may need to transfer from the current hospital to the one where your own doctor practices, or to a more specialized facility. Of course, transfer may not always be possible. For one thing, your condition may simply be too unstable, and the move would be risky at best. Only diagnostic tests and exams in the current emergency department can help the doctor decide whether a transfer would place you in danger.

Once it has been determined that a ride across town in an ambulance would not endanger your health, you must contact your personal physician so he can arrange for your arrival; without his authorization, you simply cannot be admitted. To affect this transfer, have the emergency department contact your doctor so that he or she can reserve a space for you. Then you may arrange the transfer by calling a private ambulance service or tapping the ambulance service associated with either the sending hospital or the receiving one. You will be admitted through the ED of the receiving hospital.

When it comes to discharge from the ED, you may not get what you expect. For instance, many people go to the emergency department with bags packed, thinking they'll be admitted to the hospital in no time. But it doesn't always work that way.

These days, when beds are in short supply and hospitalization is carefully scrutinized by insurance companies, admission is reserved for the truly sick.

If you are truly sick, on the other hand, you may not be released as readily as you would like. At St. Luke's recently, a woman of fifty-five with a known history of heart trouble came in after experiencing chest pain. The doctors dutifully observing her did not believe she was out of the danger zone. But the woman, whose grandson was about to get off the school bus with no one to greet him, decided she simply had to go. Doctors strongly urged the woman to stay, but when she wouldn't hear of it, they had her sign a form accepting responsibility for her actions. "You could walk out that door and die," they told her. "We don't advise it."

"What can I do?" she shrugged. "He's a little boy, and it's dangerous on the street."

"I'll be back," she told the emergency department doctors. Then she signed the form and left.

No one wants to leave a child alone on New York streets. But in fact, this woman had taken her life in her hands. Indeed, one recent study reveals that numerous preventable deaths can be attributed to patients who, unwilling or unable to stay, leave the ED before receiving treatment or a formal release. Under virtually any circumstance, this is a dangerous course of action. If doctors or nurses tell you to stay for further tests or observation, you must make every effort to comply.

SOME SHAGGY DOG STORIES

When asked to describe the "heart and soul" of the emergency department, head nurse Eleanor Mulligan, a fixture at Roosevelt for the past quarter of a century, brought up two dog stories, both unlikely but true tales.

The first involved an elderly gentleman whose hip was broken one weekend during a mugging in Central Park. "He'd been with his dog, an old animal that was very, very big," Mulligan explains. "The dog, the man's only companion, jumped up on his stretcher to say good-bye right before surgery." When Mulligan came in to work on Monday morning, she found the dog in her office, where the nursing staff had placed it the night before. Throughout the day, a brigade of nurses walked and fed the dog until the staff social worker found a temporary placement for the animal: a kennel in Rye, a suburb of New York City. "When the man came out of the hospital, he brought the dog back to visit us to show to everybody," Mulligan recalls.

In Mulligan's second dog story, a small boy rushed into the ED to say his dog had been hit by a car. "We brought him into the hospital," Mulligan says, "and then someone from the staff got into a cab with the boy and rushed the dog to a vet. We took up a collection so the dog could stay in the animal hospital, in intensive care."

Who would have thought? Actually, Dr. Lynn is skeptical: "Do people really want to read these dog stories?" he queries. "We don't have to print everything." Yet, in a way, the anecdotes are germane. The emergency department can seem so forbidding and cold to visitors, it's comforting to know that behind all the high-tech medicine is an undercurrent of humanity, oftentimes masked by the urgency of the situation, but there just the same.

Chapter 6

The St. Luke's–Roosevelt Guide to Emergency Tests and Treatments

Now that you have a feel for what to expect and how to behave the next time you must visit the hospital with a medical emergency of any kind, we offer some additional details in list form. You will find an explanation of the complaints most likely to bring you to the emergency department, along with probable treatments; a list of diagnostic tests you may need; a thorough description of the most common emergency procedures; and a summary of medicines most often prescribed by emergency physicians. You may want to read all of the pages here thoroughly, or you may want to use them as a reference for particular problems or procedures when they become issues for you.

What to Expect in the Emergency Department

What can you expect if you go to the ED with a laceration, severe abdominal pain, or a neck injury? With shortness of breath or a broken bone? Here are the probable tests you will undergo and the spectrum of treatment you might receive for thirty-one of the most common complaints presented at emergency departments throughout the country. For tips on recognizing these emergencies, on first aid, and on the ambulance experience, you may refer to previous chapters. But for a review of what will happen in the ED and some tips on follow-up care at home, read on.

Cuts: Emergency department staff will clean cuts with saline solution. A doctor will note the location, length, and depth of the cut and query the patient as to how it occurred. Was a dirty tool, which could cause tetanus, involved? Could foreign bodies like pieces of metal and glass be embedded deep inside? If so, the doctor will work to remove those first, then will check to see if the nerves, muscles, and tendons are working well by testing for range of motion and sensation. He will examine for color and warmth to determine whether veins or arteries have been damaged. If the cut needs suturing, the doctor will first irrigate with lots of fluid under pressure, then anesthetize the area and either hold skin together with adhesive "steri-strips" or take a needle and stitch. If the patient has not received a tetanus shot in the past five to ten years a tetanus booster will be given. Finally, a dressing and bandage will be applied.

At home: Look for signs of infection, including pain, fever, redness, puffiness, or lack of motion or sensation. Return to the emergency department or your private physician to have sutures removed and wound rechecked in five to ten days.

Profuse external bleeding: The patient will be taken into the trauma room, where the bleeding area will be cleaned and examined under sterile conditions. Doctors will apply pressure to make the bleeding stop. If the wound is on an extremity, the extremity will be elevated. If the bleeding doesn't stop, physicians will reevaluate by looking for the source. Depending on the source of the blood, additional techniques will be used: A blood vessel may need to be sutured, or even more pressure exerted through use of an arterial tourniquet. If the bleeding still does not stop, the patient may be sent to the operating room for exploratory surgery.

At home: Look for signs of additional bleeding under the skin, usually obvious because of excessive swelling, bruising, or discoloration. If internal bleeding is a possibility, rush back to the ED.

Puncture wounds: The area will be cleansed under sterile conditions. The doctor will note the depth of the puncture and enquire as to how it occurred: Did something break off in the wound? Is the instrument inflicting the damage a known entity, and if so, what is it? The doctor will also check to see if the nerves, muscles, and tendons are working well by testing for range of motion and sensation, then will examine for color and warmth to determine whether veins or arteries have been damaged. Finally, the wound will be irrigated with a saline solution and, if the patient has not received a tetanus shot in the last five to ten years, a booster will be given at this time.

At home: Look for signs of infection, including pain, fever, redness, puffiness, or lack of motion or sensation. Return to ED or private physician to have the wound rechecked in three to ten days.

Bruises: As far as injuries go, the straightforward bruise is relatively minor. In the emergency department, physicians check bruised areas for signs of deeper injury, especially dangerous internal bleeding under the skin. They also look for damage to the musculoskeletal system, including sprains and broken bones. An X ray may be indicated. Expect to be examined for color and warmth as a check on the circulatory system, including the integrity of your blood vessels. And expect to receive a motor-sensory exam, so that doctors can make sure all your moving parts are in working order.

   At home: Look for excessive swelling, numbness, or severe pain. With the advent of any of these symptoms, return to the ED.

Amputation: First, ED staffers will query as to the mechanism that caused injury: Was that finger severed while chopping lettuce? Did that hand get crushed by an oncoming train? They will also attempt to classify the injury as to location: How far above or below the elbow, say, or the knee. If the severed piece is available, and if it's been kept cold and sterile, it may be reattachable, though the more distal the better. That is, it's easier to reattach a finger than a hand, and easier to reattach a hand than an arm. If reattachment is to be attempted, the hospital will gather a team of microsurgeons on-site or, more likely, send the patient to a facility specializing in such procedures. If the severed part cannot be reattached, the patient will be sent to the hospital's own operating room, where surgeons will remove any other skin and muscle no longer viable because they have been crushed or otherwise destroyed, and then close the site of the amputation. Victims of amputation will almost always be admitted to the hospital.

Burns: Virtually all burns other than the most minor are seen promptly by the emergency department physician. The doctor will first attempt to determine the mechanism of injury: fire, boiling water, electricity, the sun? There will be careful assessment of the burn: How extensive is it? What part of the body is it on? Has it damaged nerves or blood vessels? Depending on the severity of the burn, the age of the victim, and any prior medical condition, doctors may either release, admit to the hospital, or transfer to a regional burn center. If the burn can be managed at home, it's usually treated with a topical antibiotic cream or gel that is simply smoothed on. If the burn requires surgical intervention, including skin grafting, that is done after the patient leaves the ED, when surgeons and burn specialists are called in.

At home: Elevate burned extremities, change dressing, and apply antibiotic cream twice a day; return to the ED upon any sign of infection, including pus, redness, swelling, or fever.

Breaks, tears, and sprains: At first glance, symptoms for breaks, tears, and sprains may be virtually identical. The treatment path is the same to a large degree as well. To diagnose, the emergency physician will ask the patient to describe how the injury occurred, and will conduct a neurological exam to make sure the nerves, arteries, muscles, and tendons of the extremities work. If there is a break or sprain to the elbow, the doctor will examine the wrist and fingers: Can they move? Do they have feeling? Are the fingertips pink and warm, indicating normal blood flow? If possible, physicians will also feel for a pulse. The doctor will evaluate the intensity of the pain as described by the patient, and will examine the injury directly to see if unusual bony movement can be detected under the skin and if the joints are stable or abnormally lax. (For instance, the knee normally bends just to the front and back, not right or left; if it does move right and left, a tendon or ligament may be torn.) Usually an X ray is in order and will be the ultimate determiner of whether a fracture or break has occurred. Either way, some sort of splint or cast is usually indicated. Emergency department doctors are well trained in creating splints and casts, though patients may sometimes need to see an orthopedist.

At home: Look for signs of neurovascular compromise, including cold, numb, or painful fingers and toes. Elevate the injured extremity and avoid using the area as much as possible. Follow up with your personal orthopedist if symptoms and pain persist for more than a day or two, or if your bones and muscles have been badly broken or sprained.

Joint pain: Though not a life-or-death problem, severe joint pain often brings people to the emergency department. Upon meeting with the doctor these patients will be asked to describe the problem: Does the pain afflict one joint or several? Has it happened before? How intense is it? Does the patient take medication? The physician will carefully examine the joint, in the process seeing if it can go through its complete range of motion. The doctor may study the joint with the help of an X ray, or examine it for the presence of fluid through arthrocentesis, a procedure by which a fine needle enters the joint area. Sometimes fluid is aspirated out and analyzed for infection. Some patients have joint injuries, generally indicated in their description of the ailment—they'll tell the doctor the joint started hurting after a twist or a fall. Injured joints are immoblized with an elastic bandage or splint, and patients are asked to limit use. Other times, patients are diagnosed with joint disease and will leave the ED with medication for arthritis or gout. In cases where patients have been diagnosed with a condition called septic arthritis, infection is so severe it requires admission to the hospital for intensive antibiotic therapy.

At home: Make sure your joint gets plenty of rest, take your medication, and return to the ED or your private physician if problems persist.

Multiple injuries: This patient will almost always arrive via ambulance, and will be placed in an acute care or trauma room at once. A team of doctors and other ED staff will take vital signs, place the patient on a cardiac monitor, and establish IV lines. Most of the time, such patients have already been stabilized to some degree by Emergency Medical Service: That means they will probably be wearing a cervical collar to prevent movement of the neck and will be tied to a backboard to prevent movement of the spinal cord. Emergency physicians will examine patients without removing these supports. The doctor will first ask a series of questions: What happened? Where does it hurt? The questions will serve not only to pinpoint injuries, but also to see if the patient has suffered any alteration in consciousness. The patient will be examined from head to toe to see if significant or serious injuries have been sustained. X rays will be taken; CAT scans, essentially 3-D X rays, are often indicated as well. Blood pressure and pulse will be checked frequently to make sure vital signs stay stable.

The main intent of the emergency department in this situation is to keep the patient stabilized and alive. If there is profuse bleeding, doctors will do all they can to stop it. If the patient has sustained a chest injury or is having trouble breathing, he may be given supplemental oxygen and intubated with an endotracheal tube to support breathing, a chest tube to expand a collapsed lung, or a bladder tube to remove liquid while the kidneys are too traumatized to work. If the patient has lost a great deal of blood, he or she will receive a transfusion while in the ED as well.

After bleeding has been stopped and vital signs stabilized, the patient will often be transferred out of the ED to a critical care area of the hospital. In the case of continued profuse bleeding or dangerous damage to heart, lungs, or other vital organs, the patient will be rushed into the operating room. Specialists, including orthopedists, neurosurgeons, plastic surgeons, and others will be called in to consult on an as-needed basis.

Head injury: Patients with head injuries will be assessed by a doctor as soon as possible. Much of the exam will take the form of a Q&A, as the physician attempts to assess any neurological damage. The patient will be asked if he has lost consciousness at any point during or immediately following the incident. He will be asked to move, walk, speak, and think, sometimes extensively. Patients can get annoyed at what they perceive as irrelevant questions, but thorough ED physicians will persist until they're sure the patient is OK: Can the patient hear the words? Can he understand and respond? Can he use his muscles in a normal fashion? Can she shrug her shoulders or make a fist? Does he have tactile sensation: Can he feel the physician tapping his right shoulder, or his left? Does the patient have a sense of balance: Can he stand on his toes or his heels?

Physicians will also check patients out physically from top to bottom, beginning with the head. They will look for bumps or bruises on the head; for internal bleeding or injury in the ears; for ability to focus the eyes. Finally, victims of head injury will be checked out carefully for other injuries elsewhere on the body. Since brain injury is of primary concern, patients will generally be asked to have a CAT scan and will be observed in the emergency department for three to six hours before being released. Though the patient and his family may feel little is being done, in fact, the hospital staff is constantly checking him out to make sure he is neurologically intact.

If a problem is found, ED physicians will call on a neurologist or neurosurgeon to enter the picture and assume responsibility for the patient's care.

If the patient passes muster, she may be discharged—but ideally, only in the company of another responsible, alert adult who can stay with her for twenty-four hours.

At home: If, within a day of release, the patient suffers loss of consciousness, fainting spells, inability to use muscles, seizures, loss of sensation, severe headache with persistent nausea and vomiting, or sleepiness or drowsiness, he or she is to go back to the emergency department.

Neck injury: Since nerves travel from the brain through the spinal cord in the neck to the rest of the body, this injury is potentially devastating. Neck bones supporting the spinal cord are subject to injury, and any injury to those bones has the potential to damage nerves and obliterate responsiveness and sensation for any part of the body below the injury. Therefore, a patient sustaining neck injury through a fall, whiplash, or direct trauma is always at risk for damage to the spinal column as well. So that injured bones in the neck do not sever these nerves, paramedics and emergency medical technicians will always stabilize the neck with a rigid cervical collar.

In the emergency department, physicians may carefully loosen the cervical collar and examine the neck to check for spots of pain. As with a head injury, doctors will also conduct a thorough neurological exam: The patient may be asked to bend her right arm or make a fist or push against the doctor's arm with a foot. The doctor will also check for reflexes and tactile sensation. If serious damage is a possibility, ED doctors will order an X ray or—rarely—a CAT scan. If these pictures reveal any sign of damage to the bones or nerves, the patient will be admitted to the hospital until the cervical spine is stable and the danger zone is past. Sometimes the patient will be referred to the operating room for surgery to restore stability of injured vertebrae in the neck.

At home: Most often the patient will be sent home with instructions to take it easy and stay on the alert: If reflexes seem slowed, if there is inability to use muscles or there is loss of some sensation, the patient is to return to the emergency department.

Chest injury caused by trauma: This patient will usually come in by ambulance after paramedics have stabilized with a backboard and cervical collar. The patient will be seen immediately by an emergency physician, who will first check the rib cage and breastbone for pain, then will listen carefully to both sides of the chest to make sure the lungs are filling with air. If any diminution of sound is detected, the doctor will check for a collapsed lung. If a lung is wholly or partially collapsed, it will be treated by insertion of a chest tube under local anesthesia to remove accumulated air, fluid, or blood. The doctor will also check the rhythmic motion of the chest, which normally moves up and out in a synchronous pattern with each breath, but which may become irregular if bones or ribs are broken; will listen for abnormalities in the heart, which can be bruised like any other organ in the body; and will perform an electrocardiogram as well. Almost always, the patient who has suffered chest trauma will be X-rayed to determine whether bones have been broken, whether a lung has collapsed and whether there is bleeding inside the chest cavity. If injuries to bones, lungs, or heart are significant, the patient will be admitted to the hospital, possibly to the intensive care unit.

At home: In cases where patients are just bruised or have suffered broken ribs (not set in casts of any sort), they may be sent home with pain medication and instructions to return to the ED with any difficulty in breathing or significant increase in pain.

Chest pain: Patients with chest pain are brought into the emergency department immediately and put on a cardiac monitor to measure pulse rate. They are generally given oxygen through a nasal cannula or mask and set up with an IV line so drugs can be delivered rapidly, if needed. Hospital staff will perform an electrocardiogram, which may reveal damage or injury to the heart. Reading the EKG, emergency physicians will know whether the pain may be attributed to myocardial ischemia or angina (inadequate blood supply), myocardial infarction (heart attack), a disturbance in the heart rhythm, or something else. In a nutshell, the EKG may tell doctors how much damage, if any, has been done to which part of the heart muscle. Patients will also be given a blood test to measure an enzyme known as CPK, for creatine phosphokinase, which may be elevated in those with damage to the heart muscle. It often takes several hours to get the blood test results, although, of course, doctors may not wait for blood test results before treatment begins.

Patients with mild short-term chest pain diagnosed as angina are treated with the heart drug nitroglycerine. Generally, after the episode is over, if the EKG is normal or unchanged, the patient will be released with instructions to return to the emergency department if subsequent use of nitro doesn't help or the pain gets worse. If the angina is new, the patient may be asked to come in for tests.

If physicians find the patient has had a heart attack, on the other hand, they will often strive to help blood flow through clogged arteries with intravenous drugs known as thrombolytics, which work to dissolve blood clots. Patients with slow heart rhythms may be given a temporary pacemaker. Finally, if a patient has gone into cardiac arrest, physicians will use the defibrillator and numerous medications to get the heart going again and may intubate the patient to assist in breathing.

Patients who have suffered damage to the heart muscle will generally be admitted to the hospital, often to cardiac intensive care. If doctors find that chest pain is due to something relatively benign, say indigestion, they may treat it with a simple antacid. If the pain is due to pneumonia, flu, or bronchitis, the patient will be given an antibiotic and sent home or admitted to the hospital, depending on the severity of the problem.

At home: If released, the patient will be advised to return to the ED upon any recurrence of chest pain.

Difficulty in breathing: Those with labored breathing or shortness of breath are generally brought into the emergency department's cardiac area immediately and set up with a cardiac monitor as well as an IV line. The patient will be treated just like the patient with chest pain—except that doctors may also order X rays and a blood gas test to see if the blood is sufficiently saturated with oxygen. If the patient has suffered cardiac damage, the patient will be treated like the patient with chest pain, but will also be given medication to reduce the shortness of breath.

If the individual has a history of asthma, however, he may be sent to a noncardiac room and asked to blow into a peak flow meter to test lung capacity. If the lungs are found to be weak, or if the patient is wheezing, he may be placed on a nebulizer, which works to open the breathing tubes by delivering medicine in the form of a mist. If the wheezing persists, the patient may be given a shot of epinephrine or steroid treatment, in addition.

Patients who have neither heart problems nor asthma may have an upper-respiratory infection. In that case, hospital staff will monitor vital signs to check for serious illness. If none is found, the patient may be given a cough medicine and released.

At home: Ease breathing with humidified air, hot liquids, and rest. Return to the ED if labored breathing or wheezing persists.

Abdominal pain: These patients are generally brought into the emergency department and placed in a private room lying down. The physician will take a long history: When did the pain start? How long has it been going on? Is it localized in any particular part of the abdomen? Is bowel function normal? Is there nausea, vomiting, or diarrhea? Blood in the vomit or stool? Vaginal bleeding or discharge? Has the patient had any gastrointestinal or stomach problems or abdominal surgery in the past? Is there pain with urination? After eliciting answers, the doctor will examine the chest and abdomen, listen for sounds in the intestine, palpate the abdomen for presence of an abnormal mass or pain, and conduct a rectal exam. Depending on the findings, an X ray and blood tests may be necessary.

Based on this extensive check, the doctor may come up with a diagnosis, which may require further tests for confirmation. The possibilities include:

· Gallstones or kidney stones: Ultrasound tests may be needed to confirm. If the pain is severe or unremitting, the patient may be given pain medication and possibly admitted to the hospital. The patient will be kept in the ED until the episode ends.

· Appendicitis: In this case, the pain, which starts in the center of the abdomen and then travels to the right lower quadrant, has usually persisted for between six and twelve hours before the patient arrives at the emergency department.

· Virus or food poisoning: Diagnosis by exclusion; the patient will be sent home.

At home: For virus or food poisoning, the patient will be told to rest, and will be instructed to return if symptoms grow increasingly severe or if blood appears in stool or vomit.

Acute pain in the side: Physicians will attempt to figure out whether the patient is passing a kidney stone, suffering from a kidney infection, or having back problems, including strained back muscles or a malfunction of the aorta, the main blood vessel going down the back. The patient will be asked to lie down on her back. The doctor will do a back exam, running fingers along the bony part of the vertebral column. The doctor will ask the patient to raise legs, then will palpate the side, hips, and back to test for pain. If the problem is a kidney stone, doctors will give the patient pain medicine in the emergency department until the stone passes or until it's clear so that it won't pass. If the problem is a kidney infection, the patient will get antibiotics and, depending on the severity of the problem, may be admitted to the hospital or released.

At home: Patient will be asked to return to the hospital upon recurrence of pain.

Back pain: The patient will be asked to lie flat on his back. The emergency room doctor will then run fingers along the spine and exert pressure to see where it hurts, and will also palpate the rest of the back to look for muscle injury. Muscle strength, reflexes, and sensation will be carefully checked. The patient will be asked to walk so physicians can evaluate motor function, and may sometimes get an X ray or CAT scan. If doctors suspect the problem is a herniated disk, they may even order the sophisticated scan known as MRI, magnetic resonance imaging.

At home: Most back patients are sent home with instructions to rest, apply heat, and sleep on a flat surface. In cases of herniated disk, the patient is either referred to a specialist and released or admitted to the hospital.

Sudden, unexpected pain in the groin: The male patient will be brought into the emergency department quickly and asked for a urine specimen. Doctors will palpate the area to pinpoint the pain. Is the pain in the testicle? Is there sign of an injury, infection, or hernia? If the exam suggests no external injury or illness in the face of severe testicular pain, a urologic surgeon will be called to evaluate the testicle for a twisting known as torsion. If the testicle is found to be twisted, the urologist may attempt to untwist it in the emergency department. If that isn't possible, the patient will be rushed into surgery.

Weakness or numbness in part of the body, usually one side: After reporting symptoms indicative of a stroke, the patient will be examined by an emergency physician, head to toe. The doctor will check motor function, reflexes, and the ability to perceive sensation. A CAT scan may be ordered. Aside from the occasional prescription of high blood pressure medicine, there will be virtually no treatment in the ED. The patient will usually be admitted to the hospital.

Loss of consciousness: The loss of consciousness might be due to an injury, a drug, a past history of neurologic or cardiac disease, or no discernible reason at all. The patient may or may not be able to give a history. If the patient wakes up, doctors will ask questions to test mental status. If doctors believe a drug has induced the coma, they will establish an IV line to deliver glucose (for nourishment) as well as narcan (reverses effect of narcotic) and, perhaps, other antidotes. If loss of consciousness continues, the patient will be admitted to the hospital.

At home: If the patient is released, he will be asked to stay on the lookout for dizziness, memory loss, lethargy, confusion, or other signs of impaired mental status. If any neurological signs return, the patient must return to the emergency department.

Convulsions, fits, or seizures: Since seizures usually last just twenty to thirty seconds, the patient is no longer in seizure by the time she or he gets to the emergency department. The most common cause of seizures is failure to take prescribed medicines, so emergency physicians generally start by taking a detailed medical history: Has the patient ever been diagnosed with epilepsy? Has the patient been medically evaluated for seizures in the past? Does the patient have a prescription for seizure medication? Has the patient taken such medication in the past? If so, the hospital may perform a blood test to help determine the appropriate amount of the correct medication. The patient will be given the medication along with a prescription, and released.

If the patient has had no history of seizure, however, ED physicians will order CAT scans and other tests, and may admit the patient to the hospital to determine the cause of the problem.

At home: The patient who is released will probably be warned to avoid driving and the operation of heavy machinery, since seizing in such situations could be deadly.

Headache: The triage nurse will attempt to evaluate the severity of the pain. Is it relatively mild or the worst headache of the patient's life? How long has the pain persisted, and, has it gotten worse? If the headache is intolerable, the patient will probably be brought to the emergency department rapidly. Doctors will perform a neurological assessment to determine whether the patient can answer questions, use muscles and nerves in an appropriate fashion, and respond to commands. The doctor will take a medical history and record all medication in use, and will look for other, associated symptoms, including visual changes, stiff neck, fever, or injury, all signs of other problems, including bleeding, infection or tumor in the brain. In an effort to diagnose such emergencies, ED doctors may perform a spinal tap to analyze spinal fluid or order a CAT scan of the brain. The patient who is found to have one of these serious problems will be admitted to the hospital or sent to the operating room, depending on the situation. If the headache turns out to be related to migraine or stress, the patient will receive appropriate medication and referral to a specialist outside the ED and will be released.

Violent, suicidal, and delusional behavior: The patient will be taken to a special psychiatric area, where the emergency physician or psychiatrist will conduct an interview, asking about past psychiatric problems, current medications, treatment, and family history. If there is concern that the patient is suicidal, the patient may be asked whether he has just made an attempt on his life. Depending on the severity of the situation—specifically, whether the patient is a danger to himself or others—he may be admitted to the hospital.

    At home: If released, the patient may be given medicine and a referral for outpatient care.

Extreme allergic reaction: This may be a potentially life-threating emergency in which the patient may suffer severe respiratory distress or even succumb to shock. In the emergency department, physicians first stabilize the ABC's of airway, breathing, and circulation, and also monitor vital signs. The doctor will look for blotches, an itchy rash on the skin, or a swelling of the throat. He will listen to the chest, since this sort of attack is often associated with asthma. The physician will carefully assess the airway and the vital signs. Patients may be treated with an antihistamine like Benadryl or with Adrenalin. The most severely ill will be admitted to the hospital and given steroids.

    At home: Milder cases are sent home with prescriptions for antihistamines and asked to stay away from food or other substances that might have provoked the attack. Victims of extreme allergic reation are also referred to an allergist for further care and may need to carry self-administered epinephrine.

Red blistering skin not caused by sunburn: This patient is seen by a doctor quickly. If the patient has simple impetigo, a common skin infection, she will be given an antibiotic and released with instructions to use separate towels and washcloths to avoid infecting other members of the family. Sometimes, however, the problem will be a serious bacterial infection. In this case, doctors will treat with an antibiotic either orally or, if the infection is bad enough, intravenously. The patient may be released or admitted to the hospital, depending on the severity of the infection.

At home: The patient watches for further sign of infection—including redness, temperature and pus—and returns to the doctor if the infection persists.

Bites: The bite will be assessed, irrigated with a large amount of sterile saline or salt water, and thoroughly cleansed. A neurological exam will determine whether muscles or nerves in the area of the bite have been injured. The patient will need a tetanus booster if the last shot was received more than five years earlier. Bites are usually not sutured, since the wound area is likely to be dirty and infected. Doctors will ask about the source of the bite: If the attacker was an unknown dog, cat, raccoon, bat, fox, or skunk, the patient will require rabies vaccine—the first is given in the emergency department on the spot and subsequent vaccines are given later, either at the ED or the office of a private physician.

At home: The patient will generally be sent home with antibiotic medication and instructions to soak the wound area a few times a day, and to return to the ED at any sign of infection, including redness, swelling, or pus.

Poisoning or drug overdose: If the poison is on the surface of the skin, the patient will be decontaminated in the emergency department shower, specially designed for that purpose. If the poison is in the form of pills, medication, or some other ingested substance, physicians will attempt to identify the offending chemicals. If the substance will not damage the esophagus or feeding tube, doctors may empty the stomach with the drug Ipecac, which causes vomiting, or with a stomach pump. If the poison is a toxic substance known to damage the esophagus or feeding tube (Drano or lye) doctors may try to bind it up with charcoal so it doesn't enter the blood stream. Emergency physicians may call the local poison control center for guidance as well. The poisoned patient will either be admitted to the intensive care unit or released from the hospital, depending on the poison ingested, the patient's condition, and the amount of time that passed before treatment.

Alcohol-related disease: If the primary problem is intoxication, emergency department doctors will first examine the patient for injury. They may test to see how much alcohol is in the blood. If alcohol has compromised the ABC's, doctors may have to intubate to assist respiration. If the patient is going through alcohol withdrawal, or delirium tremens (the DTs), doctors will monitor vital signs, especially blood pressure, temperature, and pulse, and treat with sedatives. Once the patient has been physiologically stabilized, he or she will generally be admitted to either the intensive care unit or detoxification department of the hospital.

Problems in pregnancy: The patient will be taken to an examination room with an OB/GYN table—generally a private space behind closed doors. The hospital staff will check vital signs. The physician will take a detailed medical history, asking about the date of the last menstrual period, previous pregnancies, any existing health problems, and other pertinent information. The patient will be asked to describe the pain: How intense is it? Where is it localized? How long has it gone on? Can you describe the extent and duration of any bleeding? Depending on the problem, doctors will conduct a pelvic exam or do an ultrasound test to determine the length of the pregnancy or to make sure all is normal. If emergency physicians find that the pregnancy is stable and the mother healthy, the patient will be released. But if anything is amiss, an OB/GYN specialist will be called in immediately. If the pregnancy has advanced beyond the fourth month, patients will generally be sent to the labor and delivery area of the hospital for treatment by OB/GYN specialists in that department.

At home: The released patient will be told to return if pain intensifies or the bleeding resumes.

Fever: Doctors will take a history and conduct a complete physical. They will search high and low for the source of the fever, be it an ear infection, a urinary tract infection, or strep throat. The temperature will be taken again and blood tests may be conducted. With a fever of 105 and above or 95 and below, the patient will usually be admitted to the hospital. If physicians think the patient has a serious infection such as meningitis or pneumonia, they will establish an IV line and admit to the hospital.

At home: If the problem seems to be a flu or virus or some other infection treatable at home, the patient will be given the appropriate medication and told to drink plenty of fluids.

Severe flulike symptoms (Include some combination of headache, dizziness, weakness, disorientation, cough, and fever): After reading the vital signs, ED personnel will look for problems potentially more serious than the common flu. For instance, flulike symptoms along with a stiff neck could indicate meningitis. Symptoms might also be due to an ear infection. The patient will generally be sent home for some rest.

At home: The physician might give the patient Tylenol and, if a bacterial infection has been found, an antibiotic.

Diagnostic Tests and Procedures You Can Expect in the Emergency Department

Imaging Tools in the ED

X ray: Every modern hospital has an X-ray machine. In the ED, the X ray—a picture of the inside of the body—is crucial to diagnosis of a large number of injuries and categories of disease. X rays can unequivocally show broken bones, enlarged hearts, collapsed or fluid-filled lungs, and blocked bowels. X rays can also reveal the presence of a foreign object in the body, be it a copper penny, a bullet, or a piece of glass.

CAT scan: Computer axial tomography is, in essence, an elaborate X ray. A CAT scanner takes X-ray pictures throughout the body, then reconstructs them by computer to create essentially three-dimensional images of the area in question. The major difference between the CAT scan and the X ray is that the scan reveals details that the X ray can't. The X ray will diffentiate between bones and soft tissue, for instance, but one requires a CAT scan to differentiate between the liver and the intestines or between different parts of the brain. If one wants to diagnose broken skull bones, X rays will do; but to pinpoint a soft-tissue injury within the gray matter of the brain, only a CAT scan is appropriate.

MRI: Magnetic resonance imaging is similar to the CAT scan, but can generate images with even more definition and does not involve any radiation. The technology may be particularly helpful in diagnosing brain and spinal cord injuries. This technology has two disadvantages: It is very costly, and it can be rendered inaccurate by metallic objects in the body, from replacement joints to pacemakers.

Ultrasound, or sonogram: This technology generates an image by bouncing soundwaves through the body, much like radar and sonar used to track airplanes or submarines. While the most common use of ultrasound is tracking the healthy pregnancy, in the emergency department, sonograms are particularly valuable in diagnosing soft-tissue injuries, especially gall bladder disease, kidney stones, abdominal aneurysm, and gynecological problems, including ovarian cyst and ectopic pregnancy. The technology is also useful in diagnosing heart disease and, in that context, is called an echocardiogram.

EKG (or ECG): An electrocardiogram is employed to see if a patient has suffered heart disease. Physicians also measure the heart's activity with this invaluable machine. An EKG is indicated whenever a patient is significantly ill, has chest pain, or complains of weakness, dizziness, fainting, or heartbeats that are irregular, either too fast or too slow. Leads from the EKG machine are attached to the body—one on each leg and arm, and six on the chest, right across the heart. Don't worry, nothing comes out of the machine to hurt you; it's simply a device that measures the current passing through your heart, thus revealing the rate and regularity of the beat as well as any areas that have suffered injury or, for some other reason, are just not working well.

Five-Minute Mysteries: Quick Diagnostic Tests in the Emergency Department

"Crit": Short for **hematocrit,** this test is used to measure the red blood count and keep track of potentially dangerous blood loss. The whole test takes a minute or two. To do the test, ED personnel either draw a full blood sample, or, more commonly, prick the tip of the finger and take a drop of blood. (In young babies, blood for this test may be drawn from the heel.) The test is conducted whenever there's been a loss of blood, either through a wound, through rectal or vaginal bleeding, or through internal injuries.

Blood sugar test: Used to measure blood sugar in those known to have diabetes, or in those who feel dizzy or faint, this test is done by drawing a full blood sample or pricking the finger and taking a few drops. Results are usually available within minutes. In general, blood sugar goes down when people don't eat, or, in the case of diabetics, when they take too much insulin. When diabetes is out of control, blood sugar surges rapidly.

Urinalysis: This test is conducted after patients have provided a urine specimen (in a container used in the emergency department lavatory). To do the test, ED workers take a plastic stick covered with chemical reagents and dip it into the urine sample. The reagents will cause the stick to change color, depending on whether the urine is acidic or alkaline, whether it contains abnormal protein, and whether red or white blood cell counts are out of whack. Urinalysis is usually done for patients with symptoms of urinary tract or kidney infection, and in those with trauma to the abdominal area to rule out injury to the bladder or the kidneys. Results should be available within minutes.

Urine pregnancy test: This test, performed by analyzing a urine sample, is conducted in the emergency department for many reasons. A young woman comes in with vague complaints of abdominal pain. Could she be pregnant? Or, could she be suffering the effects of a pregnancy gone awry? For instance, if she has an ectopic pregnancy, in which the fetus is rooted in the fallopian tube instead of the uterus, her life may be at risk. Pregnancy tests are also performed in the ED to make sure a patient is *not* pregnant before receiving drugs or treatments (such as X rays in the first trimester) that could be harmful to the fetus.

Quick strep test: To test for strep, ED staffers may take a cotton swab and brush it along the lining of the throat to collect some throat cells and strep germs. The collected tissue is analyzed and, within ten or fifteen minutes, doctors will be able to determine the presence of strep.

The Diagnostic Armory: Other Common Lab Tests Performed in the Emergency Department

CBC, or complete blood count: Measures the total red blood cell *and* white blood cell count. The white blood cell count is critically important in determining the presence, absence, or severity of infection: the higher the white blood cell count, the more infection present in the body. The CBC can also measure blood platelets, crucial for clotting. Blood for this test is drawn in tubes and sent to the hospital lab. Results are usually reported within fifteen to thirty minutes.

Blood chemistry panel: Sometimes the ED will draw a quantity of blood and order a whole series of tests from the hospital lab. Specific parameters to be tested depend on the patient's symptoms and the probable diagnosis suspected by the doctor in charge. To conduct a panel of tests, doctors or nurses will, of course, have to draw a quantity of blood from a vein, not a fingertip. Specific elements analyzed in the blood chemistry panel may include blood sugar (a measurement of glucose level); electrolytes (including sodium, potassium, and chloride), which must all be in balance; and carbon dioxide, which can indicate the blood is too acidic or too alkaline. As part of the basic blood chemistry panel, the lab will also generally test for what's known as BUN, or blood urea nitrogen. BUN is a test of kidney function: When the BUN goes up, it usually means the kidneys are not working well.

Taken in large numbers of situations, the blood chemistry panel can tell ED staff whether the patient is appropriately hydrated; whether medications have created problems; or whether the patient's body chemistry has become too alkaline or too acidic. Physicians generally ask the lab to look at just five or six different blood characteristics, but could request twenty or thirty different measurements, and even more, if the situation warrants it.

Bilirubin and amylase: Measured in the blood, these two elements are generally tested together when doctors suspect liver disease, pancreatic disease, gall bladder disease, or injury to the upper abdomen. Alcoholic patients who may have damaged livers or inflammation of the pancreas will often be given this battery of tests. Abnormally high levels of bilirubin may suggest damage to the liver. Abnormally high levels of amylase may suggest damage to the pancreas.

ABG, or arterial blood gas: While all other blood tests are done with venous blood, the ABG requires arterial blood which, obviously, must be drawn from an artery as opposed to a vein (while veins carry blood to the heart, arteries carry oxygenated blood from the heart to the body). Blood for the ABG is usually drawn near the wrist, in the spot where you might be able to feel your radial pulse, but it may come from groin or elbow regions as well. Because ED personnel must pierce an artery, this test is generally more painful than a venous blood test. It measures the acid-base balance of the body, and the oxygen content of the blood. As a result, it's a good indicator of the heart's ability to pump and the lungs' ability to ventilate. This test is appropriate for patients with blood clots, collapsed lungs, pneumonia, or severe breathing problems.

CSF, or cerebro-spinal fluid: Spinal fluid is collected from the body with what's known as a lumbar puncture or spinal tap. To execute a spinal tap, doctors stick a needle through the back into the spinal canal and draw out the fluid. Spinal fluid is analyzed for signs of bleeding or infection, and is frequently used to diagnose meningitis as well as hemorrhaging in or near the spinal cord or brain.

Toxicology screen: Done by analyzing blood or urine samples, this test screens for a spectrum of toxic substances, measuring the quantity in the blood. Substances that can be detected and measured include alcohol, aspirin, acetaminophen (or Tylenol), barbiturates, and theophylline (a stimulant found in asthma medications). In addition, physicians, when asked to do so by law-enforcement authorities, can test for a wide range of illegal drugs, from amphetamines, to heroin, to cocaine. When a patient is unconscious or exhibiting bizarre behavior and the cause of the problem is unclear, the toxicology screen may be a tool of choice.

Type and cross: This blood test enables doctors to determine blood type and then match with blood stored in the blood bank. In the emergency department, this essential screening may be important to avoid reactions between maternal and fetal blood at childbirth or during miscarriage.

Cultures: A sampling from any part of the body (i.e., the throat or the site of a wound), blood, stool, sputum, or urine is collected and allowed to grow bacteria in the lab. Cultures must grow for forty-eight hours before lab technicians can examine or otherwise test for microorganisms that may be causing infection.

CPK: The initials stand for **creatine phosphokinase**, the enzyme that is elevated in those with damage to the heart. The test is given to most who come to the ED complaining of chest pain. It can take up to six hours to get the results.

Special Procedures and Surgeries You Can Expect in the Emergency Department

Suturing lacerations: Almost any cut or laceration greater than about a half an inch (or a centimeter) in length probably needs to be stitched. The doctor will initially evaluate: How deep is the laceration? Is anything stuck in the laceration? Has a nerve, joint, tendon, or artery been injured as a result of the laceration? After assessment, doctors will cleanse and sterilize around the site of the laceration, often irrigating with large amounts of normal saline, or salt water. They will then inject a local anesthetic—usually lidocaine—in the vicinity of the wound to make the area numb, and will put in the stitches, or sutures—generally of black nylon—with a curved, C-shaped needle. Physicians may sew one stitch or many, depending upon the length of the laceration. Afterward, doctors cleanse the area once more and apply a sterile dressing to cover the wound. At home, the patient is told to keep the area clean and dry and to look for signs of infection, including heat, temperature, pus, and redness. In most cases, the patient can go back to the ED or to a private doctor to have the stitches removed between five and ten days after they have been put in. While the sutures may be associated with some pain, patients are asked to avoid aspirin-containing drugs, which may encourage bleeding. Medicines like Tylenol, with an acetaminophen base, or ibuprofen, however, are acceptable.

Draining abscesses: An abscess—a boil or a carbuncle—is, in reality, an infection, a collection of pus underneath the skin. Though abscesses can occur anywhere, people most often get them around an infected tooth, around the fingernail, or in the underarm area or the groin. To treat abscesses, doctors cleanse and anesthetize, and then make an incision, enabling the pus or the infection to drain out. At home, patients are asked to soak with warm water several times a day so the infected material can continue to come out. Sometimes antibiotics are prescribed and cloth packing may be left in the abscess cavity to allow the infection to drain easily.

Inserting chest tubes: Chest tubes are often utilized in the treatment of collapsed lungs. Inserted through the skin and muscles of the chest into the lung cavity, chest tubes generally suck air or fluid from the space surrounding the lungs, allowing them to re-expand. The procedure requires sedation, as well as a local anesthetic to numb the skin. Doctors cut a small hole in the anesthetized area with a surgical knife and then insert through it the clear plastic tube attached to a suction device.

Conscious sedation: In any number of situations, emergency procedures will be painful: A fracture needs to be set; a chest tube must be inserted; complicated lacerations must be sutured. To calm patients down so the procedure can be performed, and to relieve pain, doctors may turn to conscious sedation. To administer such sedation, ED staffers first establish an intravenous line and provide the patient with supplemental oxygen. They attach the patient to a heart monitor. Then the sedative—often a mixture of a sedative like Valium and a narcotic—is dripped, via catheter into the vein. Within about ten minutes, the patient becomes much more comfortable and sedate, though still awake and able to respond, and the procedure can begin.

Intravenous line (IV): Emergency department staffers start IV lines for two basic reasons: One is to provide the dehydrated patient with more fluid; and the other is to administer medicine rapidly and directly into the bloodstream. To start an IV line, the doctor or nurse must first find an appropriate blood vessel, usually somewhere on the arm or hand. A tourniquet is tightened around the upper arm so that the veins bulge and become more visible. The ED staffer will then sterilize the skin around the chosen vein, usually with some combination of alcohol and iodine, and will pass a very small needle with catheter attached through the skin and into the vein. The catheter is then covered with a clear-plastic tape, for easy visualization, and connected to an intravenous tube which is connected to a bag of fluid. The fluid bag hangs above the level of the patient, generally on a movable metal pole. Gravity causes the fluid, which may contain a basic salt solution or appropriate medication, to drip down into the vein. Sometimes, the rate of flow is controlled by a device called a flow control monitor. The very sickest patients may have IV lines in two or three different places at once.

Central venous line: In some situations, an IV line must be put into a large or central vein of the body. A central venous line enables physicians to pass a larger catheter that carries more medicine or fluid rapidly and directly into the vicinity of the heart. A central venous line also provides a route into the body when, due to shock or cardiac arrest, circulation has become so poor that ED staffers can no longer easily see the smaller, peripheral veins on the extremities. Central lines are usually placed in the vicinity of the collarbone or the neck. In some circumstances they may be placed in the large vessels in the groin. (Note that vessels used to establish a central line are not ones that the doctor or nurse can see or feel; rather, they know where these large, central veins are based on their knowledge of anatomy.) To insert a central line, the general area is numbed with local anesthetic. Then the needle is passed through the skin and muscles into a very large vein that may be as thick as an index finger. The needle may sometimes be threaded inches into the body so it sits alongside the heart. As with a more conventional IV line, a long plastic catheter is passed through the needle into the vascular system, and the needle itself is then removed.

Nebulizing: If you have asthma you're familiar with the hand-held dispensers that spray a mist of medication into your mouth and lungs. Take a deep breath, and the drug enters your lungs and the rest of your body, loosening the restriction gripping your chest and enabling you to breathe. In the emergency department, this process is made more potent by utilizing a nebulizer. The mouthpiece of the nebulizer, resembling somewhat the mouthpiece of a clarinet, is held between the lips. As the patient grips the mouthpiece it dispenses medicine that has been nebulized, or dissolved, directly into the air and then is breathed into the lungs over a prolonged period of ten to fifteen minutes. For those patients who are very ill, the nebulized medication may be delivered through a mask; to be effective the treatment must sometimes be repeated two or three times.

Supplemental oxygen: Oxygen is given to a large number of patients in the emergency department—patients who are short of breath or otherwise having difficulty breathing, including asthmatics and those with emphysema; patients with heart disease; patients with collapsed lungs; and to all patients whose oxygen level is deemed inadequate after measurement with an oxygen saturation device. While oxygen is crucial to sustain life, it makes up just 21 percent of the air we breathe. In emergency department delivery systems, however, the concentration of oxygen may be drastically increased. The simplest oxygen-dispensing device is the nasal cannula—a clear-plastic tubing with two tiny prongs that sit in front of the nose. As concentrated oxygen is released near the nasal passageway, the patient gets a boost. To deliver oxygen even more directly, hospitals also use an oxygen mask—a clear-plastic mask that fits around the nose and mouth, drawing oxygen from a plastic reservoir and shunting it directly to the patient's nose and mouth.

Intubation: A procedure used to assist patients in breathing. The emergency department staff passes a plastic endotracheal tube through the mouth into the lungs. This procedure, which can be painful, is usually performed in people who are sedated or unconscious. First, a metal device is used to push the tongue aside so the trachea and air passage can be directly visualized. Then the physician will pass the tube through the vocal cords into the windpipe. A small balloon at the end of the tube is blown up to seal it in place, and then either a breathing bag—often called an "ambu bag"—or a ventilator/respiratory device is attached to blow air and oxygen into the lungs, causing the patient to breathe. In unusual circumstances, the endotracheal tube can be passed through the nose.

Tracheotomy: Also called crichothyroidotomy, this is a surgical approach to the airway. When the patient cannot breathe, and intubation is not possible, doctors apply a local anesthetic and make a small incision through the skin in the front of the neck, passing a tube directly into the trachea, or windpipe.

Nasal packing: When a nosebleed cannot be stopped by routine means—applying pressure to the bleeding area or blood vessels underneath—the emergency department team may literally pack the nose with gauze. For nasal packing, the patient will be seated in an upright position and sedated. Then the inside of the nose will be sprayed with a local anesthetic and the work will begin. A long, moistened piece of gauze, usually soaked in Vaseline, will be inserted into the nose until almost all of the nasal cavity is filled. It's the pressure inside the nose that stops the bleeding at last. Such packs are left in only a short period of time—usually overnight and rarely more than twenty-four hours. Patients must return to the ED or a personal physician to have the pack removed. Patients with nasal packing may also sometimes receive antibiotics to reduce the risk of infection.

Removal of object from eye: After the surface of the eye is anesthetized so the patient can keep it open, the emergency department doctor will visualize the eye by looking directly inside and scouting around for the invading speck of dirt or other irritant. If the invasive object cannot be found this way, the doctor will ask the patient to focus eyes up very high and down very low so that the eyelid can be peered under; it may even be necessary to turn the upper eyelid inside out. If still unable to pinpoint the debris, the doctor will use a machine called a slit-lamp microscope, which magnifies the area so the problem comes into view. Once found, the invasive material can be removed through irrigation; with a damp cotton swab; or, if it's stuck in the cornea, with a tiny needle sometimes called a spud.

Defibrillation: This procedure serves to correct the life-threatening condition of ventricular fibrillation, in which the heart beats in a completely irregular and uncoordinated fashion, (resembling a quivering bowl of jelly) and loses the ability to propel blood through the body. The standard treatment of defibrillation is to place the paddles of the defibrillator on the surface of the chest near the heart. One is usually placed just to the right of the breastbone underneath the collarbone, and the other, just to the left of the heart, on the patient's side. The defibrillator machine itself stores an electrical charge, and when released, it passes that charge between the two paddles, in the vicinity of the heart. The electrical energy actually changes the heart's rhythm, and, if it's effective, it changes that rhythm back to a normal, regularly beating heart pattern. Defibrillation is generally performed on patients who are comatose and in cardiac arrest.

Cardioversion: Similar to defibrillation, cardioversion is brought to bear on patients with regular, but extremely rapid, heartbeats—a condition that may result in shortness of breath, shock, or chest pain. As with defibrillation, emergency department personnel use paddles for cardioversion. But this time the discharge of energy is carefully coordinated with the patient's own heartbeat to slow it down. Unlike recipients of defibrillation, most cardioversion patients are alert and must be sedated before the procedure begins.

Temporary pacemaker: If the heart is beating too slowly, and if routine medication doesn't help speed it up, emergency department physicians may use a temporary pacemaker. In one technique, doctors attach the external pacemaker device to the chest via electronic leads in the form of foam rubber pads. Sensing the heart rate, the pacemaker will then stimulate the heart to beat by delivering energy through the pads. Using another strategy, instead of foam rubber pads, doctors sometimes insert the pacemaker "leads" internally; the lead then, is a catheter passed through a central venous line directly into the heart. In the emergency department, these temporary pacemakers are often utilized until heart surgeons can implant a tiny, permanent pacemaker inside the body.

Intracardiac injection: Sometimes epinephrine will be injected directly into the heart through the chest as a means of stimulating cardiac muscle, but this is performed only in life-and-death situations.

Bladder catheterization: For patients suffering from heart failure and pulmonary edema (water on the lungs), it is important to give a strong diuretic such as Furosemide to aid the excretion of fluids. To capture the strong surge of urine, a catheter, or tube, is attached to the urethra through the penis or vagina. The bladder may also be catheterized to open the blockage caused by an enlarged prostate gland.

Stomach pumping: If the patient has ingested poison, emergency department staff may need to pump his or her stomach, usually with what's called a "nasogastric tube" or "stomach hose" that runs through the nasal cavity into the stomach.

Medicines You May Receive in the Emergency Department

Note: Most books on prescription drugs present an alphabetical listing. Our summary of medicines commonly dispensed in the ED takes a different tactic. Hoping to emphasize the medical complaint, we place all medicines in categories that pertain to use. As you read through our list, you will learn how medicines compare and contrast with others in their category, and will get a sense of some potential side effects as well. Where brand names are given, the word is capitalized (Demerol, for example); others, all lowercase, are generic chemical names (ibuprofen, for example).

For Pain and/or Sedation

Narcotics: Used to sedate and/or relieve severe pain. The most common narcotic medications are morphine and Demerol. Both can be given either intravenously or via injection through the intramuscular route. There are also new narcotic medications that act more rapidly, including Fentanyl and sufentanyl. Patients treated with narcotics include those with migraines, those with heart attacks, and those with broken bones that must be set in painful procedures. Patients passing kidney stones are sometimes given these powerful painkillers as well. Since narcotics may, on occasion, lower blood pressure or suppress respiration, patients who receive narcotic medications in the emergency department require monitoring for at least several hours after the last dose. One last note: A single dose of narcotic medication given in the ED is *not* addictive.

Nonsteroidal anti-inflammatory drugs: Used to reduce pain and swelling.

Among them are ibuprofen (Motrin), Advil, or Nuprin, Naprosyn (now marketed without prescription as Aleve), and Toradol. Toradol, which is not available over the counter, may be given intravenously or by injection; the others are taken orally. Also in this class and frequently dispensed in the ED are ordinary Tylenol and aspirin, which may be given in the form of a pill, a liquid, or a suppository, depending on the situation. These two medications relieve pain and are also especially effective at reducing temperature. Tylenol and aspirin are sometimes mixed with codeine, a narcotic, to ease pain that is particularly severe. Available in pill form, the Tylenol/codeine combination comes in a series of strengths with number notations: Tylenol #4, for instance, is stronger than Tylenol #3.

The major difference between such medications in the emergency department as opposed to those taken at home is that the emergency physician may prescribe them in stronger doses. These medications may sometimes irritate the stomach, but carry none of the more serious side effects occasionally seen with narcotics.

Local Anesthetics for Painful Procedures

When doctors must make an area numb so they can suture it, they rely on local anesthetics, the most frequently used being lidocaine or Xylocaine. Delivered by injection into the skin, these drugs cause almost instant anesthesia and last for about thirty minutes to an hour. The only major complication is very rare allergy.

Antibiotics for Bacterial Infection

Used to fight bacterial infection, antibiotics may be given intravenously, by injection, or by mouth. Broad-spectrum antibiotics are used to fight common infections of the ear, the throat, and the skin. The most common of these antibiotic groups is penicillin. There is pure penicillin and many drugs that are related to penicillin, including ampicillin, amoxicillin, and Augmentin. This antibiotic family covers a broad spectrum of diseases, and is frequently used to treat strep throat, ear infection, and urinary tract infection. The only potential problem here: 5–10 percent of patients are allergic to penicillin, and for those patients, other antibiotics are used.

One possibility: the cephalosporins, including Keflex, Velosef, and Ceclor, as well as cefoxitin, cefotetan, and cefoxurime. The first three—Keflex, Velosef, and Ceclor—are given by mouth. The others are generally given by intramuscular or intravenous routes, and *only* in the hospital. These broad-spectrum antibiotics are frequently given for cuts and scrapes, infections of the hand, and sometimes for earache. Though a small percentage of those allergic to penicillin will be allergic to these as well, these drugs have almost no other potential problems.

Other broad-spectrum antibiotics you may receive in the hospital include Gentamicin and amikacin, both particularly effective against infections that begin in the abdomen, though they may cause problems with kidney function. Also prescribed is erythromycin (frequently given to those allergic to penicillin) for sore throats, skin infections, and earaches. About the only side effect of erythromycin is the potential for upset stomach.

Still other antibiotics are prescribed specifically for urinary tract infection. The two most common are the sulfa drugs Septra and Bactrim. Also used for urinary tract infections, and sometimes upper respiratory infections, are two relatively new antibiotics called Cipro and Noroxin. Few people are allergic to these medications and they have virtually no complications.

Emergency physicians may prescribe the antibiotic tetracycline for sexually transmitted diseases, and the antibiotic Flagyl for bladder or vaginal infections; these medications only rarely provoke allergic reactions and are associated with few side effects.

One final note: Emergency physicians have in their versatile medicine chest more than a hundred antibiotics. For those not on our list, do ask about potential side effects.

Asthma Drugs

Generally delivered via nebulizer in the emergency department, the most common asthma medications are Alupent and Proventil pumps, sometimes used to treat croup and bronchitis as well. There are few side effects, but if used too frequently, they cease to be effective and may cause problems.

If ED physicians find these first-line drugs don't help, the next step may be an injection of epinephrine, a form of the hormone adrenaline. This drug may give the patient a jittery sensation or cause the heart to beat faster. It shouldn't be given to people with high blood pressure or heart disease.

Another class of drugs used for asthma, as well as allergy, are the steroids. These powerful anti-inflammatory drugs include Prednisone, usually given by mouth; Medrol, also given by mouth; and hydrocortisone and Decadron, generally given intravenously. For asthmatics, these drugs work to reduce inflammation and swelling of the breathing tubes; in some cases, however, they are given to victims of head and spinal injury to reduce swelling in those areas as well. Over the short term, in the ED, steroids will not result in any complications. However, if taken over a period of weeks or months, they could cause puffiness about the face and other, more significant complications. Check with your primary-care physician.

For Allergy Relief

The most common medication used for severe allergy is epinephrine; in the case of extreme allergic reaction, it can be given either intravenously or by injection. If the allergy is deadly, as in anaphylactic shock, the epinephrine is delivered directly into the body either intravenously or via the endotracheal tube.

For mild allergic reactions like hives, ED physicians prescribe antihistamines like Benadryl. Benadryl can be delivered orally, intramuscularly, or intravenously, depending on the situation, and may cause drowsiness.

Rash Preparations

Hydrocortisone, a white, topical steroid cream, is effective against many rashes, particularly itchy rashes caused by poison oak or poison ivy.

Cough Medicines

Expectorants: These syrups make it easier to clear out the lungs, enabling the patient to literally cough out the infection. The most common expectorant, Robitussin, is a red liquid; patients are asked to take a teaspoonful once every four hours until the coughing stops.

Cough suppressants: On the other hand, these liquids suppress the cough. The most widely used form of cough suppressant is dextromethorphan, or DM. (When you buy Robitussin DM, the initials tell you it's a suppressant.) The other extensively used cough suppressant is codeine. When a cough is what doctors call "nonproductive"—a dry hack that expels no phlegm but merely irritates and exhausts the patient—a cough suppressant may be prescribed.

To Reduce Stomach Acidity

Drugs used to treat such problems as duodenal ulcer pain, gastritis, and gastric reflux (in which the acid seems to drift into the chest area), include liquid medications like Maalox and Amphojel or pill formulations like Zantac and Tagamet.

Maalox and Amphojel work, quite simply, by neutralizing the acid the stomach produces. Possible side effects include diarrhea for Maalox and constipation for Amphojel.

Zantac and Tagamet, on the other hand, actually stop or reduce the stomach's ability to produce acid. These medications must generally be taken long term, three or four times a day.

To Relieve Stomach Cramps and Nausea

Commonly used for stomach pain is Compazine, which can either be given by injection, pill, or suppository. Emergency patients may sometimes receive Reglan instead.

To Relieve Diarrhea

Often given for diarrhea relief is Kaopectate, which, as a fiber substitute, literally binds the stool; Imodium and Lomotil, which reduce the contractile ability of the intestines, are used as well.

Blood Pressure Medications

Medications used in the emergency department to treat hypertension include hydralazine (through injection or IV) and sodium nitroprusside, trimethaphan camsylate, diazoxide, or labetalol, all delivered via IV. These drugs all require careful monitoring in the ED and long-term follow-through by a physician after the patient has been discharged. Often, physicians will provide other medications long-term for patients suffering from high blood pressure.

Heart Medications

Perhaps most common among heart drugs is nitroglycerine, the small white pill you put under your tongue in case of chest pain. Use of this drug, which may make users feel lightheaded, must sometimes be repeated within minutes. Sometimes, patients come into the emergency department complaining that their own nitro simply has not worked, only to learn the impact of the drug was drastically weakened because the cap of the pill bottle was left off, or just loose. Another related drug sometimes dispensed in the ED is Isordil. Major side effect: These drugs may sometimes cause headaches or low blood pressure.

In the event of a heart attack, physicians will often strive to help blood flow through clogged arteries with thrombolytics, which work to dissolve blood clots and open the blocked blood vessels to the heart. The two in current use are streptokinase and tissue plasminogen activator (tPA). These drugs, delivered intravenously, break up the blood clots that may be blocking arteries, preventing the heart from working as it should. Patients with clogged arteries may also receive another drug called heparin, which literally works to thin the blood over a longer period of time and prevent new clots from occurring. The only problem with these drugs is that they may sometimes work too well, causing the patient to bruise or bleed easily; in some instances, they may induce bleeding in the brain, causing a stroke. Thus, these powerful medicines, while lifesavers for many thousands of heart patients, are contraindicated for those with hemophilia or a past history of stroke or recent injury, surgery, or bleeding.

Diabetes Drugs

The most usual medicine for a person with diabetes is insulin, given only by injection, either intramuscularly or intravenously. It comes in different forms, usually described as regular, which acts rapidly and is effective for a short period of time; and NPH, which is slower acting and effective for a longer period of time. In the emergency department, insulin is given to patients who have high blood sugars, with diabetes out of control. The main complication is that insulin may sometimes work too effectively, reducing blood sugar so much that people feel lightheaded and weak or even suffer blackout spells. In the event of complication, patients are treated with glucose by mouth or by intravenous line.

Antiseptics to Kill Germs

The antiseptic typically used in the emergency department is iodine, the familiar brown liquid that stings when applied. Some patients may have allergic reactions to iodine, so EDs have other antiseptics on hand too. These include peroxide, which doesn't sting like iodine and bubbles when coming in contact with the wound; and alcohol, most often used to clean an area of skin before giving an injection or establishing an intravenous line. Alcohol may be applied directly in liquid form or via presoaked paper pads.

Vaccines to Fight Infection from Injury or Bite

The medication most commonly used in the emergency department is a tetanus booster to protect against the deadly infection of tetanus, generally contracted when a deep cut, puncture, or laceration is infected with germs. If the patient has received tetanus immunization more than five or ten years earlier (depending upon the severity of the wound), he or she will get a tetanus booster. If the patient has never been immunized against tetanus, he will receive a full-fledged vaccination called tetanus immune globulin, which creates immediate immunity to tetanus. (A reminder: Since three injections are required for complete immunity, the patient who has never been immunized before will have to return to the ED or to a personal physician for two additional injections during the next eight months.) Only very rarely do people have an allergic reaction to the tetanus vaccine, though sometimes, when people receive tenanus shots more frequently than they should, the arm will swell at the site of the injection.

The emergency department is also in the business of dispensing the rabies vaccine to those who have been bitten by animals that are potentially rabid. If you have been bitten by a dog, skunk, raccoon, bat, or fox, and if the animal cannot be brought in for testing or you don't know whether the dog has been vaccinated against rabies, you will need the shot. Years ago, the rabies vaccine was notoriously painful, but now rabies shots are no more painful than a shot of penicillin. Patients require a single shot at the time of infection and then a series of five more shots over a period of three weeks. While the old rabies injections were known to provoke strong allergic reactions, the new injections are associated with only minor allergy complications.

Burn Salve

A white cream called Silvadene—actually a sulfa antibiotic drug—helps relieve the inflammation and itch of burns and fights infections.

Eye Medications

Antibiotics like erythromycin, sulfa drugs, and gentamicin, in the form of drops or ointment, may be put in the eye to halt the spread of infection. Drops are usually easier to get into the eye, but stay put for a lesser period of time. Ointments are somewhat stickier, messier, and harder to get in the eye, but once in, have staying power.

An anesthetic agent called tetracaine is often used to numb the injured eye so doctors may examine it or remove foreign bodies without inflicting pain. In the case of a scratched cornea, patients are unable to open eyes for examination or application of antibiotic unless they have been anesthetized. The anesthetic also provides patients with some needed relief from unremitting pain.

Seizure Medications

Dilantin is given to seizure patients in the emergency department. A capsule that's taken three times a day, this drug has virtually no complications—except when users forget to take it, and then suffer a seizure.

Poison Antidotes

There are two drugs that the emergency department regularly dispenses to victims of poisoning. The first, Ipecac, rarely used, may help induce vomiting, thus causing the stomach to empty. The second, activated charcoal, literally attaches to the poison inside the body so it cannot leave the intestinal tract and be absorbed into the bloodstream.

Chapter 7

The Littlest Patients: A Look at Pediatric Emergencies

He was just getting over an ordinary stomach virus when he awoke in the middle of the night, itchy and uncomfortable. When his parents walked into his room to ease him back to sleep, they were shocked by what they saw: Huge red blotches covered the expanse of his body, including his face, arms, and legs, even his palms and soles. "This wasn't just an ordinary rash," his mother recalls. "It was as if someone had beaten him up. The condition had the purplish tinge of black-and-blue marks, as if he were bleeding inside." Though it was three in the morning, the frantic parents called their pediatrician and then rushed to the emergency department. Doctors conducted an elaborate series of tests, eventually concluding that the boy had a rare but noncritical reaction to the virus leaving his system. Fortunately for this child, age six, their diagnosis was correct. Despite the horrific appearance of this frightening rash, it disappeared, without consequence, in a week.

Another child wasn't as lucky. A member of the town swim team, he'd been working out in his local pool. Lifeguards on duty were more than surprised when the ten-year-old, known for his water skills, went under and disappeared. Though he was quickly pulled out of the water, his breathing was shallow and his pulse faint. Lifeguards, and then the paramedics who were summoned, performed cardiopulmonary resuscitation. The child was rushed by ambulance to the nearest ED, where emergency physicians aided his breathing with an endotracheal tube and respirator and, with the help of a CAT scan, finally diagnosed the problem: A burst aneurysm (a weak spot in an arterial wall) at the base of the brain. The boy was rushed to the operating room, where pediatric neurosurgeons were able to drain the blood from the region, stop the internal bleeding, clip the aneurysm, and save his life.

When a child gets sick or hurt, emotions can run high. The worry we may have for friends and relatives is greatly magnified when the victim is a child. And when medical emergency hits a child, the problems are often frightening, indeed. At the St. Luke's–Roosevelt Hospital's pediatric emergency department, for example, children come in not just for colds, flu, and tummy aches, but also for head injuries, burns, severe lacerations, broken bones, and asthma. Recently, a sobbing, wheezing sixteen-month-old with asthma was so sick, doctors had to admit him to the hospital, where he was given a bed in pediatric intensive care. Automobile and bicycle accidents, drownings, and poisonings are also common, as is child abuse. Shockingly, doctors say that assaults and even shootings have increased not just among adults, but also among children.

What's more, children, like adults, are subject to a range of mysterious ailments which, at first, are hard to diagnose. At St. Luke's recently, one newborn boy, just twenty-one days old, had been in and out of the hospital with an enigmatic series of symptoms, including small lesions on the abdomen, an *E. coli* infection was detected by blood culture, and a constant low-grade fever ranging between 101 and 102 degrees Fahrenheit. Bent on solving what he called a "medical mystery," one of the emergency department's attending pediatricians, Dr. David Kroning, the assistant director of the pediatric ED, oversaw a battery of lab tests in his search for subtle clues. Finally narrowing in on a probable diagnosis, he suggested the child might have an immune deficiency. With his problem no longer in the domain of emergency medicine, this child was admitted to the hospital for further tests and sent to a room upstairs.

The importance of the pediatric ED is underscored by the statistics: Accidents are the leading cause of death in children, claiming twenty thousand lives a year of those nineteen and younger. And for every death from accident, forty-two additional children are hospitalized. Some thirty thousand children a year suffer permanent disability from head injuries alone.

Children Are Not Small Adults

While accidents and serious ills afflict adults as well as children the medical particulars—the rules of diagnosis and treatment—can be a world apart. Children, after all, are not just small adults. They have different diseases, and these diseases require substantially different treatments. Moreover, even when children do get diseases common to adults, symptoms may differ in the extreme. In fact, medically speaking, the differences between child and adult are so enormous that they exist across the board in virtually every organ system, body part, physiological process, and disease syndrome.

It only makes sense, the experts say, that when children come to the emergency department, treatment by practitioners trained in pediatric emergency medicine confers a clear and crucial edge. Children's lungs, for example, are smaller and more fragile, so during cardiopulmonary resuscitation, they require gentler thrusts. Provide a child with the same CPR effort required for an average-size adult, and his lungs might literally collapse.

The list of danger zones, in fact, is extensive. Children have faster heart and respiration rates than adults, so what may look like normal adult rates can actually be a sign of serious trouble in a child. When a child goes into cardiac arrest, it's generally a sign of breathing problems; but a doctor who is not trained in pediatric emergencies may not know this, since cardiac arrest in grownups overwhelmingly indicates the presence of heart disease.

Children also have different presenting symptoms when it comes to shock. Adult victims of shock experience a gradual decrease in blood pressure over time. For children, on the other hand, blood pressure stays virtually normal during the precipitous descent into shock, and decreases rapidly right before death, when recognition of the problem is almost always too late to do any good.

Even when it comes to diagnosing ordinary ear infection as opposed to deadly meningitis, those not schooled in pediatric emergency medicine find it difficult to differentiate between the two.

In the hospital, children require specialized care and equipment because of their size. Their bodies are smaller, so they need medicine in correspondingly smaller dosages. Yet, in some ambulances and emergency departments, drugs are usually prepackaged in single adult doses, forcing emergency personnel to recalculate the correct amount for a child, based on estimated weight and age. Children's veins and tracheae are smaller, so they require smaller intravenous needles and intubation tubes (used to assist breathing). Adult-size blood-pressure cuffs slip off little arms, and even the collars used to keep youngsters with spinal injuries immobile are too large, often obscuring their faces and even impairing ventilation.

Doing Your Homework

To ensure that *your* child receives the best care emergency medicine has to offer, you must do your homework. Long before emergency ever strikes, find out to which hospital your pediatrician admits patients. Is that the hospital your pediatrician recommends your child go to in the event of emergency? If so, contact that facility and find out whether it has a devoted pediatric emergency department or an emergency medicine specialist in the emergency department.

According to Dr. Ilene Kaufman, head of Pediatric Emergency Medicine at St. Luke's–Roosevelt, emergency departments connected to hospitals with pediatric inpatient units are best. Often these facilities will have a separate pediatric emergency department with pediatric nurses and pediatric emergency doctors, who have been specially trained in two fields: emergency medicine *and* pediatrics. "If you live in a city like New York, a lot of EDs have this specialty," Kaufman states, "and you can have your pick. If you have access to a specialized pediatric emergency department, one that exists apart from the adult ED, that's best."

Remember, if you have the choice of taking your child to an emergency department with staff both trained and experienced in pediatric emergencies, or to an ED without a specially trained staff, where your own pediatrician happens to have privileges, you will always do well to choose the pediatric ED. After all, your child's personal pediatrician is just a phone call away and can be called from anywhere. In the middle of an emergency, however, your child's fate rests with the doctors who are treating her, not the one on the phone.

In some areas, notably suburbs and rural regions, specialized pediatric EDs cannot be found in abundance. However, as a medical consumer, do check to see if the emergency department you plan to use offers full-time pediatric emergency services within the walls of the ED. If you can find an emergency department staffed with experienced, board-certified pediatric or general emergency physicians on a twenty-four hour basis, that is best.

Unfortunately, many people don't have access to EDs with pediatric emergency specialists in-house twenty-four hours a day. If you must take your child to a general ED staffed exclusively with practitioners specializing in the treatment of adults, do ask these additional questions: Are emergency department doctors and nurses trained in emergency medicine, including the full gamut of pediatric emergency techniques? Have they taken special courses? Does that hospital have a pediatric intensive care unit? Does the hospital have a separate in-house department devoted to pediatrics? Does the hospital have child-size equipment in the emergency department or anywhere in the building?

Finally, suggests Dr. Kaufman, ask how many children the emergency department sees per day. The pediatric emergency department at St. Luke's, for instance, treats one hundred children a day, but Kaufman places the critical mass for true experience at about twenty: "If an emergency department treats twenty children a day," she says, "that facility probably has sufficient experience with children. All things being equal, choose the ED that sees twenty children a day over the ED that sees one or two."

If the emergency department you must use does not meet even minimum suggested standards, do proceed with care. Of course, in life-threatening situations—if your child has been poisoned, is suffering from severe asthma, or has gone into cardiac arrest—survival may depend on getting to any emergency room *fast*. In fact, in cases of extreme emergency, training in emergency medicine is far more important than training in pediatrics. If your child has been hit by a truck, an emergency physician trained and experienced in trauma can do more to save her life than a pediatrician without emergency training. If your child's not breathing and emergency physicians are about to insert an endotracheal tube to deliver oxygen to her vital organs and brain, the last thing you want to do is stop the operation while you scout out a pediatrician in a hospital across town.

And one last tip: Do not be shy about calling the various emergency departments in your area to do your homework in advance. We have found that when faced with such questions, ED staffers tend to be honest and up front, and generally do everything they can to steer patients in the right direction. One anonymous call made to a New York area hospital not known for pediatrics, for instance, elicited this response from a nurse who picked up the phone: "This is not our specialty. We do not advise you to take your child here unless there's no choice." The nurse then proceeded to provide a list of three other, more appropriate, hospitals known for pediatric emergency care. She provided addresses and phone numbers as well. Other hospitals also willingly described their equipment and capabilities over the phone to anonymous prospective patients. If the hospital you are investigating comes up short, do look into other, better equipped facilities.

Ready for Anything

Once you locate appropriate emergency facilities, do a few test runs from your house. Make sure you can drive to the emergency department quickly without any confusion. You may even want to write the directions out on an index card and place them in the glove compartment of your car.

As with adult emergencies, there are many steps you can take to prepare yourself to be better equipped to deal with problems that may emerge. For instance, make sure you have posted a list of relevant numbers on the wall by the phone. These include: your pediatrician; the ambulance; the emergency department; and poison control.

Also make sure to list your child's relevant medical documents and vital data. Create a medical packet and keep papers handy—by the phone, above the sink, or some other spot where you can grab them without a lengthy search. Relevant documents include insurance information; your child's immunization record (including date of the last tetanus shot); a list of allergies, especially allergies to medications like penicillin; a list of any ongoing or current medical problems; and a list of all medications your child regularly or intermittently takes, ranging from psychoactive agents like Ritalin to over-the-counter products like Benadryl or Tylenol. Also be sure to include the name and phone number of your child's pediatrician, and if your child has ever been hospitalized, reference the hospital, the date, and the problem. If doctors can access old X rays or blood tests, they may be able to make more accurate diagnoses far more rapidly.

Kaufman suggests that if your child is taking a particular prescription medicine, for instance, an antibiotic, you take the bottle itself to the emergency department. "People will tell us, 'He's taking the pink antibiotic,'" she relates. "But they don't realize they're all pink. We have to know which one."

Finally, she states that if you walk in to find your two-year-old walking funny and acting drunk—or just out-and-out unconscious—you may want to take your whole medicine cabinet, load it into a bag and take it to the ED with your child. "If I know what's in the house, then I know what to think about," says Kaufman. "Is somebody taking blood pressure medicine? Antidepressants? Cardiac drugs? You don't know how many times parents under stress will forget the exact name of the prescription, and then, it's just more difficult for us to determine what's wrong."

Since waiting time in the emergency department can often be lengthy, try to keep a bag of children's books or games easily accessible as well. You may grab these before you leave. If you think your child may have to stay in the hospital, take along a best-loved teddy bear, doll, or toy.

If your child is in school or with a baby-sitter, make sure that under virtually any circumstance, you can be reached. If you work in an office make sure your current office number is posted on the wall by your phone and is on file with the school. If you are traveling and will not be in one particular spot, make sure you have a phone answering machine with a remote feature or an answering service, and call in every hour or two to get your messages and make sure things are OK.

These days many parents carry cellular phones. If you can afford it, and if your work or lifestyle carries you away from a wired phone for any length of time, it's something to consider. Not long ago a group of parents and children were traveling to visit a campsite when the bus rolled off the road and into a ditch. In this deserted country locale, it seemed as if no one was around for miles. But two parents pulled cellular phones out of their bags and were able to summon help, including ambulances and police backup, at once. The same phones make these parents accessible while commuting to work on the train, while shopping in the supermarket, while making the rounds of clients, or while taking a summer walk.

Also make sure, no matter how accessible you may be in general, that you have a backup. In case of medical emergency, is there anyone else besides you who can meet your child at the hospital, provide comfort, and talk with the doctors? Most schools ask parents to sign a medical consent form, enabling them to authorize medical or surgical procedures in your absence.

But some parents also appoint one or two "medical guardians" to act on their behalf if, for some reason, they can't be reached. To do so, write one or two letters granting such "guardianship" to trusted individuals, such as grandparents, baby-sitters, or close friends. Address the letters "To whom it may concern," and grant permission to a specific individual, by name, to authorize medical or surgical procedures for your child when you cannot be reached. Write an original letter for each such guardian to keep in his or her possession. Have the letters notarized, distribute to the appointed guardians, and place copies on file with the school. (Keep copies for your files, too.)

It's also not a bad idea to have the letter available for baby-sitters when they come to your home. If you have a few regular sitters, it might be wise to prepare letters with their names in case an accident occurs.

A sample guardianship letter appears on page 206.

CONSENT-TO-TREAT FORM

(DATE)

TO WHOM IT MAY CONCERN:

I (we) authorize

_____

(CARETAKER'S NAME)

_____

TO CONSENT ON MY BEHALF FOR ANY NECESSARY MEDICAL EVALUA-
TION, TREATMENT, OR SURGERY FOR

_____ ,

(MINOR'S NAME)

MY/OUR SON/DAUGHTER IN MY/OUR ABSENCE.

_____   _____

(SIGNATURE(S) OF PARENT(S))

_____   _____

(PARENTS' NAMES, PRINTED)

NOTARY PUBLIC'S SEAL

_____

(WITNESS SIGNATURE)

_____

(WITNESS SIGNATURE)

While such letters can generally grease the wheels of medicine, they may not always carry the authority of the parent. The reason: The blanket consent granted by the letter is not the same as informed consent, in which the parent has heard all the pros and cons of a given treatment and agreed. The result, many times, is that the hospital will perform lifesaving treatments for such problems as asthma, internal bleeding, and shock, but may wait until the parent can be reached before doing anything else. Physicians, fearful of being sued, may decline to suture a laceration on the face or set a broken bone—they may wait for hours, even though the delay may result in impaired healing or worse scars. But, in most cases, a note like this one will allow the treating emergency physician to make important decisions on your behalf.

Another important part of planning is to prepare your child for an experience at the emergency department long before a trip is ever made there. For a child suddenly injured or seriously ill, the stress of the emergency department will be multiplied without prior information on what to expect. For younger children, we recommend children's books such as *Curious George Goes to the Hospital* by H. A. Rey; and *A Visit to the Sesame Street Hospital* by Deborah Hautzig. For older children, a discussion based on the information in this chapter would be helpful. You may also wish to request a school trip to visit an emergency department or explore the inside of an ambulance. Call your local emergency department or ambulance/EMS service; they will be glad to arrange a visit. The St. Luke's–Roosevelt ambulance is well known at our local kindergarten and first-grade classes, and fourth to sixth graders have frequently visited the emergency department.

The truly prepared parent will also have some knowledge of lifesaving techniques, including the Heimlich maneuver, rescue breathing, and cardiopulmonary resuscitation. For a quick lesson in applying these skills to children, we suggest you study the instructions provided in Chapter 3. They may help you pull your child through.

Parents will be most effective if they take a course in first aid and CPR for *children*. Ideally, such a course would be a requirement for parenthood. Many a grateful parent has saved a young one's life as a result of special training.

Not long ago, for instance, a young Midwest boy was playing in a sandpit on the family farm, when a landslide of sand and boulders suddenly covered his body and head. His father dug him out, and while awaiting the arrival of an ambulance, performed rescue breathing. "My skill was rusty," the father confessed, "but I did the best I could." Though the boy ended up needing months of rehabilitation, doctors predict he will make a complete recovery, thanks in large part to his father's intervention. "His father provided minutes of oxygen to the brain," the boy's doctor commented. "Without that supply of oxygen, brain damage would have been severe."

To locate a course in your area, contact your local Red Cross, Heart Association office, or your community hospital.

Recognizing Emergencies in Children and Getting Them the Help They Need

As with adults, dire emergencies in children are always afoot when the ABC's—the airway, breathing, or circulation—are disrupted. If a child cannot breathe; if a child seems to be choking; if a child is unconscious or semiconscious; if the child is bleeding profusely; do not waste a second. Call 911 and summon an ambulance as fast as you can. Do this before you call the child's pediatrician, and even before you administer first aid.

There are, however, two exceptions: If you are the only person available to call 911 and the child has stopped breathing, help the child first by administering rescue breathing for one minute before summoning help. If you are the only person available to call 911 and you detect no pulse, help the child first by doing cardiopulmonary resuscitation for one minute before summoning help. Through these efforts, you will have delivered a minute's worth of oxygen to the child's brain and other vital organs. You can then rush to the phone and call 911 as expediently as possible. Having called the experts, rush back to resume your lifesaving efforts until the ambulance arrives. Remember, after four minutes without oxygen, the brain and other vital organs will sustain permanent damage and start to die.

Dr. Kaufman points to other true emergencies that warrant a visit to the emergency department as well. If your child seems so sick that you intuitively feel he's crossed the line into serious illness, based on your knowledge of how he usually responds to things, even when ill, the ED may be an option for you. Any time your child is doubled over with so much pain that you feel you could be putting her at risk by waiting, get to emergency.

Other problems, injuries, or symptoms that may signal extreme medical emergencies in children include:

· Wheezing or respiratory distress, symptomatic of asthma, bronchitis, or other lung disease. If the child's breathing or wheezing is particularly heavy or labored, call 911. Emergency Medical Services can begin treatment at once.

· An extremely rapid heart rate. While Dr. Kaufman says this symptom is usually *not* indicative of emergency in children, occasionally it can signal the onset of a condition known as supraventricular tachycardia, a heart disorder that requires immediate treatment. Usually the problem is accompanied by feelings of weakness. Since it is impossible for parents, or even doctors, to diagnose the condition without the backup of hospital technology, it's important to get to the ED at once.

· Severe pain to the right lower abdomen, which could be a sign of appendicitis. This may also be accompanied by vomiting or appetite loss.

· Blood in the stool or vomit. Diarrhea and vomiting are signs of sickness, of course, but they can usually be handled by your family doctor or pediatrician. However, if your child is excreting blood with the diarrhea or vomit, you must get to emergency at once. And remember, a bloody stool may be red or black.

· Any injury to the eye.

· Loss of a whole, permanent adult tooth, including root and shaft. "If the whole thing comes out," says Kaufman, "it can be reimplanted provided you get to the ED in thirty minutes." For the older child, she advises, "you can have him place the tooth in his cheek so it's bathed in saliva. For the younger child, place the tooth in milk." Then, it's best to hop in a cab or your car and get to the ED. Do not call 911; for this particular problem, EMS cannot do a thing.

· Hives, swelling, flushing, or respiratory distress that erupts after eating a meal, receiving an injection, or sustaining an insect sting. This may be an allergic reaction. Do not waste time getting to the emergency department yourself. Instead, call 911, so treatment may begin in the ambulance on the way to the hospital.

· Complications related to underlying illness, including sickle-cell anemia, heart disease, cystic fibrosis, or endocrine diseases like diabetes. Generally, these children have been diagnosed early in life, and parents will stay on the lookout for life-threatening problems that they have discussed with their pediatrician in advance.

· Thoughts of suicide or violent behavior. Such psychiatric emergencies in children, even those as young as seven, are more common than most people realize. If you have time to get your child to a personal clinician, that is best. But if your child is truly a danger to himself or others, get to the emergency department.

· Poisoning. Accidental poisoning is a grave problem often seen in the pediatric emergency department. Kaufman advises that parents first call their local poison-control center and follow its advice. (Do remember to post the number of the local poison-control center on the wall by your phone. At the St. Luke's–Roosevelt Emergency Department, we call the New York City Poison Center at 212-P-O-I-S-O-N-S. You may call it or your local poison center.) Depending on what the experts tell you, you may call 911 or go directly to the ED. If you do not have access to a local poison-control center, call an ambulance. This is one situation, advises Kaufman, in which your private pediatrician does not need to be part of the loop—at least not until after you've followed the directions of poison control or arrived at the hospital.

Dr. Kaufman also points to situations she defines as urgent. "They don't necessarily need to be treated in the ED," she says, "but they do need to be treated urgently—within hours." If your personal pediatrician can see you immediately, you can visit that office. But if it's the middle of the night or your own doctor is unavailable for any reason at all, go to the ED at once.

These situations include:

· Any fever at all in infants under two or three months. Kaufman defines a fever as anything greater than 100.4 degrees Fahrenheit.

· Any fever greater than 105 degrees Fahrenheit in a child of any age.

· Severe persistent headache, especially if it's associated with fever and neck pain. Your child might have meningitis.

· Severe, persistent vomiting or diarrhea.

· Any fall that results in vomiting or temporary loss of consciousness.

· An arm that has come out of a socket or hurts so much that the child won't use it.

· A fall or accident that results in extreme swelling, especially of an arm or leg. If the limb has been broken, it should be set as soon as possible, Kaufman advises, since "it will become increasingly swollen and difficult to set as time goes on." If you can get to an orthopedist immediately, that might be the option of choice—if that orthopedist has his own X-ray machine. Otherwise head for the emergency department. Advises the doctor: "If the child appears to have broken a leg and is too big to be carried without inflicting pain, call the ambulance to transport her to the ED."

· Seizure, recognizable when the eyes roll up, the body stiffens, and there's some kind of rhythmic shaking, often accompanied by drooling or excessive saliva. Common in children, especially between the ages of six months and five years, seizures can often occur as the result of fever, and are usually benign. However, if your child has never had a seizure before, or if the seizure has followed an accident, especially a head injury, get to a doctor right away. Likewise, if your child does not resume a normal state of consciousness within thirty minutes, emergency medical help is required; such symptomology could signal a diagnosis of meningitis or brain injury.

· Feeling of weakness accompanied by an inability to take in fluids or urinate. The child may be seriously dehydrated.

· Long, deep, or dirty lacerations: These cuts are not life-threatening, but they will need to be sutured. If the cut is on the face, you may want the services of a plastic surgeon. But especially if the laceration has become dirty or in some way infected, it needs to be treated as soon as possible. If it isn't cleaned out within about twelve hours, bacteria will start to multiply and doctors may not be able to suture for fear of locking the bacteria—and a dangerous infection—inside the wound. The laceration will still heal, but without stitches, the scar will be obvious and possibly unsightly.

There are times when, despite the discomfort, your child is not that urgently ill. While she may need a doctor, if it's three in the morning, you can wait until the sun comes up before going out in search of medical help. As long as your child receives treatment in twenty-four hours, things should be fine. For instance, even a terribly painful ear infection will hold until morning. "Just give your little one some Tylenol and she'll probably sleep through the night." says Kaufman. In general, the same holds true for sore throats, ordinary stomachaches, and the flu.

In attempting to determine whether a visit to the emergency department is appropriate, many parents consult their pediatrician first. If you know for sure the situation isn't life-threatening, this is a good idea. If your child has a fever, or just doesn't look right, your doctor can often assuage your fears. If the situation warrants, your doctor can call the ED, alerting the staff that you are on your way.

However if your child appears so ill that you are frightened for her life, if you have the sense something dangerous is afoot, get to the emergency department first. Your pediatrician, after all, is not operating an ED, but is a doctor in an office, and like the internist or urologist, can sometimes be hard to reach. Waiting for your pediatrician to call you back, trekking down to a doctor's office for evaluation, and waiting for an assistant to send you through to the doctor may eat up minutes and even hours of vital time. Besides, he might not have the X-ray machine or suturing materials and tools your child's case demands. While the triage nurse in the emergency department is schooled in recognizing dire medical problems in children (especially if it is a pediatric ED), the receptionist manning the phones and desks in the pediatrician's office usually is not. Speak with a sampling of parents, and you'll hear all too many tales of the time the pediatrician's receptionist wrote them off as pests unwilling to wait their turn, when, in fact, their children were desperately ill. In the event of a bona fide emergency—if your son has fallen out of a window, say, or if your daughter's not breathing—viewing your pediatrician as the gateway to the emergency department can be a costly mistake. Take your child to the emergency department *first,* and then, by all means, call your pediatrician. When time is of the essence, the ED will be there for you.

EMERGENCY THROUGH THE AGES

Neonatal Emergencies

These days, with mothers and newborn babies regularly released from hospital maternity wards in as little as twelve or twenty-four hours, babies are not observed as thoroughly by professionals for as long a period of time as they were in the past. That's why the neonate—the newborn infant less than two weeks old—has a higher chance than ever of showing up in the pediatric emergency department.

Of course, babies born prematurely will be kept in the hospital for close observation. But healthy, full-term infants may develop problems that require immediate medical intervention. While in the past these babies were routinely treated in the hospital for a few days, today's new parents must be on the lookout for symptoms themselves.

If you notice any of the following problems in your neonate, get to hospital emergency at once:

· Hard, swollen abdominal area, sometimes accompanied by vomiting or absence of bowel movements for a day or two. The problem is probably constipation, but it could also signal a serious intestinal problem.

· Blue-tinged skin that persists over time. The baby might not be getting enough oxygen, and requires immediate medical attention.

· Persistent coughing or choking whenever the infant is fed, which could indicate a problem with the lungs or digestive tract.

· Yellowish cast to the skin, indicative of the condition known as jaundice. In jaundiced babies the blood contains too much bilirubin, formed as red blood cells break down. If the bilirubin level becomes very high, the nervous system may be damaged. After a blood test to determine bilirubin level, the infant may be placed under flourescent lights for a day or two until the liver is able to handle the bilirubin load.

· Unusual lethargy. All newborns sleep most of the time. Still, a newborn baby should have periods of alertness and should wake up on her own to eat. If she does not she could be sick and must be seen immediately at the emergency department.

· Pus, red skin, or pain associated with the area around the naval might signal infection where the umbilical cord was severed. This condition must be treated at once.

· Respiratory distress in a newborn must be treated in the ED immediately. In the neonate, signs of respiratory distress include rapid breathing (more than sixty breaths in a minute), flared nostrils, grunts, bluish skin, and a behavior called "retraction," in which the baby sucks in muscles so that ribs protrude with each and every breath.

On the Home Front

For young children, life-threatening emergencies can stem from preventable injuries around the home or in the community. The worst problems, according to emergency room physicians, emerge when:

· Small parts from toys for older children are left around the house, where they are swallowed by younger siblings.

· Children don't wear seat belts or ride in infant car seats.

· Children don't wear bicycle or roller-skating helmets.

· Parents strike out at children.

· Children are burned by stoves, cigarettes, steaming cups of coffee, boiling water, or other household hot spots.

· Poisons around the house are not locked up.

· Electrical appliances are left plugged in, particularly in dangerous places like the bathroom, where there's plenty of water around. One four-year-old girl was tragically killed recently when she grabbed her mother's hair dryer, turned it on, and took it in the bath with her. Her three-year-old brother, also in the tub, was critically injured as well.

Children in Trouble: Signs of Sexual Abuse

Recognizing child abuse can be one of life's most upsetting realizations. Unfortunately, it is a skill that the staff of a large emergency department may utilize every day. When it comes to physical abuse, excessive or unusually placed bruises and wounds are often telltale signs. However, detecting sexual abuse requires a finer, more astute eye.

No matter how protective a parent you are, it may sometimes be difficult to know whether your child has been subjected to sexual abuse. If you suspect sexual abuse, the best thing you can do is take your child to the emergency department. You may also wish to review our list of indicators. If you notice any two physical indicators, or several of the other indicators, take action at once.

Physical Indicators of Possible Sexual Abuse in Children

Difficulty walking or sitting

Torn, stained, or bloody underclothing

Genital or anal itching, pain, swelling, or burning

Genital or anal bruises or bleeding

Frequent urinary tract or vaginal yeast infections

Pain on urination

Vaginal or penile discharge

Poor sphincter control

Venereal disease

Pregnancy

Chronic unexplained sore throats

Frequent psychosomatic illnesses

Behavioral Indicators of Possible Sexual Abuse in Children

Sudden change in school grades

Destructive to self and/or others

Extremes in behavior, such as aggressivity or withdrawal

Poor social relations

Refuses to change for gym

Behaves seductively and has sexual knowledge beyond age

Sexually acts out or attempts to force other children to be sexual

Regressive behavior

Complains of soreness or moves or sits awkwardly

Wears clothing that covers the body when not appropriate

Depressed, apathetic, or suicidal

Adult Perpetrator Indicators

Possessive or jealous of child

Accuses child of promiscuity

Socially isolates child

Believes child desires sexual contact

Confuses sex and affection

Poor relationship with spouse

May have history of being an abused child

May be in an abusive relationship with another adult

Drug or alcohol abuser

Please remember that none of these signs alone or in combination are *always* signs of childhood sexual abuse. Nonetheless, you must err on the side of caution. If you have *any* concerns, seek the help of your pediatrician or emergency physician early.

Adolescent Emergencies

Emergencies afflicting teenagers are often in a class unto themselves. Physically, doctors treat teenagers much like adults. They require the same equipment, for instance, from IVs to endotracheal tubes. And the dosage for various medicines depends upon the teenager's size and weight which is generally comparable to that of an adult.

Yet certain medical emergencies do strike the preteen and teen population with greater frequency. Be on the lookout for the following.

Severe scrotal or testicular pain in preteen and teenage boys: These children may be suffering a condition known as testicular torsion, in which a testicle has become twisted. Emergency physicians are well trained in the technique of recognizing this very painful and significant problem, in which blood supply to the testicle is literally cut off. If not treated within twelve to twenty-four hours, the testicle will die.

Delusional or psychotic behavior: True psychoses such as schizophrenia rarely manifest in teenage years. These mental illnesses are more likely to rear their ugly heads in the early twenties. However, virtually identical symptoms, including visual and auditory hallucinations, incoherence, and violence to self or others, may signal drug abuse. Get your teenager to the emergency department at once if such psychotic symptoms are exhibited.

Suicidal behavior: Persistent withdrawal and unhappiness with life, leading to talk of suicide and an actual suicide attempt warrants emergency department help.

Sports injuries: Breaks, sprains, cuts and bruises may be more likely in the teen years. Often more active and more physically competitive than at any other time of their lives, teenagers may also tend to take fewer precautions, such as wearing bicycle helmets.

Eating disorders: Adolescents are particularly prey to anorexia (refusal to eat for fear of gaining weight, resulting in drastic weight loss) and bulimia (in which the individual induces vomiting after a meal). If undiagnosed and untreated, the teenager may suddenly become so sick that vital signs are threatened, resulting in a trip to the emergency department.

In the Pediatric Emergency Department: What to Expect When You Arrive

Entering the pediatric ED, you'll find a scene quite different from the one you may remember as a child yourself. Back then, children went to what was called the emergency *room* under suspicion of a burst appendix or broken leg; when they had suffered some obviously terrible injury and were bleeding profusely; when they had been cut by a razor and needed stitches; when they lost consciousness; or when they screamed in excruciating pain. In other words, they went to emergency under dire circumstances, indeed.

Today, on the other hand, many parents, disenfranchised from the medical system and lacking primary-care physicians or pediatricians, take children to the emergency department for basic care. As a result, you may see a waiting room filled with sore throats, ear infections, and run-of-the-mill bruises and bumps. In the hustle and bustle of the pediatric ED waiting room, it's easy to forget that the original purpose of the facility was to treat the urgently injured and ill, not those with tummy aches and colds. Of course, for those without the means to secure a personal doctor, the emergency department is the safety net—for some of these children, the only medical safety net our society provides. With nowhere else to turn, these children are, of course, part of the ED's accepted clientele.

But for those with true emergencies, this new trend can extend the waiting time beyond the comfort zone and make it just a bit more likely to get lost in the shuffle. In one rural area, for instance, a mother reports that she took her four-month-old son to the hospital with blood in his stool—a sign of a significant problem in anyone, especially one so young. The mother waited two hours as the bleeding got worse, and still, no doctor saw her child. Finally the mother stood up in the middle of the waiting room and screamed for help. A doctor rushed out, took one look at the baby, and sent him up to surgery immediately.

Generally, it doesn't come down to this. If the hospital's triage nurse is top-notch, she will recognize such serious problems and send the patient through. As a parent or caretaker, therefore, it behooves you to understand what the triage nurse does when dealing with children. In this way, you will have a better understanding of when it is appropriate to ask that you be seen sooner, and when it is appropriate for you to wait your turn and hold your peace.

"At St. Luke's–Roosevelt," Dr. Kaufman explains, "the triage nurse will ask the parent and child questions, look at the child, take vital stats like blood pressure and temperature, and finally assess that child as to urgency. There are three basic categories that determine when the child is seen."

In the most serious category—the "emergent" cases—children are considered at risk for immediate damage or death, and they are seen at once. These true emergencies include children experiencing problems with their ABC's—the airway, breathing, and circulation; children with asthma; children who may have heart problems; children with such signs of internal bleeding as black diarrhea; those who have lost consciousness; and those with such severe pain that they may have appendicitis or other problems requiring aggressive intervention at once.

The next step down—the "urgent" cases—must be seen within twenty to thirty minutes, Kaufman says. These seriously ill children may be suffering from any number of problems, including gastrointestinal trouble, apparently broken bones, or severe lacerations.

The third category, which Kaufman calls "routine," includes those children who have run-of-the-mill childhood illnesses and injuries, from ordinary scrapes and bruises to fever and ear infections. Notes Kaufman: "In the ED these routine cases will have to wait their turn. They will be seen after emergent and urgent patients, in the order in which they arrive. Depending on which ED you go to, the wait could be twenty minutes or longer."

In short, when you go to the emergency department with an asthmatic child who can't breathe, expect to be seen promptly so that treatment can begin at once. If your child has an ear infection and a fever of 103, even if the child is in pain, you may have to wait until those who are more seriously ill are seen.

When the doctor sees your child, she will ask questions and perform an exam. Depending upon the circumstances she may also order blood tests, urine analyses, and X rays, much as the doctor would do in the adult ED. After all questions are answered and all tests results and X rays have been received, the doctor will render a diagnosis, and treatment will begin.

Often, you'll find treatment meets your expectations, with procedures resembling those you've seen at the pediatrician's office or the emergency department for adults. Occasionally, however, your child will require techniques for which you are unprepared. For instance, children, like adults, must sometimes be sedated—especially when pain causes the child to cry, scream, or move so violently that treatment is otherwise impossible. Setting a badly broken leg, for instance, can be excruciatingly painful. Intravenous delivery of Demerol and Valium, however, can reduce pain, anxiety, and even the memory of the procedure itself.

Likewise, children who cannot stay still may have to be restrained with what doctors call a papoose board; in essense, the child is wrapped up like a mummy so the doctor can apply sutures, dress a wound, or examine a painful area as skillfully as possible.

You may sometimes also find your child's problem is due to an object or pieces of food stuck in the nose or ears. One child in the St. Luke's emergency department was brought in because a foul-smelling substance was oozing out of his nose. Looking inside, Dr. Kaufman found the culprit: a pickle from a Big Mac; she was able to remove it with forceps. She also used a small suction catheter, in another child, to penetrate the nasal cavity and vacuum out a black-eyed pea.

How to Advocate for Your Child

If your child has a routine problem, it will do little good to demand he be seen right away. This is the emergency department, after all, and, in accordance with rules of triage, the sickest go first. Accept the fact that you will have to wait your turn. And expect to be treated caringly and conscientiously when your turn comes.

But, if, like the mother whose baby had black diarrhea, you are convinced he may be in danger, by all means, speak up. We do not, of course, advise that you stand in the middle of the ED and scream. In most cases a pointed question or statement to the triage nurse will be all the prodding needed.

Ask the nurse to explain why your child has been put "on hold." Perhaps she has a good explanation: Even though the laceration will need stitches, she may inform you, waiting a few minutes will not affect the result. Even though your child has scarlet fever, you may be told, the antibiotic regimen he will undoubtedly be given will work just the same if he starts an hour later.

On the other hand, perhaps your questions will prompt the nurse to reassess your case. Does he realize the baby is vomiting blood? Does he know that your child's fever has soared since you arrived just twenty minutes ago? Or that her heart has begun to beat very fast? You know this child and the triage nurse doesn't. To you she seems to be fading in and out of consciousness, and she's not alert.

Most of the time, if your child does need aggressive treatment, your firm but polite questions will do the trick. If the triage nurse has been overwhelmed with the sheer volume of children arriving just when you did, if your child's condition has worsened or changed, your questions will make that clear.

As you move through the emergency department from triage, to the inner waiting room, to the doctor's care, make sure you communicate with the nursing staff and ask questions every step of the way. Ask doctors to explain the reason for each and every test your child will receive. Ask them to explain the reason for their diagnosis and all of the elements of the treatment plan. Ask why your child is being kept for observation, or being released. And by all means, if your child's condition changes, let someone know.

Also make sure you get instructions for follow-up care. And do write them down. If anything is unclear to you, ask the doctor to explain again. Do not be put off if the doctor is abrupt or distracted; he or she may have many responsibilities in the emergency department, and must meet the needs of children who may be gravely ill. Nonetheless, your questions are important to you and will be important to the doctor. If the doctor must go elsewhere, you may want to wait until he returns so instructions are clear.

If at any point you feel that the care has not been adequate, follow advice presented in Chapter 5: Ask to see another doctor in the ED, preferably the attending physician in charge. Ask for a specialist as procedures become more complex or invasive; moreover, do inquire as to the particular doctor's credentials in performing the task. Request a meeting with the patient representative, social worker, or staff member who can serve as liaison between you and the medical staff.

The mother of Miranda Privette, profiled not long ago on the television "news magazine" *20/20,* wishes she had. The Rock Hill, South Carolina, girl, age five, was playing in her yard when her mother noticed something wrong. "She was just like almost turning blue on me," Brenda Privette says, "and she got enough of a breath and told me she had swallowed a sunflower seed."

Brenda did the Heimlich maneuver on Miranda and she started to breathe again, but the seed didn't pop out, so she took Miranda to the closest hospital. The emergency department doctor saw from the X ray that the sunflower seed was still in Miranda's airway, resting on her vocal cords. Even though it wasn't posing an immediate danger, the seed could move and block Miranda's airway again. Something had to be done. So a pulmonologist, who specialized in treatment of the airway, was called. Miranda's parents agreed to let him try and remove the seed, though they didn't realize—didn't even think to ask—that he was an adult pulmonologist and had treated relatively few children. He used an optical tube known as a flexible bronchoscope to peer into Miranda's airway and locate the seed. Then he inserted a "basket retrieval device" through the tube in his effort to grab the sunflower seed and get it out. But though she was sedated, Miranda was agitated, and in her struggle, the seed only moved farther down her airway, almost out of reach.

At this point the pulmonologist withdrew, claiming his instrumentation—and experience—were obviously wrong for the job. Miranda needed a pediatric specialist, he claimed, so the hospital arranged to send the child to another facility for care.

But during the twenty-six-minute ambulance ride to the second hospital, Miranda began having seizures. She went into respiratory arrest and then cardiac arrest, and finally she died. Most experts agree that results would probably have been different had Miranda been treated by a pediatric emergency physician or a pediatric pulmonologist in the first place. Such a specialist would never have inserted something as large and invasive as an adult bronchoscope down the airway of a five-year-old.

As your child's advocate, you have every right to know whether Dr. X has ever performed procedure Y on a child, and whether this procedure is accepted as part of the pediatric armamentarium today. If you have doubts, you also have the right to request consultation with another emergency physician or a specialist. If there is time, and if your child is stable, you may also request that he or she be transferred from a general emergency department seeing mostly adults to a pediatric facility with the special expertise to treat kids if one is available in your neighborhood.

Pediatric specialists can come with a wide array of pedigrees. Depending upon your situation, you might need a pediatric cardiologist, a pediatric neurologist, a pediatric urologist, a pediatric gastroenterologist, or a pediatric intensivist. The ED will call in such experts when needed.

Even when life doesn't hang in the balance, a request for a specialist may be key. For instance, in the case of a laceration on the face, it might be in your best interest to secure a plastic surgeon for your child, even if the emergency physician states he or she can suture quite as well. It's your child, and you and your child should have a choice.

Of course not all situations require a specialist, even if the parent requests one. Kaufman notes that parents frequently request she call an otolaryngologist—an ear, nose, and throat specialist—for simple ear infections. "These specialists simply are not appropriate for that," she says. "If you feel the ear infection requires the scrutiny of an ear, nose, and throat specialist, you will have to make an appointment to go to his office yourself."

In the same way, if your child has had a standard febrile seizure, she really does not need to be seen by a pediatric neurologist. If it is three in the morning, it is doubtful that the pediatric neurologist on call will get out of bed to see your child, even if requested to. On the other hand, if your child is in seizure or fading in and out of consciousness as the result of a head injury, the pediatric neurologist on call will probably come down to the emergency department in a flash, no matter what the time. Likewise, if your child has suffered a laceration on her knee and requires a single stitch, you probably will not need to drag the plastic surgeon out of bed in the middle of the night. The emergency physician can certainly suture that wound with all the competence you'll need.

Although you are your child's greatest advocate, the stress of the situation can sometimes cause you to overreact. In fact, there are times when, due to your own high anxiety, your presence may hinder your child's treatment. And in that case, doctors recommend that it's best for you to leave the room; they may ask you to do so in your child's best interest.

In one recent case, for instance, a five-year-old girl was brought in with electrical burns on her hand, caused when she tried to plug Christmas lights into a socket. The burns were so severe that her hand had broken out in white blisters and the doctors suspected possible nerve damage. In the worst-case scenario, the hand might have to be amputated.

To help the girl make the best possible recovery, doctors determined they would have to perform neurological tests and call in a surgeon to remove the dead skin from the hand. Before that could be done, however, the child would have to fall asleep. Doctors had already begun delivering an anesthetic and sedative to the child intravenously, but her parents, attempting to calm her fears, would not stop talking. The result: The girl could not fall asleep and treatment could not begin.

Finally, knowing that the parents were trying to be helpful and had no desire to hinder their daughter's care, the ED doctor asked the parents to step outside the room. Afterward, even the parents admitted their own anxiety had initially prevented their child from getting the care she so desperately needed.

Dr. Kaufman points out that another procedure—the spinal tap—while more routine, can cause high parental anxiety as well. Because the procedure is so delicate—a needle is inserted directly into the spinal canal—physicians may also feel more comfortable without the eagle eye of a parent watching and questioning their every move. Removing the stress of such scrutiny, she adds, can contribute to the doctor's success. "If I need to do a spinal tap on your child and I don't feel comfortable having you in the room," she states, "chances are high that I'm not going to perform as well if you're there. It may not be in your child's best interest for you to demand to stay."

A mother herself, Kaufman is deeply sensitive to parents' anxiety: The procedure can be so upsetting to parents, she explains, she has had a few try to grab the spinal needle directly out of her hands.

You can be a tremendous support to your child in the emergency department. Usually, you will be more effective in that role than anyone else. However, sometimes your anxiety can get in the way of effective care. This is particularly true in serious cases, when delicate or complex procedures take all the focus a physician can muster.

"In general, children derive comfort from their parents. And in general, parents should advocate for participation," Kaufman concludes. "But on rare occasions, it's better if parents leave: If it's a question of life and death and seconds count; if the sight of blood makes you faint or if you get hysterical; if your child is well behaved with others but as soon as you enter the room ten people have to hold him down; if your *vibes* tell you things would go better were you to leave."

When you leave the room, do not feel guilty. You love your child and are acting in his or her best interest. Your only desire is to facilitate treatment and recovery as best you can. Before you leave, get agreement that the emergency physician will contact you in the waiting room as soon as it is appropriate.

Finally, before you leave the emergency department, it would be in your child's best interest to request that the ED doctor call your private pediatrician to fill her in on what occurred. In that way you keep the lines of medical communication open, and ensure your child will receive the best possible care after returning home.

A Guide to Serious Illnesses and Symptoms Treated in the Pediatric Emergency Department

Problem: Asthma

Symptoms: Persistent cough, labored breathing, feeling of suffocation, wheezing, and blueness around the lips if wheezing is severe.

Pediatric considerations: 5–10 percent of children reportedly have asthma. This sometimes inherited condition can be activated at any age, but for the majority of young children, the first attack is provoked after exposure to inhaled irritants.

Treatment in the ED: Children are given aerosol medications. These bronchodilators, delivered as mist through a nebulizer, serve to open the bronchial tubes. If the asthma is severe, patients also receive steroid medicine.

Follow-up at home: Faithfully administer medicine prescribed by your pediatrician or the emergency physician at the hospital. A humidifier may help as well.

Problem: Bronchiolitis

Symptoms: Wheezing and difficulty breathing. Frequently follows upper-respiratory-tract infections. May start with cold symptoms, including nasal congestion and runny nose, and then progress to coughing and wheezing. Other signs include rapid, labored breathing, nasal flaring, irritability, and sleeplessness.

Pediatric considerations: This condition generally appears in babies less than a year old. Far more common in fall or winter, it is caused by a viral infection in the small lower airways called the bronchioles, which are especially tiny in babies. This is the third-leading cause of death in children between two and twelve months of age, and occurs more in those born prematurely. Children with chronic problems like heart disease are at greater risk for complications.

Treatment in the ED: Part of the treatment includes reducing the symptoms and, like asthma, involves delivery of aerosol bronchodilators. Treatment may also include special antiviral medications or supplemental oxygen. In the worst cases children will be hospitalized, but most of the time they can be sent home.

Follow-up at home: Expect bronchiolitis to get worse for three or four days before it starts to improve. As with asthma, humidified air will help. Call the doctor or return to the emergency department if, after treatment has begun, the child continues to have problems breathing or eating, or if you notice a sucking in of the flesh between the ribs with breathing.

Problem: Croup

Symptoms: Wheezing and croaking cough, labored breathing, blue or grayish cast to the skin.

Pediatric considerations: Generally a disease of childhood, croup occurs when already-narrow air passages become inflamed and filled with mucus. Problems that may lead to croup include bronchitis, laryngitis, and the common cold. The illness most often appears in winter or early spring, and may begin or get worse at night.

Treatment in the ED: Doctors will generally treat these children with humidified air to ease breathing. If the symptoms are not severe, the child will be released. But if the child is very ill, physicians will treat with special medicine, including steroids, aerosilized racemic epinephrine, or vaponephrin, and admit to the hospital.

Follow-up at home: The child with croup must rest and receive humidified air. If the child still exhibits noisy cough, lack of appetite, or other symptoms despite this intervention, he must be taken back to the doctor or emergency department.

Problem: Epiglottitis (infection of the epiglottis, the flap that closes over the windpipe)

Symptoms: Sore throat, fever, and, because of the inability to swallow, noisy and labored breathing, drooling, and inability to talk.

Pediatric considerations: In this deadly form of sore throat, most victims are children between the ages of six months and six years. Children can die if the throat becomes so swollen that breathing is impeded.

Treatment in the ED: To confirm the diagnosis, the emergency physician may order an X ray of the neck or send your child to intensive care, where the airway may be examined under general anesthetic through a procedure known as laryngoscopy. Doctors will pass a tube into the windpipe to view the obstruction and make a diagnosis while ensuring that the airway will not close up. Under extreme emergency conditions, doctors may be forced to perform a tracheotomy, making an incision in the neck and temporarily inserting a tube below the blockage to facilitate passage of air until the infection is resolved. Emergency department physicians will also establish an intravenous line to deliver antibiotics. This child will be admitted to the pediatric intensive care unit of the hospital, and will not be sent home until fully recovered.

Problem: Whooping cough

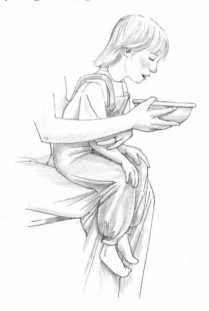

Symptoms: Initially presents as the common cold with accompanying cough. Soon evolves into incessant coughing with a telltale "whoop" as the child struggles to inhale; vomiting and sleeplessness are caused by the coughing.

Pediatric considerations: Because whooping cough causes narrow airways to become clogged with mucus, this bacterial infection is one of the most deadly childhood illnesses. Whooping cough is rare today because of vaccination; it's the *P,* for *pertussis,* in the DPT vaccination you and your child are familiar with. But when the disease occurs, it is especially dangerous in children under twelve months of age. Do remember: Not *all* children are routinely vaccinated. And even when vaccinated, there is still a tiny chance your child might contract the disease.

Treatment in the ED: In the early stages, doctors may prescribe antibiotics. In more acute phases, physicians will hydrate the child via intravenous drip, and deliver oxygen through a mask or nasal cannula, or tube.

Follow-up at home: Care at home includes sitting your child in an upright position, head and neck bent slightly forward. A bowl should be handy so your child can spit up phlegm. After fits of vomiting, provide your child with small quantities of food and drink so that something may stay down. Child must be kept quiet and still, with active play restricted, and parent must sleep in child's room so someone is always there to assist through coughing.

Problem: Pneumonia

Symptoms: Difficulty breathing and dry cough accompanied by pains in the chest area, fever ranging up to about 102 degrees Fahrenheit, vomiting, and diarrhea.

Pediatric considerations: In children, pneumonia is usually caused when upper-respiratory infection from flu or the common cold spreads to the lungs. Children with asthma and cystic fibrosis are particularly at risk.

Treatment in the ED: Treatment varies depending upon whether the child has walking pneumonia or a more severe infection. Most children presenting with walking pneumonia are given a prescription for antibiotics and sent home. Medicine may include penicillin, amoxicillin, or erythromycin, depending upon the particular combination of symptoms. If the child has problems breathing, emergency department physicians may administer supplemental oxygen through nasal cannula or a face mask. A chest X ray will be ordered to check for infection in the lungs. The sickest children will be admitted to the hospital, where intravenous therapy, supplemental oxygen, and close observation are key to recovery.

Follow-up at home: To ease breathing, prop your child up with a pillow; make sure the room has adequate ventilation; provide plenty of fluids. Humidified air may help.

Problem: Diarrhea

Symptoms: Looser-than-normal or watery stools. In more serious cases, may be accompanied by vomiting, fever, and cough. Child cannot hold anything down, and is weak and irritable. In the most serious cases, requiring immediate medical attention, the diarrhea is accompanied by abdominal pain around the navel, by abdominal cramps, by bowel movements filled with blood or mucus, and by signs of dehydration.

Pediatric considerations: In most infants and children, diarrhea is mild and will last just a few days. If prolonged, however, it can be a serious medical problem resulting in dehydration and, eventually, undernutrition. (In Africa, diarrhea is the leading cause of childhood death.)

Treatment in the ED: If the child is dehydrated, emergency doctors will start an IV line to hydrate intravenously and may consider admission to the hospital. If the child is not dehydrated, doctors will send the child home with specific dietary guidelines.

Follow-up at home: Babies should be given an electrolyte solution like Pedialyte. Older children should have clear liquids such as decaf tea and sports drinks like Gatorade as well as bland food, including bananas, rice, applesauce, and toast. (You can remember this as the B-R-A-T diet.)

Problem: Vomiting

Symptoms: The inability to hold down food usually signals a mild viral infection. However, the following accompanying symptoms may signal more serious problems: Pain around the navel and in the right lower portion of the abdomen (might be appendicitis); severe pain along with blood and mucus in the stool (could be a bowel blockage or colitis); or pain when bending the neck along with extreme sensitivity to light (could be meningitis).

Pediatric considerations and treatment in the ED: In most instances doctors will recommend a period of rest and a diet of clear fluids in small, frequent amounts. Because vomiting can sometimes signal a problem beyond the run-of-the-mill stomach virus, physicians will also check for signs of appendicitis, urinary tract infection, pneumonia, and meningitis. If the vomiting is severe, or the child is dehydrated, emergency department doctors will hydrate intravenously and may consider admission to the hospital.

Follow-up at home: Follow dietary advice given in the ED. If the child cannot keep anything down and if there is no cessation of symptoms, return to your personal physician or the emergency department.

Problem: Fever

Symptoms: On a rectal thermometer, fever is considered anything greater than or equal to 100.4 degrees Fahrenheit. (This is equal to 38 degrees centigrade.) When fever is accompanied by rapid or troubled breathing (signaling bronchitis or pneumonia) or neck pain, along with extreme sensitivity to light (could be meningitis), there is an urgent need for medical care.

Pediatric considerations: All feverish infants under three months of age must receive medical evaluation at once, as should all children with temperatures of at least 104 degrees Fahrenheit. Children with temperature less than or equal to 95 degrees Fahrenheit must be urgently evaluated as well, because an abnormally low temperature may be just as serious as one that is too high.

Treatment in the ED: Doctors will perform tests to determine cause of fever and, if a bacterial infection is found, prescribe an antibiotic. If dehydration is a problem, fluids may be replenished intravenously. Child may be given Tylenol to lower the fever.

Follow-up at home: Instructions will depend on the cause of the fever. However, if the fever goes above 104 degrees Fahrenheit and remains there despite interventions like Tylenol, the parent is advised to call the family doctor or the ED for follow-up.

Problem: Meningitis

Symptoms: Stiff neck and headache; lethargy, drowsiness, and confusion; fever; tiny blotches of purple-red rash; vomiting; and, in children under eighteen months, a bulging fontanel (the "soft spot" on the front of the head).

Treatment in the ED: Doctors will confirm the problem with a spinal tap. They will then establish an intravenous line to deliver antibiotics. Your child will probably be admitted to the hospital.

Follow-up at home: While all those with bacterial meningitis will be admitted to the hospital, those with viral meningitis may be sent home. (The spinal tap helps distinguish between the two.) For these children, any change in mental status, including confusion or diminished alertness, necessitates a return trip to the ED. In general, children with viral meningitis may be treated with Tylenol to control pain and fever, and liquids that may be tolerated by mouth.

Problem: Encephalitis (inflammation of the brain)

Symptoms: Headache and neck pain, fever, vomiting, or loss of appetite, and decrease in consciousness ranging from lethargy and drowsiness to confusion, convulsion, and finally, coma.

Pediatric considerations: In children, this terrible but rare illness is most often brought on by common viral infections like chicken pox or the mumps. Sometimes a child may have bacterial encephalitis as well. In babies, encephalitis can be fatal.

Treatment in the ED: Doctors will first perform tests, including spinal tap, to determine the stage of the disease. The child will be admitted to the hospital so support staff can monitor vital signs, and will be treated with a combination of antibiotics for infection (if that infection is bacterial in origin), steroids to reduce brain swelling, Tylenol or other medications to control fever and headache, and, of course, rest.

Problem: Overwhelming allergic reaction, or anaphylaxis

Symptoms: Redness, swelling, and itching; sudden, severe swelling of the lips, tongue, and eyes; wheezing and difficulty breathing; red, blotchy hives; severe generalized itching or rash over the whole body; weakness and shock, all in response to an insect bite, sting, exposure to a substance, or inhalant to which one is allergic. Without rapid treatment, these symptoms may lead to shock, collapse, and death.

Pediatric considerations: While anaphylaxis is deadly in adults as well as children, children have the added onus of surprise. An adult is more likely to have reacted to the stimulus before, perhaps in childhood, and so has learned to avoid it. Children, experiencing their allergy for the first time, however, are prey to violent and surprising reactions.

Treatment in the ED: Physicians will fight the allergic reaction by administering adrenaline and an antihistamine such as Benadryl; if symptoms are severe, administration of the medicine, including powerful steroids, will be intravenously. To combat difficulty breathing, the child may also receive oxygen.

Follow-up at home: If your child has had a severe allergic reaction to a known allergen (a food, insect sting, or plant such as poison ivy), avoid it. Apply ice to insect stings immediately. And, with your doctor's advice, carry a self-injector of epinephrine; also consider getting a medic alert bracelet to notify ambulance and emergency staff of the allergy in the future.

Problem: Seizures, also referred to as convulsions

Symptoms: You may note a phase of rigidity (with breath held) and then a rhythmic jerking of the limbs. At the beginning of the seizure, the child may cry out and urinate or defecate without control, and his eyes may roll backward. After the seizure, the child will often exhibit confusion and drowsiness.

Pediatric considerations: In children, seizures caused by a sudden rise or fall in temperature are common, and do not signal a serious medical problem. However, if the seizure does not stop within a few minutes, or if your child does not regain full alertness, a medical emergency could be in progress. In these situations, or if your child has never had a prior febrile seizure, seek medical help.

Treatment in the ED: If the seizure continues, the child will receive an anticonvulsive drug. If the child is under age two, if the seizure is unrelated to rise or fall in fever, or if the child does not regain alertness following seizure, doctors will perform a spinal tap to test for meningitis. Physicians may also perform a series of blood and urine analyses to test for encephalitis, epilepsy, or diabetes, other possible causes of seizure.

Follow-up at home: If the seizure has been caused by fever, work to bring the fever down by sponging the skin and administering acetaminophen.

Problem: Dehydration

Symptoms: Dehydration often results from high fever, severe diarrhea, or vomiting. Other symptoms include the inability to retain fluids, dry mouth and lips, lethargy, and urine that is dark yellow in color or no urine output at all for twelve to eighteen hours. In children under eighteen months, look for a sunken fontanel (soft spot on the forehead).

Pediatric considerations and treatment in the ED: The dehydrated child will be given essential, replenishing fluids via intravenous drip.

Follow-up at home: Check urine to make sure the deep-yellow color gives way to light yellow or clear. As the illness passes, make sure fluid intake is high and reintroduce solid foods gradually.

Problem: Food Poisoning

Symptoms: Abdominal cramps, fever, weakness, chills, loss of appetite, or vomiting, and loose stools sometimes containing blood, pus, or mucus.

Pediatric considerations: Food poisoning, which results after eating food contaminated with the toxic byproducts of bacteria, can be particularly hard on young children, whose immune systems are not fully developed. Especially in babies, the symptoms of food poisoning can lead to dehydration.

Treatment in the ED: Doctors will replenish body fluids and salts by giving the child an electrolyte solution. If the child is at risk for dehydration, fluids and salts will be administered through an intravenous drip. Doctors may give an antiemetic to prevent vomiting.

Follow-up at home: Keep child cool with a damp cloth. Be attentive to issues of hygiene: Bacteria from some food poisoning can be contagious, so make sure your child washes his hands after using the bathroom. Make sure you wash your hands after changing diapers. Make sure to hydrate your child with plenty of fluids. Reintroduce easily digestible foods such as Jell-O and soup first. Make sure to throw out any food you feel may have caused the food poisoning (frequently dairy products or cream-based foods).

Problem: Ingestion of poisons

Symptoms: Child is unconscious or inexplicably groggy or seemingly drunk.

Pediatric considerations: Children are especially at risk for swallowing medicines, household solvents, and other deleterious substances.

Treatment in the ED: Depending on the poison in question, physicians may pump the child's stomach, give an antidote, or induce vomiting.

Follow-up at home: Go through your house or apartment with a fine-tooth comb so the child never has access to this or any other poisonous substance; discard poisonous substances, cleaning solutions and all medications, or lock them carefully away.

Problem: Reye's syndrome

Symptoms: Fever, uncontrollable vomiting, altered consciousness, including delirium or drowsiness, and finally, coma. The disease, which is essentially a combination of encephalitis and liver problems, often starts as a respiratory infection from which the child seems to recover, only to be stricken days later with high fever, vomiting, and other symptoms associated with full-blown Reye's syndrome.

Pediatric considerations: This childhood illness generally occurs a few days after contracting a viral infection such as influenza or chicken pox. It affects children from two months of age through adolescence, but is most prevalent in the six–eleven age group. While Reye's syndrome can lead to permanent brain damage or death, most children make a full recovery.

Treatment in the ED: Children suspected of having Reye's syndrome are first diagnosed through blood tests and a spinal tap. Sometimes doctors must examine a specimen of liver under the microscope; they remove liver cells for this purpose by inserting a needle through anesthetized skin into the liver. Once diagnosed, children may be intubated for help with breathing and given an IV so they may receive fluid and nourishment in the form of a glucose solution. Children with Reye's syndrome will always be admitted to the hospital, where doctors can monitor vital signs and treat the symptoms.

Problem: Appendicitis

Symptoms: Look for pain that starts near the navel and travels to the lower right quadrant of the abdomen. Look for a fever of about 100 degrees Fahrenheit, loss of appetite, vomiting, diarrhea, or constipation. Appendicitis usually progresses over a twelve- to twenty-four-hour course.

Treatment in the ED: After diagnosing the problem by careful physical examination, X ray, and blood and urine tests, doctors will transfer your child to the operating room for removal of the appendix.

Problem: Cessation of breathing (apnea)

Symptoms: Chest fails to rise and fall for periods greater than twenty seconds. Also look for lack of movement, blue skin color, and pallor.

Pediatric considerations: It is normal for babies to hold their breath for ten seconds or less, especially while dreaming. However, if breathing periodically stops for more than twenty seconds, the condition is considered apnea, and might signal an underlying heart defect or some other serious health problem. If breathing stops for lengthy periods of time, the result might be oxygen deprivation—and brain damage. Babies who suffer from apnea are also at risk for crib death. Look for apnea especially in premature babies born a few months early, or in children suffering colds.

Treatment in the ED: Physicians will insert a tube directly into the airway to ventilate. If the heart has stopped, cardiopulmonary resuscitation (CPR) will be performed. After being stabilized, the child will be admitted to a pediatric intensive care unit, where a mechanical respirator will maintain breathing until it resumes naturally. Expect doctors to test extensively for causes of the apnea.

Follow-up at home: Doctors will provide parents with an apnea monitor, which will sound if breathing stops again. Parents of children at risk for this problem are advised to master the skills of rescue breathing and CPR, specifically as they relate to infants and children, through a certified course.

Problem: Diabetes mellitus

Symptoms: These may vary, but include lowered immunity, irritability, lethargy, weight loss, increased thirst, a fruity smell on the breath, and frequent urination or bedwetting.

Pediatric considerations: There are a number of reasons why a child with diabetes might need an emergency department. The first is that the problem has never been diagnosed. Symptoms, including thirst and the constant desire to urinate, might propel parents to take the child to emergency, and a diagnosis is made. The child with known diabetes might have low blood sugar because prescribed insulin intake has been too high, resulting in dizziness or even coma. The child might have high blood sugar because insulin intake is too low, resulting in the dangerous buildup of toxins in the blood. Or, the child could have a totally separate illness, such as an infection, rendered riskier because diabetes is present as well.

Treatment in the ED: Blood sugar level will be immediately assessed by taking a blood sample by fingerstick. Depending on the situation, the diabetic child might be reassured and sent home, kept in the ED for up to six hours and then released, or sent to intensive care. Any child newly diagnosed with diabetes will be admitted to the hospital so the family can learn how to handle this disease before the child goes home. As for children previously diagnosed—and presumably set up with regular treatment protocols by a diabetes specialist—treatment will depend on the nature and severity of the problem. The child with high blood sugar will usually receive intravenous fluids and more insulin. The child with low blood sugar will be given sugar. The most serious cases will be admitted to the hospital, and the rest will be released.

Follow-up at home: Parents must make sure children follow treatment protocols, including the insulin schedule—established for the treatment of this disease. Careful control of diet, scheduling of regular meals, and programmed exercise and athletic activity are important. The diabetic child who experiences any loss of alertness or loss of consciousness must be taken back to the ED at once.

Problem: Sickle-cell anemia

Symptoms: Fatigue, jaundice, abdominal pain, leg and arm pain, lowered immunity and anemia or low blood count.

Pediatric considerations: Symptoms of this genetic disease are not present at birth, but do manifest within the first six months of life. For those suffering from this condition, low oxygen levels cause red blood cells to become sickle-shape, impeding circulation and causing clotting. As a result, afflicted children experience pain wherever blood vessels are blocked, and are particularly prone to coughs and colds. Children must beware that acute symptoms may emerge if they are particularly active, especially if the weather is cold and damp, and must be protected from common childhood infections, to which they are particularly sensitive, by vaccines and vitamin supplements.

Treatment in the ED: Children with sickle-cell anemia generally go for treatment because of the pain and fever associated with their disease. Pain is often caused when sickle-shape blood cells get trapped in various parts of the body, including the legs, back, lungs, or virtually anywhere else in the body. Very young victims of the disease may also suffer what's known as a splenic sequestration crisis, in which sickling blood cells become trapped in the spleen, causing pallor and very severe anemia. (Older children don't experience this problem.) To deal with the pain of sickle-cell disease, emergency physicians administer IV fluids and pain medication. Those with sickle-cell disease are also especially susceptible to infections. Therefore, children with fever should expect diagnostic blood tests and treatment with antibiotics administered via injection or IV. Depending on the severity of the problem, these children will be admitted to the hospital after treatment in the emergency department, or released.

Follow-up at home: For the pain of sickle-cell disease, parents may give pain medication. If the pain persists, or if a fever develops, the child must return to the emergency department.

Problem: Objects stuck in ears and nose

Symptoms: Smelly, bloody, mucouslike secretions from the ears or nose.

Treatment in the ED: Doctors can usually easily remove such objects with forceps or a small suction catheter that literally vacuums the object out. Sometimes physicians will prescribe antibiotic eardrops or antibiotic medication to combat infection that remains after the object is removed.

Follow-up at home: Once a foreign object is removed it is, of course, gone. But parents are advised not to panic if they see some bleeding from the nose for a couple of days after the object has been removed. Try to prevent the child from doing the same thing again by carefully checking toys for parts small enough to fit through a toilet-paper roll; remove these toys, as well as similar size household objects.

Problem: Large open wounds or lacerations

Symptoms: A wound is serious enough to require immediate medical attention if it is gaping or very deep and bloody; if it is contaminated with dirt or a foreign body that cannot be easily removed; if bleeding continues after you have put pressure on the area for ten minutes; if it is on the face or hands; or if it takes the form of a small, deep, puncture wound.

Pediatric considerations: Parents should take the child's vaccination card to the emergency department if they possibly can. Doctors will then be able to easily determine whether or not a child needs a tetanus booster.

Treatment in the ED: Physicians will clean the wound and, if necessary, suture it under local anesthesia. Expect sutures if the wound is particularly large, or if it is on the face or hands. Doctors will work to stop bleeding by applying pressure and, if they are unable to do so, will search for a lacerated blood vessel which they will tie off, again under anesthesia. If a wound is deep or particularly dirty, and if the child has not received a tetanus shot within the last five years, a booster will be given at this time. If the wound is infected, physicians may apply a topical antibiotic or prescribe antibiotic by mouth. Finally, the doctor will protect the wound area with a sterile gauze dressing to keep out infection and dirt. Children who are very young or particularly active may have to be restrained or sedated so doctors can suture the wound quickly, cleanly, and with careful technique for a good healing result.

Follow-up at home: Parents will be asked to keep the wound clean and dry for forty-eight hours. They will also be asked to change the dressing as frequently as necessary to keep it clean. They will be asked to scout for signs of infection, including pus or redness extending from the wound, pain, or fever.

Problem: Breaks and sprains

Symptoms: Both breaks and sprains are accompanied by pain, swelling, and bruising around the injured area, and by an inability to move the injured area without pain. Breaks are sometimes accompanied by deformity at the injured site.

Pediatric considerations: The bones of children are particularly flexible and do not break as easily as the harder, more brittle bones of adults. In children, therefore, one often sees fractures in which the bone bends instead of breaks. Moreover, since the ligaments in young children are generally stronger than the bones, you do not usually see serious sprains, which tend to appear mostly in adolescence and beyond. Children's bones usually break more easily at the growth plate (epiphysis), which is present until growth stops at about age eighteen.

Treatment in the ED: If a break or fracture is suspected, doctors will take an X ray. If bones are uninjured, and if doctors subsequently diagnose a bad bruise or stretched ligament, they will wrap the damaged area firmly with a bandage. If a break is found, treatment depends on the extent and location of the damage. For a simple break or fracture, doctors will usually immobilize the bone with a cast.

Follow-up at home: Keep the injured area dry and elevated, and apply ice. Make sure the child keeps off the leg if instructed to do so. If there's a lot of pain and throbbing, or if your child has been diagnosed with a fracture or a serious sprain, see an orthopedist.

Problem: Head injury

Symptoms: Headache and irritability, alterations in mental status, including drowsiness or loss of consciousness, vomiting, and clear or bloody discharge from nose or ears.

Pediatric considerations: It's basic physiology: A child's head is much larger in proportion to the rest of the body than that of an adult. Therefore, anytime there's an accident or fall, it's more likely that the child's head will be injured from the blow. Do be on the lookout. There are other disadvantages for children as well: Their cranial bones are thinner and blood vessels in the skull more fragile. Thus, head injuries are more likely to send their brains banging against the inner skull, tearing blood vessels and causing bleeding in the process. But children's physiology also confers an advantage: Because the young skull is more flexible, it can better tolerate pressure from swelling, thus reducing the mortality rate. For very small infants under three months of age, head injury can also result in shock.

Treatment in the ED: Doctors may get a CAT scan to determine whether the brain is injured. They will suture lacerations under local anesthetic, if required. And, if your child continues to present changes in consciousness, including dizziness or confusion, he or she may be admitted to the hospital for observation.

Follow-up at home: While those with severe head injuries are admitted to the hospital, children with less serious injuries must still be watched closely at home for twenty-four hours after the accident. Caregivers will be asked to wake the child during the night to check on consciousness, and will be instructed to return to the emergency department in the event of vomiting, severe headache, seizure, loss of balance, weakness, numbness, or change in mental status.

Problem: Burns

Symptoms: Red, raw skin, blisters filled with fluid, and, in the case of electrical burns, blackened regions near the point of contact.

Pediatric considerations: Toddlers may inflict burn injuries by spilling boiling water or playing with electric cords. Preschoolers are more likely than older children to suffer burns playing with matches. And sadly, experts say that some 30 percent of all childhood burns result from child abuse. Whatever the cause, burn injuries can be particularly serious for children because they have more skin in proportion to total body volume than do adults. As a result they are more likely to suffer fluid loss—and more likely to suffer metabolic stress, placing every vital organ in danger. Also remember that in children, as in adults, burns may create unsightly, lifelong scars.

Treatment in the ED: The doctor will evaluate the extent, depth, and type of the burn, and treat the child accordingly. Procedures may include checking for other injuries; washing and wrapping the burn; starting an IV line so fluids can be replaced intravenously. A tetanus booster will be given if immunizations are not up to date. The antibiotic ointment Silvadene may be applied. If burns are extensive the child may be transferred to a special burn center or admitted to the local hospital for observation and treatment.

Follow-up at home: Parents must change dressings and apply ointment precisely as instructed. If there's any sign of infection—spreading redness, pus, or fever—parents should contact a pediatrician or return to the emergency department.

Problem: Eye trauma or injury

Symptoms: An obvious blow to the eye; surrounding area that is swollen or bruised; inability or reluctance to open the eye; tearing; pain and irritation; redness; a foreign body visible inside the eye.

Pediatric considerations: Children with eye injuries must be watched carefully so they do not touch the injured area.

Treatment: Physicians will check for the common corneal abrasion—a scratch on the cornea. Treatment for a corneal abrasion includes antibiotic medicine inside the eye lids and, sometimes, the placement of an eye patch, which holds the torn cornea together and keeps the eye still so it may heal. Referral to an ophthalmologist for follow-up care is standard.

Follow-up at home: Parents must stay on the lookout for a change in the size of the pupil, a change in vision, facial swelling, or signs of infection. If the injury is just a bruise—a black eye with no internal bleeding—treatment will consist of cold compresses for twenty-four hours. Expect the area to remain black-and-blue for one or two weeks.

Chapter 8

Female Medicine: Women in the Emergency Department

Mention emergency medicine, and the *first* thing people are apt to do is bring up the hit television show *ER*. In 1995, the most grueling episode featured a pregnant woman who died center stage, in the show's large, old-fashioned Chicago emergency room. The patient, one Jodi O'Brien, was a good-humored pregnant mom-to-be brought into the emergency room with what appeared to be a relatively benign bladder infection. But seconds after her release she collapsed in the parking lot. Her panicked husband brought her back in for an hour of medical mayhem that had pregnant women across the United States vowing they would never set foot in a hospital again.

If you've seen this episode, you can heave a sigh of relief. The good news is that this story line, in the truest sense of the word, was just a TV fiction. In fact, according to Dr. Amos Grunebaum, director of maternal fetal medicine at St. Luke's–Roosevelt Hospital, the scenario would be impossible to imagine in any real emergency department in America today.

"In all my years of practice, I've never heard of any doctor using some of those exotic techniques *anywhere,* especially in an ED," states Grunebaum. "In medical school my professors used to say it would take more than one or two mistakes to kill a patient, and in this show the doctor committed about ten unforgivable sins."

Talk about overkill: Dr. Mark Green, the show's reputed top-dog resident, first mistook preeclampsia (a life-threatening complication of pregnancy) for a simple urinary tract infection. He also failed to notice, on an ultrasound scan, a second life-threatening condition known as abruptio placenta, the premature separation of a normally implanted placenta from the uterine wall. It's not likely that a real-world emergency physician board certified in emergency medicine would miss these presenting problems. But the truth of the matter is that a real-world Jodi O'Brien would probably never wind up in the emergency department to begin with. Pregnant women who show up at the ED, hours or even minutes away from delivery, are, as a matter of course, sent "upstairs" to the delivery suite. The impetus to get such patients up there fast is even greater in the face of complications. This is the etched-in-stone protocol in American hospitals today.

But not on the show *ER*. Instead, taking a walk on the wild side, TV's Dr. Green merely called the labor-and-delivery department to request they send someone down (they never did), and decided, while waiting, to treat O'Brien himself. First he gave his patient a labor-inducing drug called Pitocin (doctors and nurses call it "pit"), something never done in the ED. When the baby's shoulder got stuck in the middle of delivery, he used forceps. "Because the baby did not have a detectable heartbeat," says Grunebaum, "this procedure would be considered so risky that only the most experienced and well-trained obstetrician would attempt it even up in labor and delivery."

Finally, when forceps delivery failed, Dr. Green performed a maneuver so life-threatening that Grunebaum says "it has never been attempted anywhere in New York State to my knowledge, nor by any obstetrician, anywhere, that I have ever known." In essence, Green decided to push the baby back into the uterus and then do a cesarean. "This is very frightening, because it could *kill* the pregnant woman, thus violating a basic tenet of obstetrics: Never threaten the mother's life to save the baby," Grunebaum states. "As a result of the C-section and her undiagnosed preeclampsia, characterized by high blood pressure, the mother developed a deadly condition called DIC [disseminated intravascular coagulation], where the blood suddenly thins. In other words, her blood lost the ability to clot, and she subsequently bled to death."

Well, we can thank our lucky stars that Dr. Mark Green practices only in TV land, where he returns to exploits of heroism week after week—and that the physicians in real emergency departments across the country have *not* been trained by the technical experts who devised Green's daredevil killer "cures."

In fact, for women with medical emergencies ranging from bleeding during pregnancy, to severe urinary tract infection, to rape, there's probably no place better equipped to deliver appropriate lifesaving care than the emergency department of a large metropolitan hospital. At St. Luke's–Roosevelt Hospital and most other modern EDs, treatment of women's health problems has grown continually more sophisticated, reflecting the "consciousness raising" of the women's movement itself. From private, well-equipped rooms devoted exclusively to women's care, to specially trained advocates for victims of rape and domestic violence, emergency departments across the country have begun to respond to the need for specialized, rapid delivery of treatment for the emergencies that afflict women in crisis.

Blood Simple: Recognizing Female Emergency

For the lay person, gynecological emergencies, even deadly ones, may be difficult to detect. Nonetheless, some conditions in this class are so dangerous that if not treated immediately, the outcome can be lethal. Because normal female conditions and functions like menstruation, pregnancy, and menopause are often associated with pain and discomfort, it is sometimes easy to dismiss symptoms that, in fact, require medical treatment at once. To help women recognize true emergencies and urgencies, we provide some guidelines.

First and foremost, pregnant or not, women should be alert to two potentially deadly signs: profuse vaginal bleeding and excruciating lower abdominal pain. Any time a woman experiences profuse, sudden, unexplained vaginal bleeding with or without pain, or excruciating pain with or without bleeding, she is in a potentially life-threatening situation requiring immediate medical attention. Given these symptoms, a woman should *not* first touch base with her private gynecologist, nor should she wait an hour or two to see "if it goes away."

Instead, instructions are clear: Call Emergency Medical Service or take a cab to the emergency department immediately. Severe pain or bleeding can signal a multitude of gynecological and obstetrical dangers, including miscarriage, infection, or a twisted ovarian cyst, to name a few. Lower abdominal pain, especially if it is localized in the area above the pubic bone, may indicate the potentially lethal conditions of pelvic inflammatory disease or ectopic pregnancy—in which the developing embryo implants outside the uterus, in the fallopian tube.

Women, whether knowingly pregnant or not, should also be on the lookout for this triad of symptoms: At least one missed period; vaginal spotting with small amounts of blood; and pain below the belly button. The problem could be ectopic pregnancy, currently one of the top three causes of maternal mortality. Most at risk are those who have had previous ectopic pregnancies, those who have used intrauterine birth control devices, and those who have had scarring of the fallopian tubes due to infection or inflammation. If diagnosis and treatment occur early, before the fallopian tube bursts, the woman will have a greater chance of surviving to have normal pregnancies in the future. After symptoms of ectopic pregnancy have been noted, a woman should visit the emergency department at once. The fallopian tube can burst at any time, threatening the woman's life as well as her future fertility.

Finally, you don't have to be pregnant to have an infection. In the case of urinary tract infection, symptoms will include a burning, pressured sensation in the bladder. Whenever a woman feels the constant need to urinate, whether she really has to or not, she may have a urinary tract infection. These infections may seem mild but they move very fast if not treated with antibiotics; a simple urinary tract infection could become a debilitating kidney infection. Research now shows that women spending just two days on a double dose of the antibiotic Bactrim (only four doses) can be completely cured; the same women, untreated, might see the infection spread to the kidneys, creating the potential for kidney problems for life. If symptoms of urinary tract infection are combined with a fever of 100.4 degrees Fahrenheit or more, the chance of developing kidney infection is greater still.

Another sign of infection is vaginal discharge *not* associated with menstruation. Obvious in the form of a small amount of brown, watery fluid or pus that stains the underwear, this discharge may indicate the presence of one of a wide range of vaginal infections or, in some instances, a vaginal injury or mass. These presenting problems require immediate attention. If the woman is not able to see her personal gynecologist within twenty-four hours, she is advised to go to the ED.

The Morning After

Pregnant or not, there are times when women may need to go to the emergency department or their gynecologist following sex. Sometimes they learn, after the fact, that their partner has had some form of venereal disease—often, one that can be treated with an antibiotic in advance, prophylactically, before symptoms set in. After learning that a sex partner has syphilis or gonorrhea, immediate treatment with an injection of penicillin will head off problems before they begin.

Women who do not wish to become pregnant may nevertheless have intercourse with birth control devices that malfunction, or without birth control at all. Where else can they go on a Sunday or before arriving at work the next day for the morning-after pill Ovral, a simple birth control pill that prevents pregnancy before it even begins? As a last resort, to their local emergency department. Sex may also result in a hemorrhage, sometimes one so severe that it may be life-threatening. Again, destination of choice is the ED.

The Perils of Pregnancy

While pregnant women should always be alarmed by profuse bleeding, intense abdominal pain, and other general gynecological problems, they must also be alert to emergencies unique to pregnancy alone. If pregnant women note any of the symptoms described below, they are urged to go to the emergency department at once. Waiting an hour or two, until a phone call placed to a personal gynecologist is returned, or until the problem fades, may mean death for the fetus or the woman herself.

If a pregnant woman notes these signs, her life may be in danger:

· Sudden bleeding from parts of the body other than the vagina, such as the mouth and the nose. Whether such bleeding starts during toothbrushing or as the result of a sneeze, the bleeder could have the clotting disorder called disseminated intravascular coagulation, or DIC. Since the end result could be death by bleeding, get to the emergency department.

· Severe headache, blurred vision, breathlessness, nausea, or pain in the upper right quadrant of the abdomen. These symptoms, either one at a time or all together, may signal the potentially life-threatening condition of pregnancy known as preeclampsia. The disorder is characterized by high blood pressure; edema, or swelling caused by fluid retention; and high concentrations of protein in the urine, a sign that kidneys are beginning to malfunction.

· Convulsions or loss of consciousness. If left untreated, preeclampsia can turn into eclampsia, characterized by extremely high blood pressure, seizures, and finally, coma and then death. Eclampsia, which can occur in the last half of pregnancy, may also be characterized by the symptoms of preeclampsia, including headache, problems with vision, and an unusual pain in the belly above the liver on the upper right side.

In addition to these life-threatening problems, pregnant women should get to the emergency department or their personal obstetrician at once in response to:

· A persistent, continuing, severe abdominal pain, obvious contractions, or any other sign of early labor. Premature labor is the predominant cause of death for about 75 percent of babies, Dr. Grunebaum says, because most women simply wait too long before getting to the hospital for help. "They wait hours and hours, sometimes overnight," he notes, "and by that time, labor may have progressed so far that they miscarry."

· Shortness of breath. This is a common problem during pregnancy. But when the onset is sudden and unexpected, the symptom may signal cardiac or pulmonary distress. If a woman was able to walk up a flight of steps one day and not the next, or if she is unable to breathe easily at night without two or three pillows, she should seek medical evaluation in the emergency department. Warns Grunebaum: When struck by shortness of breath, the pregnant woman should not wait even an hour or two before going to the hospital, since this symptom may be the first sign of heart failure.

· Exposure to chicken pox or German measles, which may damage a developing fetus. If the pregnant woman has not yet had either one of these diseases, she is likely to contract them upon exposure. However, if she knows she has been inadvertently exposed, she may be able to receive prophylactic treatment in the form of an injection of immunoglobulin at the office of her personal obstetrician or at the emergency department, thus protecting her unborn child and herself. To avail herself of such protection, however, she must seek treatment *within twenty-four hours of exposure.*

· A stream of clear water from the vagina, indicating that the amniotic sac holding the unborn child has broken and the onset of labor may begin. If the woman is near her due date, chances are the baby will now be born. If registered, she should report to the obstetrical floor. If not, in most hospitals, she can arrive via the emergency department. If the water breaks well before a woman's due date, she must get to the hospital, where she can be monitored for premature labor and infection.

· Apparent cessation of fetal movements for more than twenty or thirty minutes during the last trimester of pregnancy. If the baby seems unusually quiet, the pregnant woman should eat some food to energize the fetus and then stop everything she is doing for an hour, during which she should count for ten fetal movements (which may be hard to detect if she is working, moving around, or otherwise engaged). If the woman cannot discern ten distinct fetal movements, she should get to her personal obstetrician or the emergency department.

· Excessive vomiting. While nausea and vomiting are common in pregnancy, too much vomiting may result in dehydration, necessitating that the woman receive fluids intravenously.

Pregnant women with medical conditions that predate the pregnancy must be especially careful. A pregnant woman must get to the emergency department if:

· She is asthmatic and has an asthma attack. Without immediate treatment, shortage of oxygen might endanger the fetus.

· She has a known thyroid dysfunction and experiences the condition known as thyroid storm, with symptoms including fever, racing heartbeat, and the feeling of being hot. In this dangerous situation, her body is simply manufacturing an overabundance of thyroid hormone. Half of all pregnant women suffering thyroid storm will die if not treated promptly.

· She has diabetes and discovers, through her at-home fingerstick blood sugar test, that her sugar level has risen too high. If that level rises above two hundred and fifty, she must go to her personal obstetrician or the ED, since these levels can lead to ketoacidosis, a metabolic disturbance that may hurt or even kill the baby.

· She has chronic blood pressure problems and, through her blood pressure machine, determines her blood pressure has risen higher than 150/100. She must be treated immediately if she wants to preserve health for her baby and herself.

Private Lives: What Women Should Expect in the Emergency Department

If a woman is pregnant or has a clear-cut gynecological problem, she will be ushered to a private part of the ED. At Roosevelt Hospital, for instance, the gynecology room is set away from the hubbub of the larger emergency department. The room contains the usual equipment: heart monitor and oxygen. But some things are unique: soft lighting that may be lowered to reduce anxiety; a heated basinette for newborns; a fetal heart monitor; and special equipment for the classic pelvic exam—table with stirrups, spotlights, and vaginal speculum, an instrument that enables the physician to see the inside of the vagina. Culture materials are available so physicians can test for a range of vaginal infection and venereal disease.

Depending on the problem, different techniques and protocols will be used. For instance, the woman who describes the symptoms of urinary tract infection will be asked for a urine sample. If the emergency physician finds the presence of bacteria and many white blood cells in the urine, an antibiotic will be prescribed. The woman who says the condom broke last night may receive a morning-after pill. And the woman who complains of intense lower abdominal pain or unexplained vaginal bleeding may need an internal exam and a sonogram.

The Inside Story: What to Expect During a Pelvic Exam

It's normal to feel anxious during a pelvic exam. Even under routine circumstances, at the yearly gynecological checkup, most women approach this procedure reluctantly. This feeling is magnified in the emergency department, where patients arrive without advance warning, often in discomfort, confusion, and pain.

As in the gynecologist's office, the internal pelvic exam will generally be conducted with the doctor and one observer or assistant in attendance. It begins when a woman lies down on the examining table in what has been called the "lithotomy" position: feet up on stirrups, knees bent, buttocks pushed down to the edge of the table, and a sheet covering her body from the shoulders to knees. There's a very good reason for the posture: It provides easier access for the examiner, helps to relax the abdominal muscles, and straightens the curvature of the spine.

While the patient is in this position, the examining physician will first palpate the abdomen and then inspect the external genitalia. Using an instrument called a speculum to separate the walls of the vagina, the doctor will examine the vagina and cervix, and, when appropriate, use a long cotton swab to take cell or secretion samples for culture in the lab. The speculum comes in a variety of sizes, and the doctor will choose one that fits the individual patient. Examination with the speculum may be uncomfortable, but it should *not* be painful. If you do feel pain, verbalize it at once. You may need to change your position on the table.

The last part of the exam may involve digital examination, in which the doctor (wearing latex gloves) inserts the middle and index finger into the vagina, exploring and palpating for masses such as cysts or areas of pain. The doctor can also examine deeper structures, including the uterus, ovaries, and fallopian tubes, with the technique known as bimanual, or two-handed, examination. Using that technique, the doctor presses fingers that are inside the vagina up against the cervix, elevating it. The other hand presses down externally on the lower abdomen. As a result, the uterus can be felt between the two hands. From there, doctors can palpate to locate the ovaries on either side of the uterus.

As with speculum exam, digital exam should be uncomfortable but not painful—

unless, of course, there is a condition that generates pain upon contact. It is important to verbalize pain and discomfort immediately, since this will enable the doctor to better diagnose the problem and be more sensitive to your needs.

The final element of the digital exam is the rectal portion, in which the index finger is placed in the vagina while the middle finger is placed in the rectum. This technique is often used to help diagnose abnormal growths or other problems in the posterior portion of the vagina or rectum.

Remember that in the emergency department, the doctor's goal in conducting a pelvic exam will be diagnosing the *specific* complaint. For instance, if the physician suspects gonorrhea, she may push the urethral opening against the public bone and search for pus that can be squeezed from the glands, a sign of the disease. If the doctor suspects an ovarian cyst, he will use the bimanual digital technique described above. To diagnose candidiasis, a form of vaginitis, the doctor might view the vagina through the speculum to search for white plaques on the vaginal walls.

There's one crucial difference between internal exam in the emergency department versus the one you receive during your yearly gynecological checkup. The checkup routinely includes palpation and examination of the breast for sign of breast cancer; a pap smear for cervical cancer; a rectal exam; and a careful search of the vaginal entrance and urethra for inflammation, scarring, sores, or growths. In the emergency department, of course, these routine procedures will not usually be part of the exam unless related to the specific presenting problem. Therefore, a woman should never consider a pelvic exam at the ED a substitute for the yearly checkup with a gynecologist.

While a pelvic exam is not generally a favorite activity, there are some ways in which women can make the experience easier, and more effective:

· Empty the bladder before a pelvic exam, since this will make the experience more comfortable.

· Do not douche before going to the emergency department, since this may hinder the doctor's ability to reach a diagnosis.

· Try to stay as relaxed as possible, since tight, tense muscles will make the exam far more uncomfortable.

· *Always* speak up when the exam becomes painful. This will enable the doctor to adjust for comfort, and will provide important diagnostic information relating to your problem.

TWENTY-FOUR MEDICAL EMERGENCIES THAT TAKE WOMEN TO THE EMERGENCY DEPARTMENT

The twenty-four most common gynecological problems to be seen in the ED at St. Luke's–Roosevelt Hospital are summarized here.

Fibroid tumors: Usually signaled by heavy vaginal bleeding without the presence of pain. Doctors can actually feel these benign tumors of the muscle making up the uterine wall during a pelvic exam. They will follow up with a sonogram to look for other sources of bleeding and to confirm the presence of fibroids. Most common in middle-aged women, these tumors can often be treated with a complement of female hormones. If they are too large, however, or if the bleeding is too profuse, surgery may be required. Either way, the woman will be sent to a gynecologist for pharmaceutical or surgical care.

Ovarian cysts: Generally detected after a woman reports pain in the pelvic area without bleeding or discharge, ovarian cysts are part of the ovary, where they may expand or stretch and cause discomfort. Ovarian cysts are most often small—the size of a grape or, possibly, a golf ball. Some, however, may grow quite large; fluid-filled dermoid cysts, for instance, may grow as large as melons. To diagnose an ovarian cyst, emergency department physicians will first test for pregnancy. Then, through a pelvic exam, they will feel for the cyst or cysts— small, balloonlike masses—with their fingers. Results of the pelvic exam will usually be confirmed through ultrasound. When pain is particularly acute, doctors may suspect the ovarian cyst has twisted, creating a dangerous situation known as torsion: Blood continues to flow into the cyst, the ovary, and the fallopian tube, but cannot leave because of the twisted vessels. The accumulation of blood and the associated pressure that builds up finally results in a situation called necrosis, in which the cyst, ovary, and fallopian tube slowly die. By waiting too long, a woman might lose her ovary and fallopian tube. Treatment consists of surgery to remove the cyst. Ovarian cysts may also be life threatening when, as sometimes happens in the case of fluid- and tissue-filled dermoids, they grow large enough to rupture, filling the abdominal area with toxins and requiring surgery at once. In all cases, ovarian cysts diagnosed at the ED will be referred to gynecological specialists for further treatment or surgery.

Bartholin's cyst: This cyst may sometimes form in a spherical shape on the skin to the right or left of the vagina opening. The problem may originate when the ducts to Bartholin's glands, located on either side of the vagina, become clogged. Though the duct is clogged, the gland itself continues to produce a lubricant which eases sexual intercourse. The lubricant becomes trapped inside the body and a cyst is the result. Bartholin's cyst is generally painless and benign, but occasionally, an abscess results. Filled with fluid and pus, the cyst must be surgically drained or pain and infection will worsen. To diagnose in the ED, physicians rely on a pelvic exam. To treat, doctors numb the area with a local anesthetic, make an incision, and drain the cyst.

Foreign object in the vagina: The first sign that something is amiss may include a strange vaginal discharge or odor. Later there is infection and pain. More often than people realize, examination reveals a tampon forgotten after the last period, or a diaphragm the woman assumed she had removed. Often, the items have moved far up the vaginal canal. This is potentially serious. Emergency department physicians generally remove such items through the vagina with long forceps called a tenaculum.

Pelvic inflammatory disease, or PID: In essence, a bacterial infection involving the uterus, the fallopian tubes, and the ovaries. When severe, PID will also spread to adjacent pelvic structures. The primary symptoms are lower abdominal pelvic pain without bleeding, usually localized in the area above the pubic bone, and vaginal discharge. As the disease progresses, pain may be accompanied by fever, nausea, and a feeling of weakness. Symptoms of urinary tract infection—including burning in the bladder area and the feeling of a need to urinate—may occur as well. PID has many causes, including gonorrhea and a common germ called chlamydia. But perhaps another cause of this serious problem is the intrauterine device, or IUD, used for birth control. Upon insertion, the IUD will virtually always carry some bacteria into the otherwise sterile field of the uterus. PID can be erradicated with antibiotic therapy; however, if untreated, the disease is life-threatening. Anyone with reason to believe she has PID should get to a doctor within twenty-four hours.

Hypermenorrhea: This condition is characterized by severe cramps and extremely heavy menstrual bleeding that requires use of several pads in addition to a tampon to contain the flow. In the emergency department, women with hypermenorrhea may receive a painkiller and have their blood count checked while doctors look for the cause of the problem, which may range from an intrauterine birth control device (IUD) to hormonal imbalance. Sometimes the woman may be given hormonal medications to stop the bleeding or be sent to the operating room for a dilaton and curettage (D and C), described in detail later in the chapter.

Unprotected intercourse: If a condom or diaphragm has broken, or if one has engaged in unprotected sex, the emergency department may dispense a morning-after pill such as Ovral, a birth control pill, to avoid an unwanted pregnancy. (A visit to your personal physician would be more appropriate, if she can be reached in a timely fashion.) Ovral works, within seventy-two hours of unprotected intercourse, by preventing the fertilized egg from attaching to the uterine wall. One word of caution: If a woman is already pregnant, the morning-after pill, a potent mix of hormones, may damage the fetus. Therefore, the ED will dispense a morning-after pill *only* after the woman has had a negative pregnancy test. Women may also come to the ED following unprotected sex if they fear exposure to venereal disease such as gonorrhea and syphilis, which may be treated prophylactically with antibiotics before symptoms ever appear. (Details about sexually transmitted disease follow.)

Sexually transmitted diseases (STDs): Transmitted through sexual intercourse, STDs infect the sexual and reproductive organs and come in a variety of forms. Viral STDs, like genital herpes, genital warts, hepatitis B, and HIV, cannot be cured; however, the symptoms can be treated. These STDs should be brought to the attention of a personal physician as soon as possible. More urgent are the bacterial STDs, like gonorrhea, chlamydia, and syphilis, which are relatively easy to cure with antibiotics if caught early.

Bacterial STDs: In many women these STDs are asymptomatic or easy to miss in initial stages, so if you think you've been exposed, get to your personal physician or, if necessary, the ED for testing and treatment at once. Here's the rundown:

Chlamydia: Symptoms, appearing seven to twelve days after exposure, may include a thin white or yellow discharge, vaginal bleeding between periods, burning pain upon urination, abdominal pain, fever, and nausea. The majority of women, however, have no symptoms. This condition may cause pelvic inflammatory disease (see above) and infertility. Diagnosis in the ED is made through a laboratory test of culture taken with a cotton swab; treatment is with the antibiotic tetracycline. If the infection has caused an abscess, the patient is admitted to the hospital, where the abscess will be surgically drained and treated with intravenous antibiotics.

Gonorrhea: Contracted through vaginal, oral, or anal sex with someone who has gonorrhea; symptoms usually appear two to ten days after exposure, though most women are asymptomatic. Symptoms, when they do occur, include a thick, yellow or white discharge from the vagina; burning pain upon urination; painful periods; cramps, and pain in the lower abdomen. This condition can cause pelvic inflammatory disease and infertility. It may be passed to a baby during childbirth. Gonorrhea is diagnosed in the ED through microscopic examination of culture from the patient's vaginal secretions. Treatment is with the penicillinlike antibiotics ceftriaxone and doxycycline, similar to tetracycline. As with chlamydia, if the patient develops an abscess, she will be admitted to the hospital, where the abscess will be surgically drained and treated with intravenous antibiotics.

Syphilis: Far less common than either chlamydia or gonorrhea, syphilis is very easy to misdiagnose or miss altogether. As with gonorrhea, it is contracted through vaginal, oral, or anal sex with someone who has syphilis. This disease emerges in three progressive stages. First stage: A painless, reddish-brown sore appears on the mouth or genitals (at the site of sexual intercourse) about one to two weeks after exposure. Sore lasts about one to five weeks. Second stage: Flulike symptoms and rash appear two to six weeks after the sore has disappeared. The flu and rash eventually disappear, but syphilis remains. After a couple of years, syphilis will no longer be transmitted to a sexual partner. However, this killer disease can be passed to an unborn child in the womb. A small percentage of all infected women who remain untreated eventually pass to the third stage of the disease, which causes heart disease, brain damage, blindness, and death. Diagnosis in the emergency department involves a simple blood test. Treatment for every stage of the disease is with penicillin.

Vaginitis: This is the name given to an inflammation or infection of the vagina from a multitude of causes, including allergic reaction, a forgotten tampon or diaphragm, or, most often, bacteria or other microorganisms. Vaginitis is often signaled when a brown, watery discharge or pus appears on the underwear. Physicians in the emergency department will usually diagnose vaginitis through a pelvic exam, using the speculum to open the vaginal cavity so they can visualize the area of infection, and through a culture analyzed in the lab. Simple infections are easily recognized and treated with antibiotics. If allowed to fester, however, vaginitis infections may become severe enough to be fatal. Vaginal infections diagnosed in the emergency department can usually be traced to one of three microorganisms, each with its own peculiar subset of symptoms:

Candida: These yeastlike organisms cause the condition known interchangeably by the names candidiasis, moniliasis, thrush, fungus infection, and yeast infection. Special symptoms include intense itching of the pelvic area and a burning sensation after urination with an odorless vaginal discharge that may be either light and watery or heavy and white, with the consistency of cottage cheese. Diagnosis in the ED involves examination of the vaginal walls with a speculum and sample collected with a cotton swab and analyzed in culture in the lab. Treatment generally involves antifungal medicines such as Mycelex or Monistat in the form of a vaginal suppository.

Trichomonas: Often referred to by ED staff as "trick," trichomonas may be diagnosed when vaginal itching and burning is accompanied by a sometimes malodorous discharge that is bubbly and yellowish, greenish, or gray. Trichomonas, parastic protozoan organisms, are diagnosed through a cell culture and treated with Flagyl, an antibiotic in pill form.

Gardnerella: This is a bacterial organism that causes a "stale fish" odor and a grayish discharge that can sometimes be quite profuse. In the ED, gardnerella is diagnosed through cell culture and is treated with antibiotics such as ampicillin or tetracycline.

If the vaginitis has been traced to an irritant such as an allergen or an old tampon, removing the offending material is often all that is needed to effect a cure.

Urinary tract infection: The urinary tract infection is diagnosed in the doctor's office or the emergency department through a urine analysis and culture and treated with antibiotic. Women should seek treatment within twelve hours of noticing the burning and desire to urinate that accompanies this problem, since, once the infection travels to the kidneys, it may do permanent damage.

Contusion of the breast: When the breast becomes injured in a fight or accident, the result may be bruising or bleeding under the skin, black-and-blue marks, or even the appearance of a swollen mass. (Since it's often difficult to differentiate between a mass rooted in the contusion and a tumor, the history of the accident is crucial.) Contusion of the breast is usually treated with a hot-water bottle or heating pad and, like any other bruise, requires rest and support.

Mastitis: The most common breast problem to present at the emergency department, mastitis is characterized by redness, swelling, and pain, generally during pregnancy or afterward, during breast-feeding and lactation. In the ED, this condition is evaluated through a careful exam of the breast. Doctors will be on the lookout for serious infection or abscess. Antibiotic treatment will generally lead to a cure; however, any abscess must be surgically drained.

Precipitous, unexpected rapid delivery: Sometimes a woman will arrive at the ED ready to give birth. In that case, emergency physicians can and will deliver the baby, asking their obstetric and pediatric colleagues to join them. All EDs are staffed and equipped to manage childbirth when there is not enough time to get to the birthing room.

Abruptio placenta: Described in grueling detail in the TV scenario that opens this chapter, abruptio placenta is signaled by pain and bleeding during the last trimester of pregnancy. This condition results when the placenta separates from the uterine wall prematurely, at some point before the baby is ready to be born, causing bleeding. Both mother and fetus are evaluated in emergency by an OB/GYN expert on call, and via ultrasound. If labor begins, the mother is sent up to the hospital's labor and delivery department at once. This obstetrical emergency will usually require immediate treatment in the labor and delivery suite.

Preeclampsia and eclampsia: These syndromes, related to high blood pressure in pregnancy, are progressive in nature and, if untreated, may result in permanent kidney and liver damage as well as maternal and fetal death. If a woman experiences the symptoms of preeclampsia, including headache, blurred vision, breathlessness, nausea, swelling, and pain in the upper right quadrant of the abdomen, or of eclampsia, including convulsions and loss of consciousness, she should get to the ED at once. At the emergency department, women with these conditions will be given an IV so that doctors may deliver intravenous replacement fluids and eletrolytes as well as a vasodilator called hydralazine to widen blood vessels and lower blood pressure. The woman may also receive magnesium sulfate or Dilantin, anticonvulsant medicines that prevent seizures. Once stabilized, the woman will be admitted to the hospital. If she is near the end of her pregnancy, physicians in the labor and delivery department will begin the ultimate treatment of preeclampsia: induction of labor. If the woman has progressed to the end stage of this condition—eclampsia—and if she is at least thirty-two weeks pregnant, physicians will induce labor or immediately deliver the baby by C-section.

Breaking of the amniotic sac: This results in the release of water, and is part of the normal course of events leading up to labor. However, if the fetus is still too young to be born, this can lead to early labor or infection. When the "water breaks" at any point in a pregnancy, a woman is advised to get to the hospital at once so physicians can listen to the fetal heart and make sure the baby is OK. The ultimate destination, of course, will be the obstetrical floor, where doctors will continue to monitor mother and child for infection.

Cessation of fetal movement: Detailed instructions to pregnant women are outlined on pages 245 to 247. But, in summary, if, after the sixth month of pregnancy a woman cannot feel the fetus move ten times in an hour, she must get to the obstetrician or the emergency department immediately.

Early labor: It can often be recognized as a severe, persistent pain and is the number-one reason for fetal death. If a pregnant woman can get to the emergency department on time, she will receive intravenous or intramuscular infusions of either magensium sulfate or terbutaline, two medications that help to stop labor.

Miscarriage: A small amount of vaginal bleeding or staining is not unusual during pregnancy; sometimes, for the first month or two, the bleeding even occurs in the cyclical pattern of monthly menstruation. But a heavier flow may be a sign of spontaneous abortion, or miscarriage. If a woman suspects she may be having a miscarriage, she is to get to the obstetrician or the ED at once.

To diagnose miscarriage the emergency physician will first test urine for the signs of pregnancy and will determine blood type. A pelvic exam will then be conducted to see if the cervical opening has widened; this is something that can be felt by the doctor's finger *only* during the time of miscarriage. The doctor will also examine for "products of conception," including pink tissue fragments, and may rarely see the embryo itself.

If some fetal tissue remains in the uterus, the woman in the first trimester of pregnancy will be sent to the operating room for dilation and curettage (a D and C); in this minor surgery, special dilators are used to dilate, or enlarge, the opening to the cervix, so that the uterine lining may be scraped with a curette in a procedure known as curettage. The uterus is then cleared out with a vacuum or suction device. If the uterus is not emptied, then the bleeding of miscarriage may persist for weeks or even months, and infection may result.

If the miscarriage occurs in the second trimester of pregnancy, the woman may be given a medication to induce contractions or prostaglandins (natural, hormonelike chemical messengers) to complete the expulsion of the amniotic sac, thus bringing the spontaneous abortion to a conclusion.

If the woman who has miscarried has Rh-negative blood, she may require an injection of RhoGAM prior to release. The reason is this: Most people have an Rh factor in the blood, making them what doctors call Rh positive. Those who lack this factor are called Rh negative. If an Rh-negative woman carries an Rh-positive fetus, she may become "sensitized" by fetal blood cells during birth (or miscarriage). In response, her body will produce antibodies to the foreign Rh-positive factor. If a subsequent child is Rh positive, these antibodies will attack that child's red blood cells, inducing anemia and other potentially serious problems at birth. To prevent this tragic outcome in future pregnancies, the Rh-negative woman who has miscarried is given RhoGAM, which destroys the Rh-positive factor from the fetus before the woman's body can produce antibodies to it. To be effective, RhoGAM must be delivered within seventy-two hours of the onset of miscarriage.

Ectopic pregnancy: When the fetus implants in a fallopian tube instead of the uterus, symptoms appearing within six to twelve weeks of conception may include missed periods, bleeding, cramps, and lower abdominal discomfort. To diagnose ectopic pregnancy, emergency physicians will take urine for a pregnancy test. If ectopic pregnancy is the problem, a pelvic exam will reveal a closed cervical opening and a normal uterus—sometimes with an adjacent mass, often causing pain on palpation. To confirm the ectopic pregnancy, emergency department doctors rely on ultrasound.

Ectopic pregnancy, one of the top three reasons for maternal mortality, is an emergency because the fallopian tubes are *not* designed to stretch as the pregnancy develops. Once stretched beyond their ability, they will burst. Since the fetus will be enclosed in a placenta rich in blood vessels, bleeding may be profuse enough to be life-threatening. During an ectopic pregnancy and the surgery that may follow, a woman's tubes may be destroyed, rendering her infertile.

The woman with this condition is sent to the operating room immediately, where surgeons perform a laparoscopy. This minor surgery is conducted with a long, thin instrument called a laparoscope. The laparoscope is inserted through a tiny incision in the abdomen, enabling the surgeon to locate the ectopic pregnancy. The developing pregnancy can then be removed with instruments inserted through another tiny abdominal incision.

Women at high risk for ectopic pregnancy include those who have had a previous ectopic pregnancy; those who use an intrauterine birth control device (IUD); those who have had a tubal ligation; those who have had any type of surgery in the vicinity of the fallopian tubes, the ovaries or the uterus; and those who have had infections of the fallopian tubes.

Women's Rights: How Women Can Advocate for Themselves in the Emergency Department

Negotiating the ED is always taxing. But when the problem is personal, as most gynecological complaints are bound to be, the task is more arduous still. First and foremost, states Dr. Grunebaum, to obtain appropriate care, a woman with a gynecological problem must overcome her sense of embarrassment so that she can explain all the symptoms in full. Often this is difficult because of the fear that the physician will be judgmental. Doctors are only human and some may be opinionated; that's his or her problem—not yours. Your responsibility is to outline the problem as completely as possible so you can get the help you need. If it's difficult to talk to the doctor, perhaps a nurse will lend an ear and help you communicate the issues involved. It might be embarrassing to admit that a tampon or diaphragm has become stuck in the vagina, or that one suspects exposure to venereal disease. But if problems are not spelled out, treatment may miss the mark.

Particularly important, notes Grunebaum, is informing the ED staff that you are or feel you may be pregnant. Pregnancy is often accompanied by complications, and many symptoms can be properly interpreted only when seen in the light of pregnancy. The emergency department will not test every woman who walks in the door for pregnancy. If you are or may be pregnant, you must state that clearly.

Women should also speak up during a pelvic exam if the situation doesn't feel right. A woman has the right to a very private setting; the presence of at least two people (including a female); and a sense of comfort with the examiner during the exam. If the woman feels she has been touched in an inappropriate way, she should express that sentiment at once.

Adds emergency department director Stephan Lynn, like all patients, women with gynecological problems must remember that there are no foolish questions. "Because they feel embarrassed," he notes, "women sometimes seem reluctant to ask for information or say what's on their mind. My advice is for them is to be assertive. They are *not* bothering the doctor with their questions. They are entitled to have all of their questions and concerns addressed in full. They are dealing with health issues: This is not the time to be shy."

In the Event of Rape

There was a time in the 1970s when doctors knew relatively little about the medical treatment of rape. Susan Xenarios, a social worker at the St. Luke's emergency department at the time, was the first to throw up her hands in frustration and anger when, in 1976, a Columbia University student was rushed to the hospital after a brutal attack. The young woman had been raped on campus in broad daylight in front of eyewitnesses, but none of them did anything to help.

"When she arrived at the hospital," Xenarios recalls, "she was clearly traumatized, not just physically, but also psychologically. And we didn't know what to do."

Indeed, the physicians who first examined the woman had not been trained in the fine art of supporting the traumatized victim of rape or of collecting evidence. Their exam was cursory and incomplete. The psychiatrists who treated her later were just as unprepared for the persistent fears and depression that would not go away. "The doctors were not so much inefficient and insensitive as just scared," says Xenarios. "There was major benign neglect twenty years ago because we had no set protocols or training for the treatment of rape."

The St. Luke's staff was not alone. There had been just a single book published on rape trauma at that time, and Xenarios could not locate one rape trauma program at any hospital in the United States.

The rape at Columbia mobilized the hospital's Upper West Side community. Part of it, of course, was the timing: The women's movement was in high gear, and the anti-rape group, Take Back the Night, had already staged its marches in cities throughout the country. In New York State, laws had recently been changed to make it easier for rape survivors to prosecute.

But part of the impetus came from the rape survivor herself: While her physical injuries healed, her psychic trauma became overwhelming. Experts at the hospital and university knew they had to help.

The course was clear: They would meet as a cohesive group and learn the hard, complex facts about rape. Based on what they found, they would replace the knowledge vacuum with a medical protocol of their own.

After months of reading, interviewing, and thinking, the study group could clearly identify what experts now call the "rape trauma syndrome": the common stages and symptoms involved in recovery from rape. The first stage, the Impact Phase, lasts for about twenty-four to forty-eight hours after the assault. Here, some survivors may ride an emotional roller coaster, going from hysteria, to anger, to euphoria, and back—while others exhibit an affect that is absolutely controlled and flat. Either way, victims may suffer memory loss. During the second, Acute Phase, sometimes lasting from three to six weeks after the assault, the survivor may experience flashbacks, sleep disturbances, nightmares, emotional instability, and a sense of shame. Physical symptoms include vaginal and stomach pain, headache, backache, and muscle pain. In the third and last phase, the Reorganizing Phase, the rape survivor tends to make significant changes in her life: If she is coping well, she may end a bad relationship, change jobs, or move to a new apartment. If the trauma persists, she might become depressed, isolated, sexually dysfunctional, and even begin to suffer from such phobias as the fear of using elevators, going out at night, or being alone.

Of course, it was in the first phase where the emergency department staff could make its impact felt most. The ED staff had to help the survivor feel safe and protected and validate her feelings of violation while working to eliminate a sense of self-blame. And they would need to accomplish this while delivering medical care, providing access to police investigators and collecting extensive medical/forensic evidence, essential if rapists were to be successfully prosecuted in a court of law. This would be no easy task, Xenarios and her group discovered, since the victim could be retraumatized by the hospital experience itself. After all, given its mandate to deliver aggressive medical care quickly, sometimes to large numbers of people, and especially to the rape survivor, the emergency department could be perceived as chaotic, even assaultive. The net result, for the victim, might be a sense that she had been through two attacks, not just one.

"Ultimately," Xenarios says, "we realized that rape survivors needed help in advocating for themselves in this most traumatic of circumstances. While they had enormous reservoirs of strength, each one needed information, support, and counseling to help her make decisions for herself: Should she press charges? What should she tell the police, and when? Should she go through the extensive medical exam required for collecting evidence? Should she release results of that exam to the police, or hold off while deciding what to do? How should she deal with the possibility of pregnancy or sexually transmitted disease? What should she say to her family? Her friends? Her coworkers?

"We were told we could not do anything that cost a dime," Xenarios explains, "yet something had to be done. So we gave the hospital administration an offer it could not refuse: Tapping the enormous community concern over this issue, we would train volunteer 'advocates,' who could come into the emergency department and advocate for the survivors as well as work together with the staff and the survivor to orchestrate the elements of treatment, medical, legal, forensic, investigative, from beginning to end. Whenever a rape victim came in, the hospital social worker or, in her absence, one of the advocates, would explain the procedure to the rape survivor. These people would help survivors interface with doctors as well as police investigators, who generally wanted to talk to victims right away."

The St. Luke's team soon had its work cut out for it: During the day, well-trained social workers were available to advocate for rape victims. And each night and weekend, a different volunteer was on call for the rape survivors. The system was set up so that after the victim had been through triage, the first person to be called would be the social worker or volunteer advocate, who would be no more than fifteen minutes away.

Once the rape survivor was treated for medical emergencies, including knife wounds or life-threatening internal injuries, the advocate would step in and introduce herself. If the rape survivor accepted the services of the advocate, the first thing the volunteer negotiated would be some time and private space to present the facts: Should the survivor wish to press charges, there would be certain medical and legal steps it would be advantageous to take right away. What would police want to know? What would the medical exam entail? The advocate explained it all.

Since those early days, the original rape survivor advocacy program at St. Luke's has changed. Xenarios, now director of the Rape Intervention Program/Crime Victim's Assessment Project of the St. Luke's–Roosevelt Hospital Center, has received important recognition through numerous state and private grants. Her pioneering rape intervention program, located on the Upper West Side of Manhattan at St. Luke's–Roosevelt Hospital, is available to all New York State residents free of charge. This enables her to reach out and help survivors through all three phases of the rape trauma syndrome. She brought the volunteer program downtown, to the Roosevelt emergency department, many years ago as well. And she has integrated men into the advocate program, too. "They are coadvocates for family members, spouses, lovers, roommates," says Xenarios. "And when the rape victim is a male, which happens from time to time, the male advocate assumes the primary role."

How Rape Is Treated in the Emergency Department

While the advocacy program at St. Luke's–Roosevelt is a model of its kind, most EDs do not have such programs in place. Nonetheless, notes Xenarios, the emergency department remains the destination of choice for a victim of rape.

Even without formal advocacy programs, the awareness level of emergency personnel today is substantial. Doctors in EDs across the country have been trained in methods of evidence collection. And staff members understand that even if a woman does not *seem* emotionally distraught, she may still be severely traumatized and in desperate need of help.

Thanks to programs like the one started by Xenarios and Dr. Lynn, it is only in the ED that the treatment of rape has become a specialty unto itself. In New York State, for instance, all ED doctors must be trained in accordance with a uniform system of treatment and evidence collection. It's simply the law. New York hospitals even have on hand an official "Sexual Offense Evidence Collection Kit," and other states throughout the nation have comparable tools as well. Due to such expertise, police now escort women who have been raped to the emergency department as a matter of course.

In the event of rape by a stranger, survivors may be severely brutalized, even left on the street for dead, and an ambulance is called. More often, the physical injuries are relatively minor compared to the psychic trauma; these women are disheveled and bruised, but more or less intact.

The larger group of women, raped by known assailants, are turning to emergency department as well. "We are seeing the walk-ins more and more. These people have often waited a day are two before treatment," notes Xenarios, "and are often past the point where it is possible to collect evidence or provide much medical treatment, but they can still get information and counseling. They can still begin to take the steps required to get the help they need."

Victims of serious injury in the course of the rape will have dangerous or life-threatening medical problems treated first. Otherwise, the survivor will be sent to a private room, where she can collect her thoughts away from the frenzy of the emergency department. If she has come to St. Luke's or Roosevelt, a volunteer advocate will arrive shortly. At other facilities, nurses or social workers may assume the advocate's role.

Either way, the woman should be presented with the information she needs:

· What treatment is required so that she may take care of her own body?

· If she is interested in having the assailant caught and pressing charges, how will doctors collect evidence toward that end?

· What is entailed in talking with the police?

· How can her confidentiality be maintained?

· What if she is afraid to go home?

· Suppose she does not want to press charges now, but changes her mind next week?

For Health's Sake

"Whether or not a woman wishes to press charges," notes Xenarios, "we advise her to take care of her body in basic, commonsense ways." Indeed, since rape may result in internal damage—not to mention sexually transmitted diseases or unwanted pregnancy—treatment for the sake of health is usually advised.

The first thing doctors do is assess the woman from head to toe: They look at her entire body for scratches, bruises, and cuts. They may take confidential photographs to document visible injuries in the medical record.

Then they examine those areas where penetration has occurred. Many women will resist the notion of a pelvic exam following the ordeal of rape; it's only natural that some may perceive this to be a second assault. But Xenarios suggests that survivors agree to an internal exam even if they feel nothing is wrong. "I was with a woman who said she was sure she had not been penetrated vaginally but had been beaten very badly," Xenarios explains. "I encouraged her to have the exam anyway. They found sticks in her vagina. She did not feel those sticks because she was so traumatized and so numb."

The internal exam for injuries is followed by prophylactic treatment for potential infections. Large doses of the antibiotics ceftriaxone and doxycycline will be given to protect against sexually transmitted diseases, including gonorrhea, syphilis, and chlamydia. (There will be a wait to ensure there's no allergic reaction to the ceftriaxone.) If there's any laceration, the woman can expect a tetanus shot to protect against tetanus. If there has been anal or oral penetration, these areas will be examined, specimens taken, and treatment offered.

The victim may also want the morning-after pill to avoid unwanted pregnancy. After a pregnancy test to eliminate the possibility of a preexisting pregnancy, the survivor can, if she wants, eliminate risk of pregnancy with two tablets of Ovral as soon as possible, followed by two more tablets twelve hours later. (Some hospitals may also use the drug diethylstilbestrol, or DES.)

Although it is impossible to test for the HIV virus immediately after a rape, emergency staff will provide literature so that the individual can be alert to the risk. The rape victim will also be reassured: Chances of contracting AIDS from someone who has HIV, based on just one encounter, are statistically small.

Quest for Evidence

If the rape survivor wants to press charges in a court of law, she must, of course, have evidence. And these days, there's no place more expert at gathering that evidence than the emergency department.

Gathering forensic evidence for rape can be an extensive, time-consuming process. Physicians will search for fibers and debris on the body and clothes; DNA evidence in the form of the rapist's semen, blood, skin, and hair, often found in the victim's vaginal, anal, or oral orifices; and for other incriminating evidence found in scrapings taken from under the fingernails. First, the woman must understand what is entailed in such an exam. Then she must sign a consent form so the process can begin.

In New York State, collecting such evidence is now a science. Emergency physicians even use what's called a "sexual offense evidence collection kit," so that the protocol is followed exactly, each and every time. The kit comes prepackaged with swabs, slides, fingernail scrapers, and combs—everything in the exact quantity that the physician will need. The exam will yield more evidence, of course, if the rape has occurred within the previous twenty-four hours, if the victim has not washed, douched, or gargled, and if she is open with examiners about the intimate details of the attack.

The forensic exam includes the steps, below:

· Doctors use cotton swabs to collect material from the victim's mouth and gum pockets.

· The victim disrobes over a large piece of exam paper, which catches debris for later analysis.

· ED staff collect and seal the victim's underwear and clothing. (The emergency department at St. Luke's–Roosevelt will provide her with a new set of underwear when she is discharged.)

· ED personnel rub paper towels along the victim's skin to collect debris, including leaves, fibers, glass, and hair.

· Doctors explore the victim's body for secretions that have dried. Then they rub a wet cotton swab across the skin to pick up part of the stain.

· Doctors use wooden scrapers to collect material from beneath each nail.

· Using thumb and forefinger, the doctor pulls five hairs from each of five scalp locations (center, front, back, left side, right side) for a total of twenty-five hairs. This procedure is often particularly traumatic for victims of sexual assault.

· The doctor combs pubic hair with downward strokes so any loose hairs or debris can be collected on a paper towel. (The survivor may do the combing.)

· Using thumb and forefinger, the doctor pulls fifteen pubic hairs from various areas of the pubic region. If she prefers, the victim may pull the hairs herself.

· Using cotton swabs, the doctor collects samples from the vaginal vault. This may provide sperm or DNA evidence strong enough to stand up in a court of law.

· Using cotton swabs, the doctor collects samples from the anal area, if it has been penetrated.

· The victim provides a saliva sample by saturating a piece of paper placed in her mouth. She should not have anything to eat, drink, or smoke for a minimum of thirty minutes before this part of the exam.

Note that while more evidence will emerge closer to the time of the rape, examiners can often collect valuable forensic evidence for up to three and four days, especially if the victim has not washed.

After all treatment and tests have been administered, and after all evidence has been gathered, the emergency department staff will offer the woman some form of douche.

Finally, just because a woman has provided evidence, she does not have to release it to police. "The evidence kit may be kept by the hospital security department for as long as thirty days while the survivor decides whether or not to get law enforcement involved," Susan Xenarios says. "This option is especially important for women who know the perpetrator and are ambivalent about pressing charges. The longer they wait, the harder it will be to prosecute, but if they have had a comprehensive exam and evidence was collected and secured, it counts a lot."

Police Report

Rape victims in the emergency department may be faced with detectives and police. Remember, rape is not a mandated reportable crime in most states except when a deadly weapon is used or the survivor is under eighteen. Therefore, a rape victim can decide whether she wants to report the crime at all.

If she does, at St. Luke's or Roosevelt, it is generally a social worker or advocate who runs interference with the police. The investigator may be kept away until the victim has had time to calm down and collect her thoughts.

Police will want to hear about the attack in as much detail as possible: time, date, place, number of assailants, for starters. They will want to know the most intimate details of the rape and everything the victim can remember about the perpetrator, from his height and weight to the sound of his voice. They will also want to know whether the patient has douched, urinated, showered, or brushed her teeth before getting examined at the emergency department.

Reporting the crime can provide victims with a sense of empowerment and may prevent the rapist from striking again. But many victims feel the processes of investigation and prosecution are just too arduous given the long, stressful road to recovery ahead.

The rape survivor is the only one who can decide how to proceed. However, should she decide to prosecute, she will have to fill out and sign a detailed, written report of the crime. At this point, a case file number will be assigned and an investigation officially initiated. The decision to prosecute ultimately rests with the prosecutor, and will be made at some point in the future.

Hospital Self-Defense

The advocate programs set up at St. Luke's and Roosevelt are models. However, most of the time rape survivors will not find this comprehensive support in place. Despite the trauma, they will find themselves in the difficult position of advocating for themselves in that most chaotic of environments, the emergency department.

To fend for yourself, one of the most important things is a knowledge of basic rights. The rights guaranteed by the laws of New York State, presented here, are applicable in most other jurisdictions as well:

· The rape survivor should be taken immediately to a private room, preferably a gynecology room. The emergency department registration process should be completed in privacy.

· There should be an attendant of the same sex present during all medical procedures.

· Verbal consent should be obtained for taking of history, physicians' examination and treatment. Written consent must be obtained for collection of evidence and release of information to appropriate authorities. Such consent should be documented on the ED record.

· Sexual assault is not a mandated reportable crime unless child abuse or neglect is suspected or a deadly weapon such as a gun or knife is used. Depending on the circumstances, the patient may or may not wish to involve the police in the incident.

- Victims of sexual assault under age eighteen *must* be reported to the Child Welfare Agency.

- Though generally encouraged by hospital personnel to undergo medical examination and treatment in their own best interest, adults have the right to refuse any treatment.

- Victims of sexual assault have the right to have someone present during an interview with investigators or police.

So that the emergency department may be the first step in the healing process, not the first step in revictimization, Susan Xenarios also provides some special pointers:

- Ask emergency department staff to give you some time and space so you can collect yourself and organize your thoughts.

- Ask ED staff to provide you with a sense of safety. For different people, that may mean different things. You may want to be stationed near the ED guard, away from rowdy teenagers, or alone in the back.

- If you do not remember your rights, ask someone to explain them to you.

- Ask someone in the ED to explain the protocol for the medical exam.

- Ask someone to explain the procedure generally followed by the police.

- If you feel you are not ready to speak with police or go through the medical exam, say so. The emergency department staff will certainly give you the time you need if you ask.

- Look for advocates wherever you can find them. Xenarios points out that emergency department social workers, nurses, and physicians are usually quite sensitive and helpful to rape victims, although of course, the nurse will have to care for more than just one patient at a time. Adds Xenarios, "Cops have been known to be pretty effective advocates for rape survivors as well."

- Be aware that untrained advocates, in an effort to help, may inadvertently take over and start making decisions for you. Assert your right to make decisions for yourself. Reassuming control is the first part of healing.

- Speak to the doctor about your risk of pregnancy, and decide about the morning-after pill (Ovral) as well as antibiotic treatment for any sexually transmitted diseases you may have contracted.

· During the exam, inform the doctor of the exact acts committed, so that all medical evidence may be duly noted and documented by a medical professional.

· Make sure the doctor takes semen smears, documents all bruises or injuries, including bleeding or lacerations, external or internal, and tests you for sexually transmitted diseases.

· Ask the emergency department to put you in touch with a rape crisis center or rape hotline so you can talk by phone with someone who has had training or schedule an appointment in person.

In the Aftermath

In the end, the rape survivor will leave the emergency department. Either staff will call a cab for the patient, friends will come to get her, or police will take her home. But without follow-up, phases two and three of the rape trauma syndrome—including a descent into dysfunction—can hit hard.

That's why, at St. Luke's and Roosevelt, about 80 percent of all rape survivors follow through with counseling at the offices of the Rape Intervention Program, where Xenarios now works. With its gently flowered futon, Oriental rugs, and Diego Rivera print (a girl with braids embracing flowers), the office has the inviting, casual look of someone's home. Here, rape survivors do the difficult work of recovery, overcoming the sense of defeat, of loss of control, of disorientation, that victims often experience after this brutal crime.

Says Xenarios, "We expect nightmares, sleep disturbances, intrusive thinking, and a whole gamut of emotions that come with the territory of rape. Nonetheless, we have found that the majority of those who get here shortly after the attack can function well after five or six sessions of counseling. We then follow up in three months, and then eight months after that to mark the one-year anniversary of the rape. With counseling and support, the survivor gradually gains control, is able to trust herself and others, learns to assert herself, and puts the blame for the incident where it belongs." Xenarios explains, "Though flashbacks, fearfulness, and a sense of vulnerability are likely to last for months, the survivor is able, in most respects, to function as she did before. To me, the validation of the counseling is that the earlier the survivor comes to us for help, the more rapid and complete the recovery."

DOCUMENTING VIOLENCE: **Battered Women in the Emergency Department**

There's nothing like success to engender innovation. So in 1995, Susan Xenarios, director of the St. Luke's–Roosevelt Rape Intervention Program, has followed her pioneering effort with a similar one for domestic violence.

Women and children subject to domestic abuse have long taken their woes to the emergency department. "It's an anonymous way to get the medical care they need," Xenarios explains. "I know one battered woman who used about a dozen EDs around the city. That way, she remained anonymous because no one was able to detect a pattern, but she received treatment for her injuries through the years."

Of course, skipping from hospital to hospital after each abusive episode is no way to live. "Ultimately," says Xenarios, "battered women must learn to live violence-free. For us, the ideal situation is getting the abuser to leave."

For that to happen, women need more than medical treatment; they require encouragement and understanding, and often, a paper trail documenting the abuse, so a court of law can intervene.

Notes Xenarios, if someone is the victim of battering—even if she doesn't really need medical intervention at the moment, and even if she doesn't wish to involve the police—the emergency department is exactly where she should go. "This is the best place to document the problem, to generate an official paper trail that may be the only means of protection for this woman later on. It's a good place to begin to talk about a very painful issue with trained and caring professionals; it's an open door to treatment and counseling."

Yet, battered women in the emergency department face suspicion that is sometimes hard to overcome. "The problem," Xenarios explains, "is that many ED personnel have trouble understanding why these battered women keep going home and then returning to the ED with injuries again and again. They feel helpless to really heal them, and wish these women would just leave the situation that inflicts so much pain."

To help these women help themselves, Xenarios marshaled a two-pronged effort at Roosevelt and St. Luke's. First, she and Dr. Lynn have trained ED doctors and nurses to understand the psychology of the victim. "These women often do not *want* to take their five children to a shelter, " states Xenarios. "Jane Doe may show up in the ED on ten separate occasions with dozens of injuries before she is ready to leave the abuser. We want the medical staff to have empathy for Jane Doe, and to treat her problems with respect." To help the victims find a voice, Xenarios is also recruiting advocates—but this time, paid advocates from the community of women who have completed their own treatment after being battered themselves.

"My fantasy," says Xenarios, "is that eventually, all the biases and fears will fade. We'll see the day when battered women come to our ED as a resource and haven, and will use our facilities to document the abuse, including evidence of rape, and interface with legal authorities and police."

Chapter 9

In the Gray Zone: Emergency Care for the Elderly

If Harrison Bloom, MD, chief of geriatric medicine at St. Luke's–Roosevelt Hospital, feels anything for his patients, it is empathy. Even when the elderly are healthy and alert, he notes, their ability to comprehend and communicate may be hampered by a laundry list of problems: hearing loss, weakening vision, nerve damage, medications that fog the brain. In the nurturing nucleus of the family, or with close friends, these problems are usually manageable: A daughter may speak slowly and loudly; a long-time accountant may go over finances early in the day, before the late-afternoon blur of too much medication has begun to set in. There are hearing aids, glasses, and hopefully, an atmosphere of calm that enable the elderly to actively negotiate and enjoy their world.

But in the event of medical emergency, even the most functional octogenarian will be challenged in the high-stress hubbub of the modern metropolitan emergency department. Just picture it, Bloom explains: As paramedics hustle the patient out to the ambulance, hearing aid and glasses may be left by the bedside. In the ED, that person cannot hear; perhaps, if dentures have been left behind, she cannot even speak clearly. The proximity of other sick patients threatens her already-weak immune system, and the noise jangles her nerves. She must urinate, but cannot clearly ask for a bedpan—remember, no teeth. When she finally urinates on the stretcher (just as anyone might do), she is incorrectly labeled incontinent. Since she can't hear well enough to respond when spoken to, the hospital staff erroneously assumes she is senile, unable to understand the basic facts of her medical care. Therefore she is not consulted or advised as she winds through the confusing nexus of the emergency department. Despite that, she must somehow deal with numerous attendants, nurses, and doctors as she is shuttled to the X-ray room, as she is attached to a heart monitor, and prodded for tests. Moreover, unless she is treated by a skilled emergency physician, the symptoms of her disease may go unrecognized and undiagnosed.

The emergency department is challenging for even the sturdiest and healthiest of us. For the elderly—already often laboring under the handicaps of decreased physical and mental stamina—the experience can be a nightmare. "It may seem harsh," says Bloom, "but many urban EDs literally assault the fragile elderly physiology with noise and overcrowding. These patients are taken out of their environment quickly, not knowing what's going on, and find themselves in a foreign place, sick and confused. If they are not sick when they arrive, they *will* be within twelve hours." Add all this to the fact that when it comes to medical diagnosis, symptoms of the elderly may differ drastically from those of the younger population, and the arena of geriatric emergency medicine becomes problematic, indeed.

Like the rest of us, if the elderly don't want to succumb to trauma or disease they may, from time to time, have to visit the emergency department. That's why, in the pages ahead, our goal is to help soften the ED experience for the elderly in our midst. When should senior citizens go to an ED, and when should they contact personal physicians instead? What can they do before they have an emergency to make their stay at the ED as safe and effective as possible? How can these patients communicate clearly with medical staff when they have arrived without their dentures or hearing aid—or in so much pain and confusion that they cannot respond at all? How can they overcome the bias of ageism, found in the nation's hospitals just as everywhere else? How can their weakened immune systems fend off the crowding, noise, and rigors of many modern EDs? For answers to these questions and others, read on.

Who Is Old?

Is old age a matter of chronological years since birth, physical health, or state of mind? Is the octogenarian world traveler older or younger, and by what standard, than the sixty-five-year-old who has retired because of failing memory, dearth of energy, and arthritis in her hands?

These are all questions we must strive to answer as we deal with the "graying" of America. In the year 1900, about 75 percent of all deaths occurred in people under sixty-five years of age; most of us just did not live that long. Very, very few lived to see eighty. Today, about 67 percent of all deaths occur in people sixty-five or older, an age group comprising about 11 percent of the population. What's more, these numbers are likely to increase drastically starting in the year 2011, when baby boomers born between 1946 and 1964 begin to turn sixty-five. As medical care improves, those surviving and even thriving beyond age eighty-five will shoot up as well. The numbers are jarring: Population experts predict that by the year 2030, the United States will have fifty-eight million people older than sixty-five, and eleven million people eighty-five years of age or older.

As life span begins to push the outside of the biological envelope, and as people of all ages stay healthier longer, the answer to the question of "who is old" will become increasingly important. One point experts do agree on is that as far as medicine is concerned, age has far more to do with physiology than with the absolute number of years one has walked the earth.

We are all aging constantly, from the moment we are born. The experts say the body's organs start to decline from their peak when we reach age thirty or thereabouts, and continue their descent into oblivion at a steady pace throughout the ninth, tenth, and (for some rare individuals who last that long) the eleventh decades of life. Each individual, and each organ system within the same individual, may age at a different rate.

The Biology of Aging

Even though physiological age is not tied to chronological age absolutely, at some point, usually in our seventies or eighties, but earlier for some and later for others, we will meet the criteria for the category medicine defines as "old."

From the medical point of view, older patients, even those who are healthy, differ from younger ones in a variety of ways. First, the older heart is simply slower. The walls of the heart's chambers tend to thicken with age, making it difficult to "race" the heart, as younger people do, in response to trauma or stress, thus providing the stricken area with extra blood and oxygen. The heart's internal pacemaker slows with age, rendering the individual more susceptible to cardiac disease. Older arteries are less elastic, increasing the potential for high blood pressure.

Older lungs are different too. As the chest wall becomes more rigid, as the diaphragm falls, and as the surface area of the lungs decreases, breathing—the process of inhaling oxygen for delivery to the bloodstream—becomes less efficient.

The nervous system declines with age. For instance, lowered ability to control internal body temperature means the elderly are more prone to hypothermia in the cold and hyperthermia in the heat. And since internal signals may not work to increase blood pressure rapidly enough when the body needs more oxygen—perhaps because of a wound—the injured elderly are more likely to fall or faint.

Other organs and systems also become less efficient as people grow older. The storage capacity of the liver declines. The gallbladder produces more gallstones. The kidneys begin to weaken, causing the elderly to suffer dehydration or electrolyte imbalance more readily when stressed by excessive heat or activity. The bones, especially in women, are brittle because of calcium loss; this condition, known as osteoporosis, makes breaks or fractures more likely.

Subtle Signs: Detecting Emergencies of the Elderly

It only makes sense that as people age, presentations of illness and injury may change. "What is looked on in a younger person as a relatively straightforward, clearcut event may, in the elderly, have a different meaning and cause," explains Dr. Bloom. As is the case with children, who are not just "young adults," from a medical perspective the elderly among us are not just "old adults"—they have health and medical issues that may differ quite significantly from the bulk of people in middle age.

When it comes to detecting medical emergencies, these differences are crucially important. The reason: Emergencies, by definition, must be treated at once if the individual is to recover or survive. But because emergencies may present with different signs and symptoms in the elderly, they may sometimes be ignored. The result may be a tragedy that could have been avoided had the people involved been atuned to the signs.

For example, when a younger person falls down, we generally assume there has been an accident. The person has tripped, perhaps, or has toppled over a ledge. If the individual emerges with just a minor bruise or scratch, only the most excessive or neurotic would dream of rushing to an emergency department. An older person can and does fall down for the same reasons. However, for an older person, it's far more likely that what appears to be just a fall may actually be the manifestation of a heart attack or a stroke. Therefore, an older person who has taken a fall *should* rush to the emergency department or to a personal physician, even if there's no scratch or bruise at all.

For a younger person, the heart attack, when it occurs, will be easier to recognize because it is likely to present with classic symptoms like chest pain. For an older person, on the other hand, chest pain does not always accompany heart attack, since a number of chronic conditions associated with age tend to blunt sensory perceptions of pain: If the individual takes a lot of medicine, if dementia has set in, if conditions like diabetes have caused nerve damage, the brain may register no pain at all.

Finally, that fall, no matter what the origin, is more likely to cause the brittle, osteoporotic bones of the elderly to break. Imagine how this might play out in the event of a car crash, where broken bones with jagged edges can puncture organs, causing internal bleeding. Put a fifteen-year-old and an eighty-five-year-old in the same relatively minor accident—say, in a car crashing into a fence at fifteen or twenty miles an hour. The younger person will probably come through with just a few bruises, but the older individual could smash her chest and break a number of ribs, or fracture his legs and arms.

In the face of *any* life-threatening medical problem or injury, moreover, older folks generally have fewer reserves with which to ride out the onslaught until medical help arrives. For instance, in the event of a gastrointestinal bleed, younger people can hang on longer because their heartbeat will race up fast enough to pump blood to the vital organs, even though blood volume is diminishing as the result of the bleed. Likewise, younger lungs will be efficient enough to extract oxygen from the diminishing supply of blood for a longer period of time. The elderly, many already victims of heart or lung disease, will generally have fewer reserves with which to supply the brain and other vital organs with blood and oxygen. Faced with a gastrointestinal bleed, the older person will simply have a smaller window of time for survival before medical help arrives.

The elderly individual may be perfectly functional with his or her moderate level of heart disease or emphysema in the absence of other health problems. But enter the stress of another, unrelated problem—anything from a gastrointestinal bleed or a stomach infection to lowerered body temperature due to hypothermia or a fall—and a spiraling cascade will begin. Without treatment, of course, anyone might eventually succumb; the elderly, however, just don't have as much time.

What's more, this negative cascade into serious medical compromise and death presents itself long before the end. The younger person with the gastrointestinal bleed will come into the emergency department with mental faculties fully intact. The older individual, just on the border of getting enough oxygen to the brain *before* the bleeding began, is now not getting enough oxygen, and comes in utterly confused.

Given the unique biology of aging, how does one recognize an emergency in the elderly? Under what circumstances should an older person go to emergency?

Dr. Bloom says the answer is often complex. All the usual standards apply: If the individual has lost consciousness or is bleeding profusely, if he has had an obvious heart attack, if she has suffered traumatic injury in an auto accident, the emergency department is mandatory, no matter what a person's age.

However, sometimes the elderly must go to the ED when others should not: For instance, say your elderly mom falls against the fridge and says she'll be just fine. It was just a bump, after all, despite the nagging pain. If it happened to *you,* you would pick yourself up and go about your business without another thought. But Mom should be checked out, because at age eighty her bones are osteoporotic and prone to break. A minor fall against the fridge—even one that seems to have caused no major injury— can result in a break.

The older person with a fever greater than 102 degrees Fahrenheit must also be checked out. Since older people are actually *less* prey to viral infection than younger folk, it's likely the fever may signify a serious *bacterial* infection, which might be life-threatening if left untreated.

You've also got to get an elderly parent to the emergency department when you notice a sudden, severe change in mental or physical status that is not immediately corrected and cannot be easily explained: any sudden dizziness, stomach pain, confusion, fever, or trembling. If the older person in question is unable to express him/herself well due to dementia, or if that person is on one or more medicines, all the more reason to be alarmed.

Finally, for senior citizens who lack the support of family or friends and have become increasingly isolated from the community, the emergency department is one channel through which they may access the appropriate social services, from a home health care aide to a cleaning service.

SHADES OF GRAY: **Emergency Symptoms You Might Miss**

As with younger people, there are myriad situations with older people warranting a trip to the emergency department. In an effort to help you recognize the subtle, often unique, signs and symptoms that signal emergency for older people, we present the following listing, by disease.

Heart disease: As people age, it becomes less and less likely that cardiac disease, including heart attack, will present with the classic symptoms of chest pain, nausea, and vomiting. Instead, look for symptoms including acute confusion, abdominal discomfort, and labored breathing.

Acute abdominal illness: Abdominal illness may result from numerous causes: appendicitis, peptic ulcer, gastrointestinal bleeding, severe bacterial infection, to name a few. Diagnosis of these potentially lethal conditions may be difficult in the elderly because symptoms do not seem as severe as those reported by younger populations. In middle age these conditions will result in severe pain and fever; when palpating the abdominal area, the physician may detect a certain rigidity, and the patient will feel an associated "tenderness." For the elderly, however, the whole spectrum of symptoms is muted. The salient point is clear: For the older individual, even mild stomach pain and mild fever should be considered a clarion call to action. These symptoms signal an urgent situation, and should receive prompt medical attention, preferably through a readily accessible personal physician, but if not, at the emergency department.

Infectious disease: The most common forms of infectious disease for the elderly population include pneumonia and urinary tract infection. Given symptoms of fever and stomach pain, the elderly patient is far more likely than the younger patient to have some form of deadly infectious disease. (The younger person will, more likely, have a less dangerous viral illness, to which the older person has grown immune as a result of many years of exposure to the routine viral illnesses.)

In the face of infectious disease, the elderly are just less likely to present with common symptoms like fever or severe pain. Instead, for older patients, the first clues to infectious disease often include lethargy or confusion. Take common pneumonia. Younger people generally have symptoms including high fever, chest pain, and cough. The older person with this illness, however, may present with weakness and lethargy, but the fever, cough, and chest pain may not be there.

Neurologic and psychiatric emergencies: Often, neurological symptoms such as confusion, disorientation as to time and place, and even psychosis, may signal another, underlying medical problem. These neurological symptoms, known as delirium, may be due to a number of medical insults, including head trauma, infection, alcohol withdrawal, drugs, diabetes, brain lesions, lupus, thyroid problems, or brain hemorrhage. Delirium can become so severe that the patient hallucinates, hears voices, and has no sense of reality at all.

Delirium and other neurological problems are addressed extensively in Chapter 11. However, as far as the elderly are concerned, it's important to note the difference between delirium and dementia. Dementia, most often seen in the form of Alzheimer's disease, is related to permanent deterioration of the brain and is *not* a medical emergency. People closest to the elderly individual will often mistake delirium for dementia. The mistake can be lethal, since delirium may signal medical emergency related to an underlying injury or disease. The message is clear: If your elderly friend or relative seems quite suddenly confused or disoriented, do not just assume it's a "touch of senility" setting in. If this individual has, in the past, been perfectly oriented and alert, assume the problem is a medical emergency and get to the emergency department.

Heat- and cold-related illness: Like all mammals, we humans are warm-blooded. That means we are able to maintain a set body temperature of about 98.6 degrees Fahrenheit, even in the face of extremes of heat or cold in the outer environment. For the elderly, however, the "thermoregulatory" mechanism we so casually rely on is often off-kilter, inefficient, or impaired. This explains, perhaps, why senior citizens are so vulnerable to heat-related illness, and why the number of deaths from all causes rises so precipitously in the geriatric population during the hot summer months. Perhaps one reason why heat is so dangerous for older individuals is that all body systems, including the heart and lungs, are already functioning near the edge. When one more stress is added—in this case, heat—the older body just cannot adapt quickly enough. Other factors increasing sensitivity to heat include drugs often used by seniors, damage to the central nervous system, and infection.

For the elderly, environmental heat is an important risk factor. As temperatures rise, complaints of weakness or discomfort should be considered particularly worrisome, since they *could* be a sign that heat exhaustion, heat stroke, hyperthermia, or dehydration are at work. If so, the elderly individual may require intravenous hydration in the ED. Also note that if thermoregulation is significantly impaired, the elderly individual may suffer these problems even in moderate environmental heat.

Inefficient thermoregulation may also lead to the other temperature-related illness, hypothermia, in which body temperature plummets below about 95 degrees Fahrenheit. Since lowered body temperature may often signal other medical problems, from shock or heart attack to drug reaction, it always warrants a trip to the doctor or emergency department. If hypothermia does happen to be the primary problem, and if temperature drops too low, the patient must be rewarmed in the ED through such techniques as "airway rewarming," in which the patient inhales heated, humidified oxygen through a nebulizer.

FIVE SYMPTOMS THAT MIGHT SIGNAL MEDICAL EMERGENCY IN THE ELDERLY

For a college student or a "fortysomething," these symptoms might simply indicate it's time to take it easy. For the elderly individual, especially those over age eighty, these symptoms mean it's time to get to the emergency department.

· Confusion

· Lethargy or feeling of weakness

· Low-grade fever

· Labored or rapid breathing

· Mild abdominal discomfort

Proceed with Caution: When to Stay Home

There are times when the older person *must* receive medical attention at once. To be casual about a senior's medical trauma can be a prescription for death. However, it's unfortunate, say most experts in geriatric medicine, that this care is delivered primarily through the bustling, pressurized, noisy arena of the urban emergency department—a potentially difficult environment for the patient whose ability to communicate and tolerate stress is already compromised in the extreme. Emergency physicians and nurses must use their very special skills to diagnose and treat the elderly in the ED.

"Elderly in the ED are often treated just as they are in the larger world—they are misunderstood and misinterpreted, victimized by prejudice, shunted to the rear," Bloom states. "When they are hard-of-hearing, people assume they are demented. When they have left their dentures or hearing aid at home, and are thus unable to communicate clearly without help, people assume they have lost the capacity to make decisions for themselves, or to think. In all situations where people move fast, there is a bias against the elderly: at the supermarket, in a restaurant, and in the ED. Some emergency personnel may infantilize the older patient, and—especially if that patient has trouble communicating—cease to inform and consult with them as the diagnosis and treatment proceed."

Bloom's point of view, echoing that of his colleagues in geriatrics, is absolutely clear: Older people *must* tap emergency resources when needed. But when other avenues of care are possible, they should take those instead.

When should an elderly person visit their personal physician instead of the ED? If the individual is not deathly ill, says Bloom, and if he or she can reach a private physician who can speak with them on the phone or see them quickly, if needed, that would be best. "Sometimes," notes Bloom, "a telephone conversation with your doctor is all you need. If your physician tells you it's OK to wait until morning, take that advice to heart."

Sage Advice: How the Elderly Can Prepare for Emergency in Advance

Given the vicissitudes of the emergency department, one of the most important things an older individual can do to ease the experience is prepare well in advance. Older people should follow all guidelines put forth in Chapter 2: They should keep a list of their doctors, ambulances, poison control center, and local emergency departments by the phone, and should discuss their particular medical problems with their personal physician well in advance.

Dr. Bloom adds that there are some preparations the elderly should be *sure* to make. First, he notes, it's crucial to create a document, to be carried in a wallet or posted near the phone, that details some vital information:

· All regular medications, their frequency and dosage.

· Name, phone number, and affiliation of private physician.

· Medical history, including any chronic conditions from cardiac disease to asthma.

· Any prosthetic devices, including glasses, hearing aid, or dentures. If the elderly individual has been whisked off to the ED without these supports, hospital staff might incorrectly assume the patient cannot respond because of senility and fail to communicate the situation or defer to the patient's decisions for medical care.

· A list of implanted devices, including pacemaker, artificial hip, or prosthetic aorta.

If possible, elderly patients should carry a small photocopy of their latest electrocardiogram so doctors can have a baseline for comparison when they take an EKG again.

Elderly patients must also arrange, in advance, for a trusted friend or relative to meet them at the hospital should an emergency strike. Because older people are often on medication, says Bloom, because they tend to move slowly, and because they may have communication problems, it is essential that they take a companion who can keep them oriented and can help negotiate the terrain.

Anyone who expects to accompany an elderly friend or relative to the emergency department, Bloom adds, should prepare to stay for at least six hours and should take a supply of quarters for phone calls and money for food. If the patient has important documents such as a health care proxy or living will (see Chapter 13), the advocate should be aware of those as well.

Through the Nexus: How the Elderly Can Negotiate the Emergency Department

Once in the ED, it's important that older patients and their friends and relatives understand how to negotiate the situation. Many of the guidelines are the same as for younger people: Make sure you describe your problem in as much detail as possible; ask questions when confused about a diagnosis or procedure; and, if you feel unsure about the performance of a particular doctor, ask to speak with a superior farther up the chain of command.

But there are some guidelines which, while helpful for anyone, are particularly important for the senior set. Below, Dr. Bloom lays out some absolutes the elderly individual—or a companion—must insist on in the emergency department. While in the best of all possible worlds elderly patients would advocate for themselves, it may well fall to friends who have come along to see things through.

If at all possible, the elderly person should have his or her personal physician call in to alert the emergency physician as to the individual's physical and mental status. Is the patient completely lucid and cogent? Senile? Deaf, but otherwise totally alert? Ideally, the private physician will call and prepare the ED for the patient's arrival. The private doctor should also stay in touch with and make herself available to the ED throughout the day, as long as the elderly patient is there.

Always ask that one companion be allowed to accompany the elderly individual on the journey through the emergency department. "Because emergency departments have become so crowded," says Bloom, "hospitals often ask that visitors wait in the outer waiting room only. But this rule, while fine for most patients, is probably inappropriate for the older patient (as for the pediatric patient), whose ability to communicate and withstand stress may be severely compromised by anything from hearing loss to medication." If the ED staff asks you to wait outside, suggests Bloom, respectfully request that they bend the rule for you due to special circumstances. Remember, the elderly person will *need* someone to communicate relevant medical history or to summon the medical staff, someone to simply get a blanket or ask for a bedpan. As an older person's companion, your presence *inside* the ED is important.

Never allow an elderly patient to be placed flat on his back unless he is hypotensive (suffering from low blood pressure) or bleeding. "The position is one of complete powerlessness," Bloom states. "The elderly patient should always be propped in the sitting position unless medical circumstances indicate otherwise."

Make sure the patient's emergency physician and nurse have introduced themselves to the patient by name. If the physician and nurse have not introduced themselves, the elderly individual—or the advocate—should begin the introductions and ask for the names. Remember if the advocate does the asking, it is only to help the patient.

Ask that the elderly individual be seen as quickly as possible. Be polite, but persistent, if you feel your elderly friend has been languishing in the ED for too long, Bloom states. Of course, there's nothing like the rude, demanding family member to turn off hospital personnel. Besides, this is an ED, and if someone comes in with gunshot wounds, he must be treated first. Still, an advocate can sometimes make all the difference in the world when it comes to reminding staff that this frail, elderly individual has less stamina than others for the conditions of the emergency department.

If the elderly individual is placed in close quarters with other sick patients, ask that he or she be moved to an area with more space, if possible.

Make sure that members of the hospital staff do not infantilize the elderly patient. Often, says Bloom, the elderly find that hospital staff address the caregiver instead of the patient. But if a patient is alert enough to understand and make decisions, communication should be with the patient, not the relative or friend. States Bloom: "If you find the doctor is addressing the patient's advocate and not the patient directly, it is appropriate to ask the doctor to speak directly to the patient."

Make sure the patient is informed every step of the way—preferably directly by the medical staff.

Ask all doctors and nurses to address the elderly individual by title: "Mr. Smith," or "Mrs. Orbach." If ED personnel use familiarities like "honey," or "dear," or if they use the person's first name, do correct them, politely, unless, of course, the elderly individual has asked to be called Jim or Sally. Simply say: "This is Mr. Johnson," and that should get the point across.

Passages: A Gateway to Help

As difficult as the emergency department may be for the elderly, it is often the gateway to social services that the older individual desperately needs. Not every senior citizen comes to an emergency department surrounded by caring relatives or friends. Not every octogenarian will bring as advocate the loving son or wife hoping to get an accurate diagnosis and swift, appropriate treatment so the person can go home. Not every old woman or man has been admitted to a caring, humane nursing home with medical staff to tend their needs.

Some elderly people live alone in single-room-occupancy hotels or isolated apartments. Without children to look after them, without any close friends still living, they may stop eating regularly and suffer malnutrition; drink too much and fall prey to cirrhosis or other diseases of alcoholism; or languish sick and uncared-for because they have become too weak and disoriented to pick up the phone.

Other times, elderly individuals are subject to abuse; yes, there is elder abuse, too. Whether they have been beaten by a grown son or daughter too overburdened with their care, or swindled by a hired caretaker, the elderly, like children, are often vulnerable to psychological and physical abuse.

One of the most disturbing problems in the emergency department of the 1990s is the issue of abuse of the elderly. Staff at St. Luke's and Roosevelt often treat the elderly for what appears to be a routine fall or bruise, only to discover during the evaluation that the individual has been abused by a caretaker or family member.

Personnel at most emergency departments today have been trained in recognizing elder abuse. The first step is sensing something amiss either in the demeanor of the elderly patient or in the bruise or injury itself. Does the elderly individual look as if he hasn't been fed in a week? Is her depression due to emotional isolation? Has he been deprived of medication? Are that broken rib and black eye due to a fall down the steps or a well-placed punch? The next step is interviewing the elderly individual privately, out of earshot of the abuser who might intimidate the victim, preventing expression of the truth.

When faced with this situation, here is some advice for family and friends: Do not argue with ED staffers or attempt to intervene. If abuse is not a factor, the medical staff will reach that determination. If it is, be assured that help—for the abused, and the abuser—will be on the way.

SIGNS OF ELDER ABUSE

Your elderly father lives in the next town. As he has requested, he's stayed in the old family home, but he's just too sick to care for himself. So you have hired a caretaker who goes there each day at seven. She does the shopping, takes your dad out for walks, and makes his meals. But, you sense something is not quite right. Your father has a bruise near his eye. He says he fell, not to worry; he's lost weight. Could he be the victim of an increasingly troubling modern phenomenon: elder abuse?

Abuse of the elderly can take many forms, including:

· Passive neglect: Unintentional failure to fulfill a caretaking obligation. For instance, forgetting to feed the individual or to provide medication.

· Psychological abuse: Infliction of mental anguish by demeaning name-calling, insulting, ignoring, humiliating, frightening, threatening, or isolating.

· Material/financial abuse: Illegal or unethical exploitation by use of funds, property, or other assets of an older person for personal gain.

· Active neglect: This would include intentional denial of food and medication or abandonment. Unfortunately, elderly individuals are abandoned by their caretakers in the waiting rooms of emergency departments throughout the country every day of the week.

· Physical abuse: Infliction of physical pain or injury, including forced confinement, slapping, bruising, sexually molesting, cutting, burning, restraining, pushing, or shoving.

When looking for signs of abuse in the elderly, tip-offs may include increasing depression, anxiety, withdrawal, hostility, lack of responsiveness, confusion, injuries, recent inexplicable lack of funds or impoverishment, suicidal thoughts, vague health complaints, a desire to please, and the impulse to shop around for doctors.

Sometimes, one must examine not just the abused, but also the abuser—in the case of the elderly, their caretakers—for signs of the abuse. In caretakers, a tendency to abuse or mistreat the elderly may be accompanied by such signs as conflicting stories; mounting resentment; shifting blame; aggressive or defensive behavior; substance abuse; unusual fatigue; new health problems; new affluence; or depression.

These signs do not necessarily *prove* abuse. But, if you see these signs and feel, intuitively, that something is wrong, you must take action. If you do suspect elder abuse in any of its forms, the best thing you can do is take your friend or relative to the emergency department.

Chapter 10

Treating Athletes: The Urgent Art and Science of Sports Medicine

F or spectators, the warmth of the day was welcome. A balmy sixty-eight degrees in November, it was sweatshirt weather. Despite the on-and-off rain, the humidity, there was none of the bone-chilling late-autumn cold that had defined this event so many times before.

But for contestants, the temperature and humidity, hovering at some 78 percent, meant trouble. This was the New York City Marathon. In this 26.2-mile race through the city's five boroughs, it was coolness and dryness that would protect these 27,665 runners from the curse of dehydration and heat exhaustion, enabling them to stay the course to the end.

As it turned out, the twenty-fifth New York City Marathon, on November 6, 1994, would go down in history as the most dangerous to date. Two men died at the finish line—the second and third fatalities associated with the event since its inception in 1970. One victim, a twenty-seven-year-old French Canadian, succumbed to severe heat exhaustion and the other, a veteran of eight marathons, had a heart attack: Both were later pronounced dead at the Roosevelt emergency department. Hundreds of other runners brought to makeshift medical stations along the route were treated for heatstroke, heat exhaustion, dehydration, leg cramps, and more.

Manning a medical tent near the finish line inside Central Park, alongside the world-famous restaurant Tavern on the Green, Drs. Stephan Lynn and Prentice Steffen treated runners for all these problems and distributed hydrating fluids orally to hundreds. Many hours after the marathon, at ten o'clock that evening when Dr. Steffen, a lanky, athletic Oklahoman, walked from his Upper West Side apartment to his full-time job as attending physician at the Roosevelt emergency department, he was only mildly surprised to see marathoners still straggling in through the hospital's doors.

Though it was the late-night shift, the debilitating heat and humidity still were taking their toll. Six hours after the race, for instance, a marathon participant from Nebraska arrived at the ED in a cab. Accompanied by his sister, he was shivering, moaning, gasping, and vomiting as the result of dehydration so severe he might have died. Sent back to Dr. Steffen for immediate treatment by the triage nurse, this runner was set up with an IV line and given five liters of fluid. Four and a half hours later, after some small talk with Dr. Steffen about Big Eight College Football, the runner walked out the door.

"We had four others like him that night," Steffen recalls. "They had severe heat exhaustion and dehydration. Their livers and kidneys were out of whack. They all needed about four or five liters of fluid, and they stayed in the ED through the night."

These runners lucked out when they landed at Roosevelt and into the competent care of Prentice Steffen, MD. One of the nation's first emergency physicians to be board certified in sports medicine, Steffen knew his stuff. A seasoned bicycle racer, he had traveled the world as physician to several professional cycling teams, the American and Canadian Olympic cycling teams, and the Coors Classic and the Tour Du Pont stage races. His experience was intensely hands-on.

All one need do is listen to Steffen to understand that the art and science of sports medicine encompasses more, much more, than the traditional orthopedic tools used to mend broken bones, repair torn cartilage, and fix tears and sprains. The sports medicine expert must master everything from nutrition, to electrolyte balance, to training techniques, and must do so in the context of human performance: How do the complex and various elements of physiology and psychology work together so each athlete can play or compete at his or her best? In addition, the sports medicine specialist must learn to treat a hundred illnesses and injuries that can strike anyone, but tend to afflict athletes more than the rest.

For the runners, gymnasts, and soccer players among us, the advent of sports medicine is a welcome turn indeed. But how does this discipline fit into the emergency department? The disturbing tale of the recent New York City Marathon makes the answer abundantly clear: Athletic activities *can* result in catastrophic problems which, if not treated promptly and correctly, might cause sustained injury, permanent damage, or death.

Take the sport of volleyball. To most of us, the name conjures images of lazy summer days on the beach, or some long-ago tournament at an idyllic childhood camp. Volleyball: What could be more benign? Yet the experts will tell you that the injuries suffered in volleyball can be severe: Volleyball players have lost eyes after being struck by the ball; some have even suffered brain damage after crashing into net equipment, another player, a wall, or a floor.

Other sports cause problems as well. Tennis players spending long, strenuous hours outdoors may develop heatstroke. Baseball players struck by the ball may suffer head injury, brain damage, organ damage, loss of sight, or even death. Soccer players may suffer spinal-cord injury when failing to brace the neck properly as the ball makes contact with the head. Cyclists suffer what's known as road rash, massive abrasions on the shoulders, hips, ankles, or knees. On average, one thousand cyclists a year die of internal organ damage or injury to the head.

And then there are the so-called higher-risk sports: football, boxing, ice hockey, skiing. Stories are legion of high school football players who have been permanently paralyzed or killed; of boxers who, though successful at their sport and now millionaires, are brain-damaged and forever speech-impaired.

Because sports constitute such big business, the high-tech specialty of sports medicine has been supported by the power elite. But in recent years, this discipline, developed in large part to treat the needs of high-level athletes, has begun to spread its bounty to us all. Like the space program, whose high-tech developments have slowly trickled down to our cars, our shopping malls, and our homes, the specialty of sports medicine now benefits the weekend athlete, the high school runner, the disco enthusiast, and the hundreds of thousands of children in Little League, soccer leagues, basketball summer camps, and more.

THE MOST COMMON SPORTS INJURIES TREATED
AT THE ST. LUKE'S–ROOSEVELT HOSPITAL
EMERGENCY DEPARTMENTS

· Head injury

· Acute injury to knee ligaments (the blown-out knee)

· Heat exhaustion and dehydration

· Fracture of the wrist, ankle, lower leg, and collarbone

· Sprain of the wrist and ankle

· Lumbar back strain and tendinitis (swelling of tendon in the back)

· Tendinitis of the elbow

· Eye injuries

Dangerous Liaisons

The health problems usually associated in most people's minds with sports are the orthopedic ones: broken bones, sprains (tear or pull of the ligaments and tendons that support the joints); and strains (tear or pull of a muscle or tendon). Head injuries, spinal injuries, eye injuries, and hand injuries, to name just a few, may bring serious consequences as well.

When should you take your sports injury to the emergency department? You must seek medical treatment promptly anytime an injury causes severe pain or loss of consciousness, even if only briefly, and anytime a body part has lost function. If you can no longer move your foot, your finger, or your leg, get to the doctor or the ED quickly.

If an injury is accompanied by symptoms of dizziness or nausea, that might signal problems as well. For the athlete who has taken a bad fall or run full speed into anything from the other team's quarterback to a wall, symptoms of dizziness and nausea might indicate shock or head injury. Even if external injuries seem minor, the dazed or nauseated athlete might be bleeding internally. Evaluation by trained hospital staff is imperative, much as it would be if the person were in a car accident.

Until you are treated by a doctor, you can intervene on your own behalf by treating any injured body part with the first-aid method called RICEM—an acronym for rest, ice, compression, elevation, and medication. Your prognosis will improve considerably if you use RICEM for at least twenty-four hours after the injury has occurred.

THE "RICEM" TECHNIQUE IN A NUTSHELL

R = Rest the injured joint, muscle, or limb. Continued use could make the injury worse.

I = Ice the injured area for at least thirty minutes immediately after the injury. Wait two hours and then, for the next several hours, continue to apply ice for thirty-minute periods with two-hour breaks in between. Put a damp cloth between the ice pack and the skin to prevent cold injury. Ice causes injured blood vessels to contract, thus limiting bleeding, and swelling, at the site of the injury. The more blood that collects at the site of an injury, the longer it takes to heal.

C = Compress the injured area. Compression limits swelling, which is the accumulation of blood at the site of injury and can extend the length of time it will take for the wound to heal. Use an Ace bandage, available from any drug-store.

E = Elevate the injured area above the level of the heart. This will tap the power of gravity to drain excess blood and fluid from the injured site, speeding the healing process.

M = Medicate with an anti-inflammatory drug such as aspirin or ibuprofen.

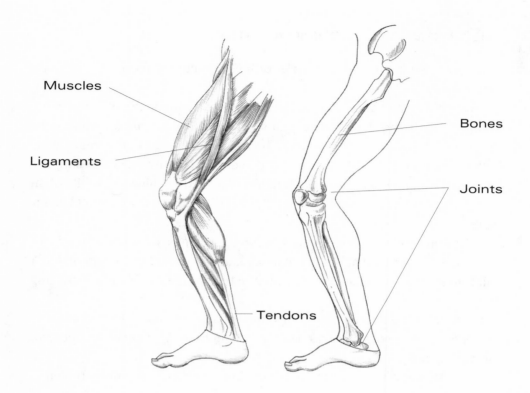

Muscles

Ligaments

Bones

Joints

Tendons

After you get to the emergency department, you may be asked to take an X ray to detect or rule out broken bones. You may be quizzed as to time, date, and your identity so doctors can determine that you are neurologically intact. You will most certainly be asked to describe how your injury occurred in as much detail as possible.

While every patient and every injury is unique, we have listed some of the most common sports injuries and their likely treatment in the emergency department. Many of these problems have been covered in other chapters, and we see no need to repeat information here. Where the specifics of diagnosis and treatment have been covered elsewhere, we will be brief. Instead, the focus will be on how these injuries relate specifically to the athlete.

Common Sports Injuries

Head injuries: These injuries are diagnosed and treated much the same way whether the individual has been hurt in a car crash or a skiing accident (see page 172 for details). For the athlete, treatment may be complicated because certain sports—for instance, football and cycling—tend to breed head injuries. With each new head injury, the athlete is more at risk for permanent damage. If you are an athlete who's gone to the hospital for head injury more than once, be sure you make note of past traumas to the doctor or other ED staff. Physicians are particularly concerned about concussions involving an alteration in consciousness, including complete loss of consciousness and amnesia, confusion, dizziness, or blurry vision. Depending on the severity of the concussion and the number of head injuries you have had in the past, you may be advised to sit out the game, the week, or the season so that you may adequately recover your health. Though different physicians hold to assorted guidelines, the American College of Sports Medicine has established guidelines that are fairly universal.

Spinal injuries: Whether the object that has fallen on you is a boulder from the cliff above or the opposing team's quarterback, you can injure your spine. Spinal injuries are treated the same way for everyone, but those who participate in sports are asked to beware of the potential for this injury, especially in contact sports like football. If an athlete is unconscious, there may also be injury to the cervical spine. Make sure the injured player is kept as stationary as possible until the ambulance arrives. Don't move injured athletes even if you think it will make them more comfortable.

Eye injuries: Diagnosis and treatment of eye injuries are the same for everyone, but people engaged in certain sports are at greater risk. The sports include basketball (fingers and elbows in the eye); baseball (balls in the eye); and racquet sports (balls and racquets in the eye). If you suffer an eye injury while engaging in your sport, see a doctor at once. Danger signs signaling true emergency include sudden decrease or loss of vision; sensitivity to light; double vision; swollen or protruding eye; irregularly shaped pupil; extreme redness in the white of the eye; the sensation of a foreign object in the eye; and, of course, extreme pain. Those suffering any such symptoms following eye injury are advised to stop all play, apply ice to the injured area, and head for the emergency department.

Broken bones: For adult humans, precisely two hundred and six calcified structures called bones serve as the body's rigid skeleton or framework. Apply enough force to any bone and it will break or fracture. The football player tackled at the thirty-yard line; the tennis player who falls and twists an ankle; the runner who pounds that leg day after day—all may come away with breaks. In the most serious of such injuries, known as acute fractures, the bone is severed. Athletes may also develop stress fractures, which result from repeated stress to a bone; such fractures may occur when a training program has been intensified too rapidly, or when the athlete runs too hard on a surface. Stress fractures are usually fine cracks, but can also be what doctors call "displaced," in which the bone fragments have moved slightly.

If you suspect a fracture, implement the RICEM technique immediately and get to your personal orthopedist or the emergency department at once. After doctors have diagnosed the injury via X ray, treatment will depend on the type and severity of the break.

If you have suffered an acute break, the two parts of the bone may well be out of alignment, and doctors will have to reduce (or set) the bone so that the two broken tips can grow back together properly. Patients requiring such realignment are generally set up with an IV and sedated intravenously. (Sometimes local anesthetic is accomplished via injection; in this procedure, known as a "nerve block," the nerve leading to the injured body part is put to sleep, but the patient remains conscious.)

In most instances, reduction is conducted in the emergency department by the orthopedic specialist on call. To set the bone, the doctor manipulates the two ends of the broken bone manually back into alignment, so they are where they were before the injury occurred.

After bones have been set in place, the orthopedist will usually create a cast to immobilize the injured bone. The cast itself consists of soft cotton tubing available in a variety of widths. The cast will then be set in place with layers of plaster or fiberglass.

Nearly all stress fractures and even most clean breaks do not need to be set, because the pieces are already in proper alignment. In these cases, doctors will simply immobilize the injured body part with a hard splint or a cast. Emergency physicians often do splinting and casting themselves without the help of an orthopedist.

While athletes can break virtually any bone, the most common injuries to be seen at the St. Luke's–Roosevelt emergency department include collarbones, wrists, and ankles.

Strains: This injury is characterized by the stretching or tearing of muscle fibers. Strains are classified in three groups. In Grade I strains, muscle fibers are stretched, and the athlete can often perform, though with pain. Signs include swelling and mild pain. Grade II strains, in which up to 50 percent of muscle fibers may be torn, involve a moderate degree of pain, swelling, and disability. The most severe strains, labeled Grade III, involve the severing of muscle fibers almost completely; with this injury the athlete may be virtually unable to contract the muscle or move the affected body part at all.

In the emergency department, strains will be treated with the requisite RICEM—rest, ice, compression, elevation, and anti-inflammatory medicine—as well as a device for protection and support. As with a broken bone, this means the physician will supply a splint and dressing to protect and support the injured area. All Grade II and Grade III strains will be referred to an outside orthopedist for follow-up.

Sprains: A sprain is a traumatic injury to the ligaments (the dense bands of tissue that attach bone to bone in physiological structures called joints) and the tendons (the end part of the muscles, which serve to attach them to bones). As with strains, sprains come in three grades: The Grade I sprain is diagnosed in patients who have torn a few ligament or tendon fibers and present with minor pain and swelling but no instability upon examination of the joint. The Grade II sprain involves more ligament and tendon tears, more pain, and more swelling, though the joint is still relatively intact. The Grade III sprain, however, is a serious injury: The ligament or tendon is completely ruptured; pain and swelling may become severe; and the joint is disabled, making it difficult to use.

Emergency physicians treat ligament injuries with RICEM (rest, ice, compression, elevation, medicine), much as they do with a strain. The injured area is supported by a splint or cast. Some Grade II and virtually all Grade III sprains will ultimately require surgery, a procedure conducted by orthopedists during scheduled operations, not in the emergency department.

Tendinitis: Overuse of a tendon may lead to this problem, whose best known sports examples include tennis elbow, golfer's elbow, shin splint, and achilles tendinitis in the lower leg. Sports that involve spinning, stretching, jumping, and throwing are most often the culprits here. To explain tendinitis briefly, tendons are strong, fibrous band-like structures connecting muscles to bones. When muscles contract, tendons are pulled, creating the ability to effect a range of motion around the joint. But if the tendon is stressed or overused, tendinitis—an inflammation of the tendon—results. Symptoms include tenderness and pain with movement. While not a true emergency, tendinitis must be treated promptly with rest, warm compresses, and a protective device such as a splint, a cast, or an Ace bandage to immobilize the joint.

Muscle contusions: These bruises to the muscle generally occur after a direct blow. The most serious of these injuries afflicts the large muscle masses, and is marked by pain, swelling, spasm, and limited range of motion in the joint above or below the injury. The muscle may actually be in spasm. In addition to ice and compression, treatment may include immobilization of the muscle in a stretched position; for the thigh and quadriceps muscles in the upper legs, this might necessitate crutches. Contusion may rarely result in a crisis; the swelling may represent actual hemorrhage requiring surgical evacuation of the blood.

Abrasions: When the skin rubs against another surface like the road, the floor, or a mat, abrasions and associated infections may result. For minor abrasions, treatment—including scrubbing, irrigation, and application of a dressing—may be carried out at home. When abrasions are severe, however, get to the doctor or the emergency department.

The Ecstacy and the Agony: When Sports Make You Sick

The athletes among us are, in general, healthier than their couch-potato peers. Their weight, blood pressure, and cholesterol are generally lower, and they face far less risk from our culture's primary killer: cardiac disease.

But sports doctors, especially those in the emergency department, can attest to the price. Because physical exertion taxes not just the bones and muscles, but also vital organs and body chemistry itself, athletes are subject to a multitude of ills. From heart attack and asthma to heat exhaustion, intensive exercise can lead to numerous systemic problems.

For instance, those who push the body too hard in heat and humidity are likely to become exhausted and dehydrated as the body sweats to keep cool. Like many runners in the New York City Marathon who stopped often for water at roadside medical stations or later stumbled into the Roosevelt emergency department, those suffering from exhaustion and dehydration had to be diagnosed and treated rapidly. In less taxing circumstances, simply resting, cooling off, and drinking some water will restore the body.

But if heat-related illness or dehydration are too advanced, they could be lethal. Indeed, in its last stages, heat-related illness is called heatstroke. And with good reason: Symptoms include complete cessation of sweating; a temperature of 106 degrees Fahrenheit or more; and delirium. Athlete or not, anyone suffering from heatstroke or severe dehydration must receive intravenous hydration and rapid cooling in the hospital at once.

Because athletes often take in so much polluted air by breathing faster and harder than the rest of us, they are more prone to upper-respiratory problems like bronchitis and asthma. Those who suffer exercise-induced asthma or bronchitis are treated like patients from any other walk of life. For acute asthma, a medicine like Proventil, delivered via nebulizer mask, is indicated. Athletes who regularly irritate their bronchial tubes are at greater risk for pneumonia as well.

Those who return to exercise after a significant downtime, especially if they have gotten out of shape, may also be at greater risk for heart attack. Any time you experience chest pains, excessive shortness of breath, dizziness, nausea, vomiting, or an overwhelming sense of tiredness after returning to exercise, do get to the emergency department. Especially at risk for heart attack during sports are those who now embrace sports as a proactive lifestyle change, but have not participated in the past: senior citizens, pregnant women, people with epilepsy, diabetes, or HIV.

Finally, truly elite athletes often suffer medical emergencies not as common in those who participate just on weekends or in a more casual way. For one thing, constant, intensive workouts may serve to suppress the immune system, leaving the athlete more vulnerable to infection and less able to fight off disease. High-level athletes who come down with a cold or the flu, therefore, must seek medical attention at once.

Athletes who travel as part of their activities are also particularly prey to viral infections and gastrointestinal problems related to changes in diet. As they travel from country to country, they are exposed to strange bacteria to which they have developed no immunity in the past. Those who fly frequently are exposed to germs through the airlines' notorious recycled air. These individuals are wise not to ignore the problem, and must seek medical attention at once.

All Juiced Up: Athletes on Drugs

Perhaps most troubling, emergency departments have been seeing more and more athletes in trouble, sometimes lethal trouble, because of their desire to improve performance with illegal drugs. Every so often, for instance, musclebound young men in their late teens or twenties will be rushed to the ED in cardiac arrest. One look at such Mr. Universe clones may tip the sports doctor off that the problem is steroids, which have bulked up the muscles—and caused atherosclerosis at the same time. Treatment will be the same as for any heart patient—but the sports physician will also attempt to educate the steroid user to the reality that anabolic steroids not only cause heart attack, but also fertility problems, acne, hair loss, depression, and mood swings. By presenting the facts, the physician hopes to ensure that steroid use stops and the patient, at some future date, will not wind up dead.

Athletes also sometimes come in to the emergency department after taking amphetamines in hopes of increasing alertness and energy. Instead, many find, their hearts start racing dangerously, requiring medical help.

Another illegal substance that sometimes takes athletes to the emergency department is human-growth hormone, which helps to bulk up muscle and reduce fat. Unfortunately, side effects may include heart trouble, arthritis, diabetes, overall weakness, impotence, and even acromegaly, in which the body produces bony overgrowth of the face, hands, and feet. Here too, a little education should go a long way.

And finally, emergency and sports physicians these days also stay on the lookout for blood doping. Dr. Prentice Steffen explains that the kidneys make a substance called erythropoietin, which stimulates the bone marrow to make more red blood cells. In recent years, this biochemical has been synthesized for legitimate use for dialysis and AIDS patients. It has fallen into the hands of competitive athletes as well. Using erythropoietin, athletes generate extra red blood cells to carry oxygen to the muscles, enabling them to work harder and longer. But if this "blood doping" is not carefully monitored, the blood gets too thick—so thick that the athlete may suffer heart attack and stroke. Sports physicians and emergency physicians like Dr. Steffen are trained to recognize the problem and treat it rapidly. For the athlete who manages to get to the hospital, treatment is vigorous IV hydration and perhaps phlebotomy or removal of blood, which is then replaced by dilute IV fluid.

Preventive Medicine

According to Dr. Steffen, part of his job as an emergency physician is educating patients before they leave, so they don't make the same mistake again—basic preventive medicine. In sports, as in any high-risk activity, the motto is classic: An ounce of prevention is worth a pound of cure. People who have suffered heat exhaustion may be told how much they need to drink before exercising—for aerobic activities in heat, one or two cups of water five or ten minutes before beginning, and then another cup of water or some other fluid every twenty minutes thereafter. Cyclists with backache are told they must change their position on the bike. Baseball players with eye injuries are asked to buy protective goggles and glasses. Those who have injured a joint running on concrete may be introduced to the virtue of running in grassy parks or on golf courses, or on that polyurethane track.

Clearly sports injuries vary with the sport; each sport comes with its own safeguards and rules. To help you recognize and avoid the problems common to your activity, we provide a sport-by-sport listing, based on advice you might get at the St. Luke's–Roosevelt ED.

BY THE SPORT

Team Sports

Football: Major injuries of this heavy-duty contact sport include sprains, strains, and fractures, as well as muscle contusions. Head and neck injuries are less common, but noteworthy, since permanent paralysis can result. When it comes to playing football, heart failure, asthma, and stroke are factors as well.

Preventive measures: Football players should acquire state-of-the-art protective equipment and clothing before venturing onto the field. Anyone playing football should have access to water on the field *during* the game. Do not participate in this sport unless you are in top condition, with special attention to endurance, flexibility, and strength.

Ice hockey: Ice hockey players are at high risk for breaks, sprains, and strains as well as eye, head, and spinal-cord injuries. This is one of the most dangerous and violent sports played today.

Preventive measures: A certified face mask is essential. Mouth guards help as well. Also important are proper blocking and checking techniques, such that the head doesn't impact first, risking injury to the neck.

Volleyball: Believe it or not, volleyball players have suffered brain damage after colliding with the net equipment and have been blinded by the ball. Another danger of volleyball is onset of cardiovascular disease, particularly in those who don't realize how vigorous this game can be. All the usual suspects, including sprains, strains, and tendinitis are there to prey upon volleyball players as well. Especially vulnerable are the shoulder, elbow, and wrist.

Preventive measures: Do not play a serious game of volleyball unless you are aerobically fit. If you fall, try to roll through the landing. Falling with an outstretched hand is the primary cause of wrist and elbow fracture. Use your arms to protect your head and face from the ball. Have water available during play, and stop when fatigued.

Soccer: This sport is more dangerous than you might think. Catastrophic injury may occur when the player fails to brace the neck before contacting the ball with the head; when two players bang their heads together; or even when tripping and falling.

Preventive measures: Players must be warned that lack of endurance training can lead to fatigue, setting the stage for injury. Players must be given adequate water during the game. In this sport, where the head is used as another vehicle for propelling the ball, the value of careful coaching must be emphasized. Players must not wear clothing that can harm other players, and should be made aware of the injury that may result when crashing into metal goalposts. Shin guards are a must.

Basketball: Look out for ankle sprain and jumper's knee, in which the patellar tendon, or kneecap, becomes stressed and overused. Other injuries include "rebound rib," a stress fracture in which the movement of the player's own muscles breaks a rib upon rebound, and heel injuries, including contusions, abrasions, and lacerations from overuse.

Preventive measures: To prevent injuries, players must be in shape so they do not get fatigued, and must respect the rules. Never play basketball on an irregular surface that could cause you to trip and fall.

Baseball and softball: Everyone who reads the paper has heard the baseball horror stories: How a Little Leaguer was hit in the chest and killed; how a high school player collided with a teammate and became paralyzed for life. These situations are rare, but baseball *can* be dangerous. Get struck by a speeding hardball and you might suffer brain damage, organ damage, or loss of sight. Collide with another player and you can break your neck. Pitch with too much thrust, and you may injure the rotator cuff in your shoulder or sprain your elbow. The most common mechanism of injury in baseball is sliding: That well-loved feet-first slide can result in injury to ankle, knee, thigh, wrist, hand, or fingers—take your pick.

Preventive measures: Obviously, baseball must be played with safety foremost in mind. The first line of defense is a batting helmet, alertness, and application of the rules. For the catcher, equipment is key. Team catchers should have a mask with padding, shin guards, a chest protector that fits snug against the throat, and a cup for the groin area.

Rowing: Rowers are vulnerable to hypothermia and heatstroke, as well as severe injuries to bones, muscles, and nerves when boats capsize or collide.

Preventive measures: Pad all protruding boat surfaces and make sure to take enough fluid along for even the hottest day.

Individual Sports

Bicycling: A distinguishing cycling injury is road rash, which occurs when a cyclist crashes. These massive abrasions—with embedded bits of "the road," tar and stones—require cleaning, treatment, and careful monitoring to promote healing. Road rash most often appears on the shoulders, hips, knees, and ankles. Also problems are acute, traumatic injuries, mostly crash-related. These include fractured wrists, fractured clavicles, fractured ribs, damage to liver and spleen, and head injuries. In fact, a rider died from head injury in the 1995 Tour de France. He was not wearing a helmet.

Preventive measures: All serious cyclists, male and female, should shave their legs. When road rash strikes, it will heal more quickly and far less painfully if there's no hair to get matted in the wound. In addition, anyone riding a bicycle should wear a helmet (currently manufactured to be light and aerodynamic). Don't worry about fashion: Some world-class cyclists avoid helmets due to the "dork factor," even though a thousand cyclists die of head injury every year. Proper maintenance of your bicycle by a qualified mechanic is essential in preventing crashes, and therefore, injuries. Protective eyewear will keep debris out of your eyes, a situation that has caused many a cyclist to crash.

Boxing: Major concerns for boxers are acute injuries, including lacerations, fractures, and head injuries, as well as chronic neurological damage. Of course, when someone is punching you on the head, face, and other places, injuries can appear almost anywhere. Also common are wrist breaks and sprains, thumb injuries, and rib fractures. (Surprisingly, boxing is *not* the most dangerous sport. It ranks eighth on the list, well after football and ice hockey.)

Preventive measures: Keep in good physical shape, and be sure to use safety equipment, including head guard, mouth guard, and groin-area cup. The safety experts say that high-top boxing shoes provide more protection than low ones.

Running: Catastrophic injury for this sport is rare except in the realm of compromise to the thermoregulatory system. Heat exhaustion, heatstroke, and dehydration are very real problems, as are overuse injuries of the relevant muscles and joints.

Preventive measures: It is vitally important to drink water at the recommended rate (see page 300) while you run. Also, if possible, run on grass, a dirt road, or a soft polyurethane track and wear appropriate running shoes.

Gymnastics: In gymnastics, injuries of the head, neck, and back most often result from falls related to fatigue and incorrect technique.

Preventive measures: Avoid gymnastics when you feel fatigued. If you feel tired, come back another day. Also, do not try an exercise like a somersault or headstand until you have been appropriately coached. A misstep can lead to serious injury.

Tennis and other racquet sports: As with running, these sports may bring on heatstroke. Twisting and turning movements may also generate joint injuries such as tendinitis and back injuries. Neck, head, and eye injuries may result if the participant runs into the net equipment or gets hit by a ball.

Preventive measures: Be sure to buy *tennis* shoes, which can handle all the pivots, as opposed to running shoes. If possible play on clay or grass, which are softer and less likely to cause injury than is a hard court. It is also recommended that you wear protective eyewear capable of withstanding the impact of balls traveling faster than a hundred miles an hour.

Golf: Due to the swinging motion, shoulder, wrist, and back injuries are especially prevalent.

Preventive measures: Many golf injuries related to the force and twist of the swing can be prevented, or at least reduced, with appropriate conditioning, including strength and flexibility training. If injuries occur despite an adequate fitness level, the golfer's swing should be analyzed by a professional golf instructor. The instructor can correct the swing, taking stress off burdened areas of the anatomy. The golf pro may also adjust length and weight of the golf clubs to maximize performance as well as health.

Diving: The major problem is misjudging water depth and hitting the bottom of a concrete pool.

Preventive measures: Divers must always check the water depth themselves before any dive.

Skiing: For downhill skiers, knee sprains and fractures are the most common of all serious injuries, though broken thumbs, broken legs, concussions, dislocated shoulders, fractured clavicles, and lacerations are also prevalent. For cross-country skiers, knee, thumb, and head injuries are common. Frostbite and cold-related problems are a given.

Preventive measures: Make sure you are in good cardiovascular shape before embarking on these activities. Strength and flexibility are key as well. If you continue to have injuries after you have become fit enough to take the slopes, have a professional ski instructor analyze your equipment and technique. Even though you will not suffer heat exhaustion on the slopes, you could become dehydrated. Make sure you have plenty of water.

Martial arts: Included are judo, karate, tai chi chuan, aikido, jujitsu, and kung fu. These can lead to bruises, contusions, sprains, and strains all over the body. When punched, vital organs, including liver, spleen, kidney, and pancreas are also at risk.

Preventive measures: Experts advise that martial arts participants use protective gear for the forearms, shins, chest, and feet as well as a mouth guard to protect the teeth and a cup to protect the groin area. Headgear will prevent most soft-tissue injury to the face, but not brain damage. Successive concussions will, eventually, lead to permanent neurological damage. If you have suffered more than one head injury while practicing martial arts, perhaps it is time to stop.

Chapter 11

Primal Screams: Coping with Psychiatric Emergencies

T he old woman had been sobbing loudly for hours when neighbors, unable to access her apartment, dialed 911. Minutes later, Emergency Medical Service workers, accompanied by police, forced their way inside. Unable to calm her or convince her to come with them, they finally placed her in restraints and carried her away.

Emergency physicians at St. Luke's examined the woman for medical problems while psychiatrists checked for underlying causes from Alzheimer's disease to schizophrenia. It turned out, however, that the woman was neither senile nor insane, just agitated because she lacked the appropriate support. Alone in her room day after day, lacking family and friends, she was too weak and depressed to clean up or even make a meal. Instead, her floor had become an open pit for garbage, with newspapers, food wrappers, and clothes piled everywhere. She herself languished on top of the heap, unkempt and unwashed, sipping Southern Comfort to soothe her nerves.

St. Luke's social worker Jorge Rey, assigned to the case following medical clearance, made a few calls. Following procedures common for social workers in most large, urban EDs, he learned the woman's apartment was an unsightly mess. Utilizing programs available free of charge to the needy elderly in New York, he deployed a cleaning service and kept the woman in the emergency department until the job was done. He also contacted some agencies and groups, including Protective Services for Adults, a visiting nurse service, and Alcoholics Anonymous. The woman would now have city workers check in on her regularly. She would receive hot meals and, if she eventually needed it, a home aide.

"What we do here," explains Rey, "is help people cope with crisis." In this woman's case, Rey's job had been done. When she left the emergency department, a day after arriving, she came home to a spotless apartment and a host of support personnel who, until then, had not known of her need.

At Roosevelt, meanwhile, a teenage boy had been brought in kicking and screaming. This frantic young man had been Maced by police, and was in pain. A truant hanging out in the subways for hours one afternoon, he was approached by transit officers who wanted him back in school. Instead of complying, however, he gave them a battle royal. As the story unfolded in the emergency department for all to hear, it ultimately took six officers—six burly men in their thirties—and a can of Mace to slow him down. (Some of the officers, bruised or bleeding from the encounter, were treated in the ED as well.)

Fearful the Mace had permanently blinded him, and convinced he would be thrown out of his school, and possibly into jail, this fifteen-year-old was beside himself with angst, and so angry he couldn't help lashing out with his feet and hands at the police as well as doctors and nurses there to help him.

Placed in four-point restraint on a stretcher in "Room 14" (the ED's "padded cell"), his hands and feet bound, he struggled helplessly, crying out, "My eyes! My eyes! How can you do this to me! I'm just fifteen!"

His anguish was met with medical attention at once. A team of doctors and nurses, finally able to approach him, rushed in to cleanse the Mace from his eyes. The attending psychiatrist, Dr. Douglas Wornell, director of the psychiatric emergency department for St. Luke's–Roosevelt, talked reassuringly to the boy, calming him down. If he could just get hold of himself, he was told, he wouldn't go to jail—just back to school.

Manic Center of the Universe

These two patients, both in obvious distress, were successfully treated in the emergency department. Troubled, but not ultimately certifiable, not so ill that they required further hospital care, these patients were medicated, counseled by the psychiatric and social work staffs, and then released.

After the teenage boy had gone, Room 14 at Roosevelt was readied yet again. Before the week was out, it would see the likes of a failed suicide who had swallowed a bottle of Valium; a psychotic college student who had begun to threaten roommates as part of his descent into the horrific netherworld of schizophrenia; and the hyper ramblings of a Frenchman who, in the throes of mania, had flown into New York on the Concorde to disrupt the kitchen staff at the Plaza Hotel.

If ever a space showed the battle scars of human misery and madness, Room 14 in the old Roosevelt emergency department was it. Though Room 14, like the old ED itself, has since been "retired," it was, when it existed, a sobering sight to behold. Branded with holes and gashes, Room 14 was host to large numbers of violent, uncontrollable, or self-destructive patients who required constant watch, immediate medication, or restraint. These days referred to in mythic sweeps of language by longtime ED staffers, Room 14 has been converted from an actual place to a dreaded state of mind.

Luckily for the manic, the delusional, the depressed, it has been replaced by a high-tech "quiet room" in the new emergency department. An acoustically sealed space covered from floor to ceiling with the soothing gray of soft padded linoleum, the new version of Room 14 is said to be indestructible. It is impossible to kick holes in the seamless, state-of-the-art tile. And, for the troubled individual looking out the window, the view no longer takes in patients agonizing over kidney stones or gasping for breath—but rather, a wall of lush, peaceful peach, Roosevelt's approximation of "Bellevue pink," a color decreed by psychiatrists the most calming shade around.

"At Roosevelt," says Dr. Wornell, "we think of the psychiatric ED as the manic center of the universe. We're right here in the center of Manhattan. Manic people from all over the world seem to converge on the city by plane, by train. They come here to spend money, to expend their energy, and some wind up right down the road, at the Plaza Hotel. Often, these people are grandiose, articulate, seemingly spectacular individuals. They fly in on the Concorde, demand the presidential suite, create an uproar in the dining room. But it takes a special situation to tip someone off that something is wrong." For instance, the manic-depressive character played by Richard Gere in the movie *Mr. Jones* was sent to the hospital after trying to fly off a girder on a construction job. "When people at work, at home, at the Plaza Hotel, realize the person is sick," says Wornell, "they phone us."

Recognizing a Psychiatric Emergency

You may not realize that whenever problems affect mood, self-control, or cognition—in short, the mind—the emergency department is one good place to turn. To utilize the psychiatric ED, of course, one must first realize a psychiatric emergency is afoot. But how does one differentiate a true psychiatric emergency from a psychiatric urgency that can be dealt with in the morning, despite the disruption and emotional pain? In some instances, says Dr. Wornell, the psychiatric emergency is abundantly clear: Your sixteen-year-old daughter has swallowed three bottles of sleeping pills. Your brother, an accountant at a Fortune 500 company, was found urinating on the living room carpet and cannot remember his name. Your college roommate, a young man of twenty-one, has begun hearing voices and seeing things; now he believes the government has placed implants in his brain, and is ordering him to jump from a bridge. A man at a Burger King throws rocks through the plate-glass windows and howls in pain.

These individuals are clearly in need of emergency psychiatric care, and pronto! They are a danger to themselves and perhaps others; they are unduly aggressive; they are disoriented as to time and place; they lack a clear notion of reality; they lack instrinsic emotional control; they are hallucinating; they harbor bizarre, inexplicable thoughts that control their actions without any basis whatsoever in the real world. They are, in short, severely clinically depressed or psychotic—delusional, or schizophrenic, or manic—and hospitalization, with appropriate medication, represents the only sure route to treatment or cure.

RECOGNIZING SERIOUS MENTAL ILLNESS

Psychiatric problems most likely to take you to the emergency department are psychoses, marked by severe disorganization and disintegration of the personality and by distorted perceptions of reality. Psychotic people may think bizarre thoughts, experience hallucinations, or act out of motivation that has no basis in reality. Severe psychiatric illness is also evident in the mood disorders, which, in their most debilitating forms—called affective disorders—may result in violence, extreme paranoia, or suicide. To help you recognize serious psychiatric illness, we provide the following review.

Schizophrenia: Those with this disease have bizarre thoughts, behaviors, and perceptions. Schizophrenics may harbor thoughts with no possible basis in fact; for instance, they may believe they are controlled by a brain implant, or a Martian, or that they are the reincarnation of some long-dead figure like Abraham Lincoln, Cleopatra, or King Henry VIII. Schizophrenics often suffer auditory or visual hallucinations, hearing voices or seeing entities. An inner voice may sustain a running commentary on the individual's activities or thoughts, or may threaten and cajole. Schizophrenics may also seem incoherent or catatonic, sustaining a stuporous state in which they are mute and immobile.

Schizophrenia is a medical phenomenon involving chemical balance in the body. It may often be treated with medicine and if doctors are successful, they may effect partial or complete remission of symptoms. But without lifelong treatment symptoms return. Schizophrenics today may sometimes be treated so effectively that they live normal, productive lives, but under current medical protocols, there is no *cure*.

Delusional disorders: Sufferers sustain fixed, false beliefs in the face of all evidence to the contrary and in opposition to beliefs held by other members of their society, cultural group, or religion. The individual's inner life and outward behavior are often governed by the delusion of extraordinary, superhuman superiority or grandiosity; of persecution by family, friends, and colleagues; of paranoia that a spouse is unfaithful or spies have bugged the office, or the house.

Manic-depression: A so-called "affective disorder," manic-depression causes swings from the height of ecstacy, in which the afflicted are voluble and hyperactive, to the depths of depression, in which feelings of deep despair prevail. This illness is sometimes also called bipolar disorder because of its two extremes. During the manic phase, signs may include increased goal-oriented activities, restlessness, distractibility, insomnia, excessive loquaciousness, a helter-skelter flow of ideas, and grandiosity. The ecstatic demeanor may quickly turn self-destructive as the manic individual drives recklessly down the highway or spends six months' worth of wages in a single afternoon. That behavior may quickly turn explosive, or sometimes even violent—a state doctors term hypermanic. Eventually, the manic phase ends in a full-blown depression, complete with thoughts of despair and even suicide. The patient cycles up and down until an appropriate medical protocol can be established.

Although medication, generally lithium, is highly effective in the treatment of manic-depression, many people with the disorder have little interest in treatment. First of all, it's fun to be manic for a while. Who wouldn't want to fly in on the Concorde or party every night for a week until dawn? Besides, the course of treatment can be unpleasant: In response to the medication, the manic individual will dip down in mood before coming back up.

When convincing a manic friend or relative to go for help, try to communicate that despite the fun of mania and the temporary side effects of drug therapy, a steady state of mind will ultimately feel best.

Depression: Also an affective disorder, depression differs from manic-depression because it exists alone, without a manic cycle kicking in. To diagnose major depression, psychiatrists look for four or five of the following symptoms: significant weight loss (without dieting); sleep disturbance; depressed mood most of the day; loss of energy; agitated or sluggish behavior; feelings of worthlessness; excessive guilt; difficulty focusing; poor memory; suicidal thoughts or suicide attempts. Less serious forms of depression are generally diagnosed when depressed mood and four or five of the symptoms above present for about two months in milder form.

SUICIDE WATCH

Perhaps the most tragic of the psychiatric emergencies is attempted suicide, the result of severe depression. It's especially important to watch for signs of potential suicide in relatives and friends since, in many instances, it's possible to prevent a tragic outcome if you know when and how to intervene.

To post an effective suicide watch, notes Dr. Wornell, it's important to tune into the "music" of depression, which often tells a story different from mere words. To comprehend the devastating melody, you must understand the "arrangement"—the sequence of stages in which depression sets in.

Depression includes four stages, one more serious than the next. In the first stage, the individual is sad, anxious, and upset. Despite the angst, this person is expressive, and the very act of "freaking out" in front of friends and relatives is a sign of residual health. In crying out for the help that is needed, this individual demonstrates that he is probably *not* about to self-destruct.

As depressive illness intensifies, the stricken individual withdraws. Often this person refuses to eat, losing up to fifty pounds quite rapidly, and may decline to get out of bed. By refusing all social interaction and psychiatric help, such individuals place themselves at great risk.

But this is not the worst of it: As the descent continues, the depressed individual may literally become psychotic, suffering delusions from extreme paranoia to extreme hypochondria. Sometimes the paranoid delusions are so extreme, the depressed individual believes others are out to get him and, in a twisted form of self-defense, may actually lash out and hurt those who care for him most.

The final stage of depression is, tragically, the suicide attempt.

While talk of suicide calls for immediate invervention, says Wornell, it's when the talk suddenly stops that the situation gets truly desperate. "As long as the person keeps discussing it, he or she may not have reached bottom," Wornell notes. "The person who comes to the emergency room to say he feels suicidal still has some degree of self-preservation, some degree of sociability, left. Sometimes, the individual stops *discussing* suicide because he or she has decided to act."

Mere talk of suicide, of course, is a medical emergency in the truest sense of the word. "That final stage—the stage of social isolation preceding the act—can come quickly, as fast as it takes to consume a six-pack of beer or inhale some cocaine." A sudden rage caused by an unfaithful spouse, or dismissal from a job, can precipitate that end-stage of social isolation as well.

That deadliest of combinations—suicidal thoughts and an asocial state of mind—is *most* dangerous in those at greatest risk. Certain factors place people especially at risk for depression and, ultimately, suicide. These include serious illness, loss of job, divorce, and middle age. If the depressed individual is a middle-aged man who has just been diagnosed with cancer, just been fired from a job, and/or just divorced, he should seek help and support at once. Adds Wornell, other high-risk groups include males as opposed to females; whites (especially those of Eastern European extraction) as opposed to blacks; those who have a personal or familial history of mental illness, especially depressive illness; a history of prior suicide attempts; or a family history of suicide completion.

"If two white male alcoholic, divorced, fired, cancer patients walk into my office," adds Wornell, "and one says he is considering suicide while the other just seems sad but says nothing at all, I would consider the silent one at greater risk."

Advice for family and friends? Do not allow that man to sit by himself and stew. You must take action to help this individual before it's too late. If you see signs of severe depression and social isolation, obtain help at once. With each special risk factor, the situation becomes increasingly urgent. Even if you don't have the knowledge or skill to intervene in a definitive way, just saying "You're important to me and I'm there when you need me" may be enough to reverse the downward spiral; it may certainly provide the depressed individual with enough time and space to seek definitive help and treatment.

Dealing with Substance Abuse

He is socially isolated, spending hours in his room playing music.

He is paranoid: Tell him he has a phone call and he thinks you are eavesdropping or that the caller is your spy.

The voices in his head tell him to pace the neighborhood streets for hours after midnight. He thinks the family dog can read his mind.

Often, when he talks he simply babbles as his thoughts become increasingly incoherent and bizarre.

This young man, age twenty-one, is just the age at which schizophrenia is likely to present. And his symptoms, virtually identical to those of the schizophrenic, make that a likely diagnosis. But perhaps luckily for this young man and his family, the problem is something else: drugs. While addiction to drugs is a devastating, potentially life-threatening problem, the drug addict, unlike the schizophrenic, can be cured. However, because the drugs themselves may be lethal, anyone suffering such drug-induced psychosis needs immediate treatment, available at the emergency department.

Those consuming too much alcohol may also suffer symptoms requiring treatment in the ED. While the disease of alcoholism, in which an individual is physically addicted to alcohol, can be cured only by long-term programs designed by Alcoholics Anonymous or rehabilitation centers, life-threatening situations must be dealt with first. But even those who are not alcoholics may suffer alcohol-related emergencies and require help in the emergency department.

Stay attuned to signs of medical emergencies resulting from substance abuse. Should you recognize a problem, call 911. In case of a true drug or alcohol emergency, you may not have time to get to emergency on your own.

Summary of Substance Abuse Data

Drug: Alcohol

Street name: Booze

Signs of use: In small quantities, alcohol dulls the reactions of the brain just slightly, producing a pleasantly relaxed feeling. In large amounts, signs include gross impairment of memory, judgment, coordination, and emotional reactions.

Associated medical emergencies: For the nonalcoholic, it is possible that consumption of too much alcohol in a short period of time may result in death if the person has not passed out first (which is usually the case). If you notice someone has stopped breathing or is breathing only with difficulty, or if you notice that pulse is dangerously slowed, call 911. For the alcoholic, sudden emergency may result after years of abuse, including: episodes of violence or amnesia; acute abdominal pain signaling pancreatic disease; exhaustion, signaling anemia, malnutrition, hepatitis, or some other infection, since immunity is compromised; congestive heart failure; and the potentially lethal condition of cirrhosis, or the scarring of the liver, signaled by yellow, or jaundiced, skin and swelling of the abdomen. The last stages of cirrhosis are marked by mental disturbances and coma.

Symptoms of withdrawal: Tremors or seizures/convulsions; agitation and restlessness; insomnia; nausea, dry heaves and vomiting; visual and auditory hallucinations; rapid pulse; high blood pressure; sweating and fever; and finally, delirium and tremors, known as DTs.

Drug: Narcotics, including codeine, heroin, morphine, opium, methadone

Street names: Fours (codeine); China white, horse, Harry, smack, stuff (heroin); hard stuff, big Munkie (morphine); Auntie, black stuff, Greece (opium)

Signs of use: After injection, needle marks may be noted, also scars and signs of thrombophlebitis, in which inflammation of veins, and possibly blood clots, leads to redness, tenderness, pain, and swelling. Also: Constricted pupils.

Associated medical emergencies: Coma with slow pulse, low blood pressure, slow breathing, and difficulty breathing caused by pulmonary edema, or water on the lungs.

Symptoms of withdrawal: Sweating, nausea, vomiting, diarrhea, anxiety, insomnia, dilated pupils, runny nose, tearing eyes, yawning, goosebumps, back pain, abdominal pain, weight loss, cold flashes, fever, rapid heartbeat, rapid respiratory rate, and high blood pressure.

Other complictions: Low blood pressure, viral hepatitis, bacterial infection, and HIV disease.

Drug: Amphetamines (benzedrine, dexedrine, methedrine, MDMA, MDEA, methamphetamine hydrochloride)

Street names: A's, bennies, benzies, speed (benzedrine); dexies (dexedrine); bonita, bambita (methedrine); ecstacy, XTC (MDMA); Eve (MDEA); ice (methamphetamine hydrochloride)

Signs of use: After injection, signs may include needle marks and thrombophlebitis, in which inflamation of veins or blood clots cause redness, tenderness, pain, and swelling. Other tip-offs to amphetamine use include extreme anxiety, hyperactivity, irritablitity, muscle tension, and dilated pupils.

Associated medical emergencies: May result in aggressive or violent behavior, paranoia, convulsions or seizures, extremely rapid heartbeat or heart attack. May also induce psychotic symptoms resembling schizophrenia, including hallucinations.

Symptoms of withdrawal: Depression and overwhelming fatigue.

Other complications: Psychological dependence.

Drug: Cocaine and crack

Street names: Bernice, big C, blow, Charlie, coke, flake, gold dust, green gold, happy dust, nose candy, paradise, snort, snow, sugar, toot, white dust

Signs of use: Hallucinations, dilated pupils, rapid heartbeat, muscle twitching, violent behavior, and damage to the nasal septum.

Associated medical emergencies: Tremors, seizures, convulsion, rapid pulse, delirium, chest pain, heart attack, cardiac arrest, and failure to breathe.

Symptoms of withdrawal: Depression, irritability, disorientation, tremors, muscle weakness.

Other complications: Psychological dependence and HIV disease if injected.

Drug: Barbiturates, including pentobarbital, amobarbital, Seconal

Street names: Yellow jackets, yellows, nimbies (pentobarbital); blue birds, blue devils, jackup (amobarbital); red birds, red devils, pinks (Seconal)

Signs of use: Slurred speech, impaired coordination, decreased mental alertness and attention span, poor memory, impaired judgment, slowed pulse rate, slow reflexes, mood swings, dizziness, dehydration, and visual disturbances, including double vision and inability to focus.

Associated medical emergencies: Suicidal behavior; a sharp and significant depression of consciousness and mental faculties; the slowing or cessation of breathing; and coma.

Symptoms of withdrawal: Anxiety, irritability, seizures, low blood pressure, increased heart rate, auditory and visual disturbances, and shock.

Other complications: Low blood pressure, physical and psychological dependence, and death.

Drug: Cannabis, including marijuana, hashish, and THC (tetrahydrocannabinol)

Street names: grass, pot, Acapulco gold, tea, reefer (marijuana); hash, heesh (hashish)

Signs of use: Slowed reaction time, dilated pupils and (don't forget this) the sweet/pungent smell of the smoke. Also: Short-term memory impairment and coughing or raspy voice similar to that of the cigarette smoker.

Associated medical emergencies: Only rarely, panic and paranoia. With THC, the user can sometimes literally seem psychotic.

Symptoms of withdrawal: None known.

Other complications: Psychological dependence.

Drug: Hallucinogens, including LSD, mescaline, and psylocybin

Street names: acid (LSD); mushroom (mescaline and psylocybin)

Signs of use: Altered perceptions, depressed reaction time, and "spaciness."

Associated medical emergencies: Characterized by the "bad trip," medical emergencies can include anxiety, frightening hallucinations, depression, and suicidal tendencies.

Other complications: Psychological dependence.

Drug: PCP, or phencyclidine (also an hallucinogen)

Street names: elephant, peace pill, angel dust

Signs of use: Confusion, fatigue, irritability, anxiety, depression, numbness, hallucinations.

Associated medical emergencies: The slowing or cessation of breathing, epileptic seizures, paralysis, paranoid or violent behavior, and coma.

Symptoms of withdrawal: None known.

Other complications: Psychological dependence and death.

Shades of Gray

A patient doesn't have to be psychotic or addicted, however, for a psychiatric emergency to occur. Many times, in fact, picking up on psychiatric emergencies is a subtle process. Indeed, mood disorders like depression are often debilitating. But sometimes the symptoms, while alarming to the professional, are subtle enough to elude the lay person.

"The main bit of advice for those trying to discern whether friends or family need urgent help," explains Dr. Wornell, "is to listen to the music, not the words." For instance, say your dad sits listlessly day after day, hardly eating, leaving his room infrequently, his eyes tearing throughout the day. Obviously, actions speak louder than words. If Dad was the sort of person who might seek help on his own, he could make an appointment with a local therapist or clinic in the morning. If he could even admit he had a problem, he'd let you make the appointment and drive him there. Treatment for his obvious depression might include talk therapy, medications like Prozac, and a plan for getting his life back on track.

But in denial, Dad's "music" speaks louder than words. If he refuses to seek help week after week, you must get him to the emergency department.

Any abrupt change in mental status may signal psychiatric emergency as well. On the top of the list is a loss of orientation as to identity, time, or place. The individual who exhibits mood swings, emoting ecstacy one moment and wild despair the next, is a candidate for the psychiatric emergency room. So is the normally energetic individual who has become suddenly and persistently sluggish, or the reserved person who, for some reason, has not stopped talking for weeks. The psychiatric emergency department is the appropriate place for the person who goes on a rampage all night, and in the morning is found sitting on the side of the road staring into space; for the individual who runs through the neighborhood naked or slashes the furniture with knives; and for the extremely depressed or obviously psychotic individual whose credo is avoiding treatment no matter what the cost.

As you listen to the music, bring your own best judgment to bear. If your teenage daughter is despondent and it's midnight, you might do well to wait and get psychiatric help during business hours. But, if you're afraid that should you fall asleep, your daughter will sneak to the medicine cabinet and swallow all the tranquilizers she can find, or slit her wrists, get her to the hospital now.

When it comes to psychiatric emergency, no one, *absolutely no one,* is immune. As

Dr. Wornell points out, "For every normal state, there is an emergency. For every thought or mood you might have in the normal course of things, there is a psychiatric emergency corresponding to the situation in which that thought or mood goes awry. From domestic abuse, to suicide attempts, to schizophrenia, emergencies in the psychiatric realm may erupt in even the most seemingly sane and balanced. Left untreated, these emergencies can result in death, much like cardiac arrest or shock. Whether the cause of the emergency is organic or inorganic, we are all potentially at risk. Given the wrong medical condition or the wrong life situation virtually anyone can become a psychiatric patient. "

When listening for that troubled "music," keep one caveat in mind: Many psychiatric problems, in fact, probably most of them, *can* hold until morning and do not necessarily require an emergency visit. Though urgent and painful, these problems will "keep" for the private psychiatrist, psychologist, or social worker who is better suited to monitor drug therapy over the long term or take patients through the painful discovery of talk therapy. If the music so instructs you, do wait until morning, when a private doctor or therapist can administer more appropriate long-term, outpatient care.

For instance, one woman decided to visit the psychiatric emergency department at her local hospital after a grueling day at home. Her husband had been fired from his job and was now so angry and depressed he was unable to talk. He was a diagnosed manic-depressive, and she feared that a cyle of depression, then euphoria, would set in once again. Her son, previously diagnosed with attention-deficit hyperactivity disorder, was alternately running amok through the apartment and staring mindlessly at the television screen. Then, her boss called to say her project was due—she had a morning deadline. She didn't dare confess the truth—that despite instructions to move forward, she never even started the work at all.

Waiting for hours in the psychiatric emergency department for someone to talk with, she saw people with bandages around their wrists; people who shouted and lashed out angrily in thin air; and those who babbled mindlessly about UFOs. When her turn finally came, the ED doctor was blunt: "I know you're suffering," he said, "but why are you here?" He wrote out a prescription for Librium, a common tranquilizer. "You're welcome here anytime," he told her, "but for your own peace of mind, next time you're in this situation, try to stick it out at home." The woman's therapist agreed. "I know how distressed you were," she said to her patient, "but you really didn't belong in the ED."

The fact remains, however, that most psychiatric problems *are* neither black nor white, but rather, a shade of gray. How can you know when you (or somewhere near to you) needs help right this minute, and whether the best place to get that help is the emergency department?

If the answer isn't clear to you, look at the guidelines below.

Get to the psychiatric emergency department if the person in question is:

· A danger to self.

· A danger to others.

· Inexplicably psychotic: hearing voices; having visual hallucinations; consistently incoherent or convinced of bizarre notions, especially delusions of persecution or grandeur.

· Disoriented as to time, place, and identity.

· Demonstrating rapidly changing mental status for no apparent reason; going from sane and sober to seemingly drunk, incoherent, or out of control within an hour.

Provided you can get appropriate help outside the hospital setting in the next day or so, you do not generally need the psychiatric emergency department if the person in question is:

· Expressing feelings of depression and would like to try some Prozac.

· Unable to sleep and is pacing the floor.

· Expressing mild to moderate feelings of anxiety.

· Demonstrating the symptoms of anxiety or personality disorder unless symptoms are so extreme that the result might be violence to self or others.

· A diagnosed schizophrenic who is out of touch with reality but is not a danger to himself or others. This individual may need long-term outpatient care so doctors can adjust medication, not an ED.

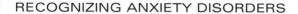

RECOGNIZING ANXIETY DISORDERS

Even those of us without psychiatric problems can recognize the pulse of anxiety: the nerve-racking feeling of apprehension caused by threat. Anxiety and fear, of course, are not the same. While fear is a specific, timed response to external threat, anxiety is that heightened sense of doom or uneasiness generated when the threat is internalized, when the problem seems to follow you around even when the specific threat cannot be seen. For instance, you may be generally anxious about losing your job because of a downturn in the economy, even if you haven't received a pink slip or haven't displeased your boss.

If, as the experts contend, every normal emotion has its corollary in emotional disorder, then normal anxiety, of all the emotions, should certainly shift from time to time to sheer psychic distress. When this distress is prolonged and exaggerated—when it becomes so extreme that it interferes with perception or normal functioning—an *anxiety disorder* is the result.

While symptoms of anxiety disorder vary with severity, in general, they include an inability to concentrate on tasks; sleeplessness; restlessness; severe increase or decrease in appetite; irritability; and behavior geared to get attention or reassurance. Accompanying physical symptoms may include dilated pupils, dry mouth, difficulty swallowing, frequent urination, rapid breathing, increased heartbeat, trembling, high blood pressure, nausea, sexual dysfunction, and cold or clammy hands.

In its most extreme form, acute anxiety can lead to a *panic attack*, signaled by difficulty breathing, chest pains, palpitations, trembling, a tingling in the hands and feet, choking, dizziness, nausea, a sense of unreality, and a fear of going crazy, dying, or losing control.

Anxiety disorders may sometimes manifest in the form of phobia, the persistent, irrational fear of a specific object, activity, or situation. Phobic people know their fears are out of proportion to actual dangers, but are unable to use this knowledge to confront the situation. Perhaps the most common and debilitating phobia is agoraphobia, or the fear of being alone and losing control in public places. Other phobias may include a fear of height, a fear of animals, or a fear of insects.

In recent years, experts have referred to a subset of anxiety disorders called *post-traumatic stress disorder*, or PTSD, defined as the anxiety resulting from an event occurring outside the range of usual human experience. PTSD has been traced to war and other disasters or traumas from rape and car crashes to earthquakes and tornados, and has been particularly identified as a problem for Vietnam veterans.

In addition to symptoms of anxiety disorder and panic attack, the PTSD victim can also experience painful emotion and thought, especially the reliving of the root event. Other symptoms might include rage, depression, or suicidal thoughts, inability to concentrate, and memory impairment.

Unless the individual cannot make it through the night, or unless symptoms of these various anxiety disorders are so severe that the individual has lost touch with reality, the problem calls for a clinic or personal therapist who can administer medication and psychotherapy on an out-patient basis over the long term. Hospitalization is not usually required.

RECOGNIZING PERSONALITY DISORDERS

Most of the time, personality disorders are *not* psychiatric emergencies. Rather, they are long-term personality traits marked by entangled, troubling relationships and inappropriate responses to people, especially under stress.

One man with a personality disorder became romantically entangled with a colleague at the office. Most of those conducting an affair behind a spouse's back would have stopped there. But this man's narcissistic disorder, marked by a false sense of superiority and a need to control *everything*, caused him to go out of his way to befriend his lover's husband. For the better part of a year, the man invited his lover and her husband, as a couple, to dinners at his home. The two couples, children in tow, spent Thanksgiving, Christmas Day, and New Year's Eve together. And, while the women talked out front, the man, posing as a sympathetic confidant, heard his new "friend" confess misery, suspicions, and the desperate sense that he had lost his wife's love. Orchestrating events like the director of a play, this man, driven by his disorder, was able to proceed for many months without guilt.

Of course, for this man and others, such disorders do not constitute an emergency, medical or otherwise. Rather, personality disorders manifest in the form of troubled love and work relationships. Such people may fail to recognize the line dividing themselves from others; may fail to feel empathy, guilt, or conscience; may perceive themselves as extremely important or powerful; and may form dependent or demanding friendships to gratify self-centered psychological needs.

Infrequently, however, a personality disorder *may* erupt into a bona fide medical emergency—especially when the disorder escalates so that hostility, lack of conscience, or self-destructive impulses cause the individual to flout the safety of self and others and to ignore society's mores. For instance, Susan Smith, the infamous South Carolina mother who sent her two children plummeting to death into a lake, may have been suffering from a potent cocktail of such disorders combined with a dose of depression. We will always wonder whether advance recognition of these problems might have translated into salvation for the children—and Smith herself.

Though most personality disorders require a good psychotherapist rather than the emergency department, it's important to recognize such disorders in the face of emergency as well. Recognition of and appropriate response to personality disorder may help you the next time you think a friend or relative needs help fast.

Some common personality disorders are summarized below.

Paranoid personality: This personality expresses excessive mistrust of others.

Schizoid personality: This individual withdraws from society.

Histrionic personality: Engaging in attention-getting behavior and dramatic displays of emotion, this person may also be subject to tantrums and suicide threats. A personality type often characterized by brief interpersonal relationships, when things become especially stressful, the histrionic person can have a conversion reaction, in which the hand or another part of the body becomes numb, and may also enter a catatonic, or dreamlike fugue state.

Antisocial personality: A range of antisocial behavior is exhibited by this person, who is sometimes, though not necessarily, violent; often, such behavior leads to court and prison.

Borderline personality: Characterized by instability, impulsivity, and periods of intense anger, the borderline personality often also has clinging, intense relationships; may project his or her problems or life experience onto others; and is capable of intermittent, self-destructive acts. Thought to represent the personality type between neurotic and psychotic, the borderline individual does not suffer chronic psychosis, but does exhibit global personality problems, including anger and lack of trust.

Obsessive-compulsive personality: Overly concerned with rules and morals, this personality type is often rigid in deed and emotion. May be overly neat or stubborn. In its most extreme form, obsession-compulsion can cause its victims to perform certain rituals: washing their hands or saying a chant again and again until the behavior is deemed psychotic.

Passive-aggressive personality: This individual displays intentional inefficiency in the personal and professional realm, thus venting anger while seeming to be merely an innocent incompetent. The passive-aggressive person might fall asleep in the middle of a "meaningful" discussion, lose the boss's papers, or consistently arrive late.

Avoidant personality: Low in self-esteem, this individual is often hypersensitive to perceived criticism or humiliation.

Narcissistic personality: Extremely self-centered, with an inflated sense of self-worth, these people feel entitled to special treatment without the need to reciprocate. They generally lack empathy for others, and have little capacity for emotional warmth.

Dependent personality: Such individuals allow others to assume responsibility for their life.

When personality disorders erupt with other factors such as depression into a full-blown psychiatric emergency, you must get the individual help as quickly and gently as possible. Remember that personality disorder complicates an already difficult situation. A person suffering personality disorder may make unreasonable or excessive demands, or become particularly resistant, angry, or defensive. Your best bet is to meet the demands that you can without endangering the individual or yourself, while waiting for help to arrive.

The Mind-Body Connection

The dangers implicit in psychiatric emergencies exist not only because those who are unbalanced may hurt themselves and others, but also because unbalanced mental states often originate in unrecognized *medical* problems. This makes sense: The brain is the most complex and sensitive organ in the body. Metabolic change affects its soft wiring, manifesting in alterations of thought and mood. Therefore, bizarre ideas and wild mood swings may indicate insult to the brain.

The set of psychiatric symptoms most often indicative of acute physical dysfunction includes delirium and dementia. Delirium, caused by a range of physical insults—including head trauma, infection, alcohol withdrawal, drugs, diabetes, brain lesions, lupus, thyroid problems, and brain hemorrhage—can result in brain death. In its mildest form, delirium can generate anxiety, restlessness, and inability to focus. Think of it as a clouding of consciousness in which perception is disordered. As the delirium progresses, often rapidly, symptoms become more extreme. The stricken individual may be unable to recognize family or friends and may even hallucinate in visual images or sound. "The patient suffering delirium certainly *appears* psychotic," explains Dr. Wornell. "But there's a difference. With delirium, the symptoms can culminate in death, often appearing suddenly and intensifying rapidly so that the stricken individual goes from stone-cold sober, to psychotic, to dead in a short span of time."

The only cure for delirium is removal of the insult. For instance, in the case of acute alcoholism, an intoxicated individual will often pass out before he or she drinks enough to die; the alcohol will be metabolized by the body before death can occur. In the case of diabetes, extra insulin, or extra glucose, can be provided before delirium results in death.

How can you tell the difference between deadly delirium and psychosis? It's not always easy, but in general, the person with delirium will at first seem to be happy, even elated, and sometimes hypersexy. These symptoms will intensify until the individual seems almost drunk: He or she may appear dizzy or tipsy, make inappropriate comments, and walk with a funny gait. Soon, the person might be vomiting, staggering, and before anyone knows what's happened, comatose, and dead.

Given these facts, it stands to reason that anyone suffering symptoms of delirium should get to the emergency department at once. In this instance you would do well to call 911 and secure the services of Emergency Medical Service instead of trying to make it to the hospital without help.

Unlike delirium, dementia does not lead quickly and irrevocably to death of the brain as a whole. Instead, those suffering dementia have suffered focal areas of insult to the brain, and the result is neuropsychiatric illness such as Alzheimer's disease. Brain regions regulating intellect or coordination are irrevocably damaged, but the brain itself lives on for extended periods of time. Also unlike delirium, dementia is a slow-moving phenomenon. When it first sets in, its signs may be so subtle that only a close family member or colleague realizes something is wrong: small lapses of memory, slight fluctuations in mood, a discernible loss of focus or efficiency. Only as the dementia progresses over months and sometimes years does the individual lose some, then more, and finally all, intellectual power and emotional control.

In primary dementia such as Alzheimer's or senility, the dementia itself is the primary disease. There are also a large number of ills that can cause what doctors call secondary dementia. Diseases including AIDS, tuberculosis, multiple sclerosis, and fungal infections can result in dementia, as can head trauma, circulatory disorders, and alcoholism. Primary dementias are always progressive, irrevocable, and sometimes deadly. As for secondary dementias, their progress can sometimes be stopped or even reversed if the original factor or disease can be treated.

If you recognize the symptoms of dementia in a relative or friend, it behooves you to get that person medical treatment at once. If the dementia is secondary in nature, depending on its cause, swift medical care can mean the difference between a normal and healthy life or a life of despair. Unless you can secure the services of a specialist within one or two days, a visit to the emergency department is suggested.

While medical problems can create symptoms that present as psychosis, psychiatric problems may sometimes reveal themselves in the form of apparent physical ills. Hysteria or panic disorder, for instance, can present as chest pain; depression can sometimes manifest in the form of flulike symptoms, including headache, loss of appetite, and exhaustion. Indeed, the experts often refer to "somatization" disorders when describing psychiatric ills that are signaled by multiple physical symptoms, none of them tied to a specific physical disease. Included are hypochondria, in which individuals persist in believing that they suffer any number of ills, despite medical evidence to the contrary; somatoform pain disorder, in which no physical cause can be found for chronic pain; and conversion disorder, in which psychological troubles result in the loss of physical functions, from body movement to sight.

How can you differentiate between a psychiatric condition and a true, physical emergency? Often, as a layperson, you can't. If your dad, known to be a hypochondriac, complains of severe stomach pain and says his appendix is about to burst, take him at his word and call 911. Like the proverbial "boy who cried wolf," hypochondriacs have been known to have real medical emergencies to which friends and relatives, long grown skeptical, do not respond. Likewise, if a friend or relative claims chest pain that you think may be related to panic disorder, don't assume the responsibility of making the diagnosis yourself. The mind-body connection is complex, and even nurses and doctors at the hospital will take an EKG and read the results before they make a definitive diagnosis.

Seeking Help: How to Approach the Psychiatric Emergency Department

If your friend or family member is violent, suicidal, or delusional, help may be needed at once. In such instances, hospitalization may be required, and the emergency department is the portal to that appropriate care.

To summon help at once, dial 911 (or the correct number in your area). If Emergency Medical Service arrives to find the patient clearly disoriented or a danger to himself or others, despite that patient's protestations, he/she will be taken to the emergency department. If EMS personnel cannot convince the patient to go voluntarily, they may summon police.

Either way, rest assured that you have acted responsibly. This individual, left to his own resources for any amount of time, might not have survived.

At other times, the situation is merely urgent. Depression or anxiety, while requiring prompt treatment, can often keep until morning. If the urgently ill individual resists help day after day, however, the psychiatric emergency department may, ultimately, be the only place you can turn. Sometimes you must force the issue by calling an ambulance. If your action is warranted, Emergency Medical Service will agree that the patient must visit the hospital and will take him there.

Of course, you take the risk that the patient may greet EMS personnel cheerfully and seem normal as can be. If the troubled individual is able to present this demeanor, perhaps sit there, seemingly sane, and say, "See, nothing is wrong with me. And I won't go," there's probably little you can do. In this instance, you must ask others trusted by the person at risk to help that individual make the difficult decision to seek psychiatric help.

Someone suffering depression, high anxiety, insomnia, or any number of other psychiatric problems may also simply arrive at the hospital alone. Such patients, who have come in voluntarily, are often less disturbed than those arriving by ambulance. For one thing, they have the ability to walk, ride in a car, or take public transportation. For another, they are aware of their problems and have decided they want the help.

Over the Threshold

What happens at the emergency department when a patient arrives? Seeking help for psychiatric problems in the ED is much like seeking treatment for an asthma attack or a broken foot. As with other problems, patients may just walk in or arrive via ambulance, often accompanied by relatives and sometimes, by police.

Like people with purely medical problems, psychiatric patients are interviewed by the emergency department triage nurse, who registers and then assesses the complaint. Whether the issue is depression, extreme anxiety, or abuse, the patient will be examined first for physical ills. The nurse will take a medical history and the "vitals," including blood pressure, pulse, temperature, and respiration.

If the patient is a senior citizen complaining of abuse by a home-care worker, examination for physical injuries and disease may take place first. If the patient complains of heart-stopping anxiety, an EKG may be ordered. And, even if the patient is a longtime psychiatric patient with a known history of hypochondria, each and every complaint will be checked out through examination and, if necessary, lab tests.

Given the intricate mind-body connection, the reasons for medical clearance, even in the face of seemingly obvious psychiatric problems, are abundantly clear. Emergency department staff *must* rule out medical emergency first.

After the triage nurse has assessed straightforward medical problems, psychiatric issues will then be evaluated as well. First and foremost will be an attempt to evaluate the severity of the problem.

At Roosevelt Hospital, no matter what the problem, psychiatric patients are ushered through a glass-brick portal to a separate suite of rooms.

Those not as urgently ill may be asked to sit in the psychiatric emergency department waiting room, a small vestibule dominated by the painting of an overarching New York City bridge. "It represents the therapeutic bridge," states Dr. Wornell, "from psychiatric illness to health."

Those deemed extremely sick, especially those clearly psychotic or of imminent danger to themselves and others, will be asked to change from street clothes and shoes into a hospital gown and slippers. Often, after clothes are removed, patients are searched for any concealed weapons and then given a yellow armband marking them as an "elopement risk." All such "elopement risks," as well as those on suicide watch, are placed under close watch.

In the most extreme cases, in which patients are uncontrollable and violent, five-point restraint will be used, in which arms, legs, and body are tied to a stretcher. The staff may then draw blood and deliver medicine, even against the patient's will, if the doctor has assessed the patient and considers it in the patient's best interest.

"In a situation in which the patient is aggressive or violent, and in which they are screaming as we hold them against their will," says Dr. Wornell, "we need about one or two hours to take control of the situation so the patient can calm down, get out of the restraints, and talk."

The Therapeutic Bridge: Inside the Psychiatric Emergency Department

As soon as a patient is calm enough, he or she is interviewed, often extensively, by the psychiatrist or emergency physician. Sometimes blood is drawn to determine whether or not a physical problem is at the root. Urine may be sampled as well to determine whether a patient is pregnant, since some medications are contraindicated for pregnant women. Patients over age forty may also require an electrocardiogram, since medications might have an impact on the unhealthy heart.

Eventually, after observation and an interview, a working diagnosis is established and treatment can begin. Sometimes, the patient merely needs advice and support. A social worker can be called in to talk, help provide services, and set up the patient with long-term support groups.

For instance, Jorge Rey, emergency social worker at St. Luke's, was called upon to help a young mentally ill man brought in by EMS. The patient had been threatening to hurt his mother and sister at home, and the family claimed they had reached the breaking point.

While the patient spoke with the emergency psychiatrist, Rey interviewed the mother, and additional elements emerged: This young man had had a long history of mental illness and had recently started using drugs, explains Rey. "He had also neglected to take his psychiatric medicine for more than a month. The mother was just overwhelmed, and she wanted him out of her home."

The upshot was this: The patient was treated by the psychiatrist and kept in the ED overnight. After just one day back on his medication, this young man turned out to be a sweet and easygoing person. Rey explains, "He was able to verbalize how guilty he felt about inflicting such pain on his family members the day before."

Rey called the family back to his office for another meeting. After informing them of the change, he invited the patient to join the group. "During this reunion the young man broke into tears and apologized to his mother and sister," Rey says. "His mother was very moved. I was able to suggest that she take her son back providing he agreed to follow up with his treatment on an out-patient basis. Both mother and son agreed."

Rey explains: "Emergency social services can educate a person about anxiety and other psychiatric problems; allow that person to grieve; validate a person's feelings; and elicit a person's coping mechanisms. They can also provide support groups for victims of crime, domestic violence, and rape."

When the problem is psychiatric instead of social, the psychiatrist or emergency physician steps in. One day not long ago, for instance, Dr. Wendy Rives, attending psychiatrist for the Roosevelt emergency department, sat chatting with her resident. All was quiet when, out in the hall, Rives heard a moan.

Long-experienced in these matters, Rives perked up her ears. Walking out in the hall, she learned that the moaner, a woman in her fifties, had been literally "run down" by a group of teenagers careening on foot through Central Park. She claimed all manner of injury and distress, but the emergency physicians who had X-rayed her virtually top to bottom and performed every appropriate test and exam could find nothing wrong (save a few bumps and bruises).

The patient told Rives she found it hard to accept that nothing serious was wrong. And in light of the doctor's findings, she added, she knew what she'd long suspected was true: She really suffered from post-traumatic stress disorder (see page 322), stemming from a prior attack that occurred while she'd been vacationing in Barbados some years back. As if to prove a point, the woman reached into a briefcase and pulled out a Polaroid snapshot of herself with black eyes, bruised mouth, and purplish skin. She said it had been taken by the Barbados police

The woman shared with Rives a lifetime of woe: Ever since the first attack, she claimed, the pain in her body had rendered her unable to work. Without a means of support, she'd spent most days wrangling with the government for disability. She couldn't go out with friends because she had no money. In fact, she was so broke she could not even visit her ailing father, who, due to lack of family support, had had to move to a nursing home. No matter where she went, the woman said, no matter what she did, people and events conspired against her.

"Nobody takes me seriously and nothing goes right for me," the woman lamented. "And my treatment in this hospital is just more of the same." As if to illustrate her point, she mentioned a sandwich that a nurse had handed her before. "Even the bread was smooshed."

"For this woman," Rives instructed her resident privately, "that statement just about sums it up." Her conclusion: The patient did not suffer post-traumatic stress disorder, as she claimed. Nor was she a candidate for Prozac, a medication she hoped Rives could prescribe. "Prozac is for depression," Rives explained, and with all her lawyers and claims against the government, this woman was hardly immobilized, which a diagnosis of depression would imply. Instead, said Rives, she had a cocktail of personality disorders, most notably, narcissism and paranoia: She believed she was continually persecuted, somehow singled out by humanity and the universe for abuse.

In the end, Rives referred the patient to a local clinic with sliding fee scales for some talk therapy. She was troubled, but without claim to a true psychiatric emergency, without need of medicine, she was provided a reference and sent on her way.

Some patients, on the other hand, must be admitted to the locked ward upstairs. The elderly gentleman suffering not only from depression but also cardiac problems and low blood pressure, for instance, cannot be placed on a regimen of medications without round-the-clock monitoring by hospital staff. The college student found wandering the streets incoherent and confused may be schizophrenic, but a diagnosis and medical regimen can be established in appropriate fashion only after observation as an inpatient for a couple of weeks. And the middle-aged woman who refused to leave her room or talk to anyone for two months after her divorce cannot just be placed on medicine and left to her own devices. Until doctors determine if those medications are effective, she must be monitored for suicide.

DRUGS IN THE PSYCHIATRIC EMERGENCY DEPARTMENT

In the psychiatric emergency department, two drugs are used most frequently: Haldol and Ativan.

Haldol, otherwise known as haloperidol, an antipsychotic medicine, is generally delivered through the mouth, muscle, or vein. This major tranquilizer, used in instances where the patient is psychotic, works by blocking the neurotransmitter called dopamine, literally blocking thought. Haldol addresses severely overworked parts of the thinking apparatus that would otherwise express themselves in paranoia or rage. As rage and paranoia go away, agitation leaves as well.

Ativan, or lorazepam, similar to Valium, is what physicians call a minor tranquilizer; it is not used in instances of psychosis, but rather, as a sedative or muscle relaxant for those suffering undue anxiety or stress. Ativan is sometimes used in combination with Haldol to control severe agitation. Like Haldol, Ativan may be delivered through the mouth, muscle, or vein.

Other medicines are sometimes prescribed in psychiatric emergency as well: Lithium is provided for manic-depressives; antidepressants such as Prozac can help alleviate depression. Such medications will typically take a couple of weeks to work, but if the emergency physicians think they're what's called for, they may provide a prescription for seven days' worth of medicine along with a referral for long-term care so the treatment can get under way as soon as possible.

Who Must Be Admitted as an Inpatient?

Those who go to the emergency department because they feel anxious or depressed and would like some help do not, in general, need to stay in the hospital. Such patients have a problem that they acknowledge. They want treatment. And unless they are violent or lacking in self-control, they can go in for treatment—usually crisis intervention—and leave. In general, these patients will receive a prescription for some medicine, be it a tranquilizer or antidepressant, and referral to a facility for long-term outpatient care.

"There's no evidence that they're insane," states Wornell. "They have come to us. They are behaving responsibly. They can be treated and trusted to follow through on their own."

On the other hand, patients who are psychotic or violent, or so disturbed that they don't even recognize they have a problem, will be compelled to stay until their health improves.

Dr. Wendy Rives mentions one delusional patient committed to the hospital who insists she owns twelve houses in Great Neck, a swanky suburb of New York. The woman, who hails from a poor, inner-city neighborhood and lives on welfare, wants to leave the hospital. But, Rives explains, not only does the patient not have a house in Great Neck, she doesn't have an apartment of her own, anywhere. "If we let her out now," says Rives, "she'll take the train to Great Neck and start ordering people out of their homes. Until she realizes she does not own houses in Great Neck and can only live by renting an apartment she can afford in another part of New York, we can't let her go. She'd be a threat to others, and she'd never survive."

Like this woman, patients often enter St. Luke's–Roosevelt Hospital's locked ward involuntarily, after a team of doctors deem they are a danger to themselves or others. Other patients commit themselves voluntarily to avail themselves of the round-the-clock treatment and scrutiny only a hospital can provide.

INSIDE STORY: Check Out the Locked Ward Before Checking into the Psychiatric Emergency Department

At hospital A, noted for its excellent care of patients suffering from depression and substance abuse, the locked psychiatric ward resembles a college dorm. The furniture is strong and utilitarian, yet homey. The carpet, of industrial quality, is a clean, friendly, dotted blue. Art and dance therapists wander about, seeking out patients interested in participating in a session or two. As for those so severely depressed they just sit and stare into space, the gentle prodding of nurse-practitioners and social workers elicits a response. Those on new medicines are monitored for blood pressure changes every four hours. And daily therapy sessions with a psychiatrist, a psychologist, or a psychiatric social worker help patients come to terms with problems and formulate future goals.

At hospital B, meanwhile, the mood of the locked ward is oppressive. The lounge reeks of street smells: the odor of food left moldering on tables; and faintly, but shockingly, even urine. The patients, highly medicated, seem mostly shell-shocked. One babbles endlessly about starships from the Pleiades, another spends hours in front of a television set, not even noticing that the volume isn't on. Nurses, when they do amble by, are delivering more medication. Doctors check patients regularly, but not to deliver therapy, just to see how they're doing on the medications.

The quality of locked psychiatric wards can differ drastically, depending upon the institution. At some, the doctors are completely qualified and even leaders in their field. Their programs are therapeutically based on the latest medicine has to offer, and nurturing to boot. At other institutions, practitioners are less well trained and experienced—well-meaning, but still learning the tricks of their trade. And the worst of these facilities may seem like throwbacks to an era supposedly gone, where the mentally ill were viewed as incurable and untreatable, pariahs not fit for the world. They may serve as mere holding facilities, places where patients are kept as calm as possible until they inevitably move on.

Therefore, before you take a loved one to an emergency department for psychiatric care, you may want to check the characteristics of the locked psychiatric ward with which it is associated. Do you have a family doctor or private psychiatrist who can recommend the best place? Do you or your friends know anyone who's ever been inside any of the local locked psychiatric wards as a patient or a visitor? They too may be able to provide some insight as to the quality of the care.

Don't wait until an emergency strikes. Gather your information now. Checking out these facilities well in advance of the time you or someone you care about shows up as a psychiatric patient is crucial.

One man we know swallowed some sleeping pills and then, in a panic, called 911. Emergency Medical Service took him to a local hospital, where he was admitted and given Prozac. Within days, he stopped talking and eating, and he lost fifteen pounds the first week. The doctors couldn't understand why, despite the medicine, he kept deteriorating.

Alarmed, his family had him transferred to the locked ward of another, recommended, facility. There, doctors quickly realized his Prozac dose was twice what was appropriate. This "double dosage," moreover, had sent his already low blood pressure plummeting. These skilled practitioners stopped all medication to clear out the man's system; treated his blood pressure problem; and then administered Prozac again, this time at the appropriate dose. Within a week— "like a miracle," his family told the doctor—the man was eating his meals, talking about his work, and reading *The New York Times.*

So do be careful about selection of a psychiatric ward. Given the complex arsenal of today's psychoactive drugs, with all their subtleties and side effects, you want the best in-house team you can find. But note that each hospital department stands or falls on its own. The hospital that overmedicated the patient in our story was renowned for its cardiac intensive care. Even if a hospital is known for its orthopedic surgery, its trauma center, or some other specialty, that doesn't mean the psychiatric service inside meets the same high standards.

With Commitment Comes Responsibility

Remember, even those patients who commit *themselves* to a locked ward can, in a flash, see that voluntary status change. A patient who has signed himself in may decide to sign himself out, only to discover that doctors do not agree. Unable to support a discharge decision, hospital psychiatrists can prevent the patient from leaving.

Of course, the patient does have recourse: He or she can make a motion to leave by putting the request in writing, at which point the hospital has three days to honor the request or to contest it. If the hospital's doctors strenuously contest discharge, the patient can be kept, or perhaps even transferred elsewhere, against his or her will.

Psychiatrists can even take a patient to court in a petition for long-term hospitalization, and the patient without the means for private care can be transferred to a state hospital which, depending on the facility, can be an intimidating and unpleasant place.

That's why anytime you, a friend, or relative decides to enter a locked unit, even voluntarily, you must remember that freedom is left on the other side of the door. True, the average length of stay inside—usually a few weeks—is less than it was just a few years ago. Still, psychiatrists are cautious when it comes to letting psychotic, violent, or self-destructive people back out. Recently, in New York City, the impetus to keep people locked up a bit longer was reinforced when a schizophrenic man, hospitalized voluntarily, walked out one day and pushed a woman onto the subway tracks, snuffing out a wife and mother's life.

For doctors in the psychiatric emergency department—the front line between life on the outside and the locked ward within—individual rights and personal freedom are always balanced against what is medically appropriate and correct. "We don't admit someone to the locked ward lightly," Wornell comments. "In an effort to balance individual freedom with the patient's best interest, we do the best we can to weed out the desperately ill at the emergency department door."

For instance, according to one psychiatrist, doctors recently worked mightily to keep a suicidal teenager out of the hospital's locked ward and in the emergency department. "This individual was brought in by his parents," the doctor relates. "We didn't want to release him, but by the same token, we didn't want to put him upstairs. It was just too intimidating. The patient was too young, and too many of the patients in the locked ward are very, very sick—schizophrenic, delusional. And even though this suicidal teenage patient was agitated and in danger of self-destructing, placing him in the locked ward indefinitely would have made things worse."

In light of the intensity of the locked ward, and the personal freedoms the "inmates" lose, it behooves you to give a friend or relative the chance to take steps to solve their problems on their own before you call an ambulance to forcibly take them to the hospital.

Think long and hard. But if, in your heart, you feel the person must be dragged kicking and screaming for help, make the call.

To make that decision, Wornell advises, "Listen to the music, not the words." For instance, a schizophrenic may tell you how happy he is in the midst of his wonderful hallucinations. But if he has no friends or job, if he's dropped out of school, or if he persists in such bizarre behavior as urinating on the floor, he clearly needs help. These signs—the music, so to speak—are functions of illness. The problem is, the person can't describe the illness because the describing apparatus itself is sick.

Once you take action—once you enter that valley of the shadow—be prepared to feel some guilt. How can you know for sure, after all, that you have not unleashed still more trouble and angst?

Wornell's advice for the guilt-afflicted is this: "If someone you care for is in trouble, don't feel too guilty about calling for help. After all, the healthier person would walk in and get help himself, but your friend cannot, so you must do it for him."

RIGHTS FOR THE COMMITTED

The patient involuntarily committed to the psychiatric ward of a hospital must, de facto, relinquish many of the rights American citizens take for granted. These patients lose the right to determine their own medical treatment; to decide who they meet with and when; and, perhaps most dramatically, to control if and when they may leave.

However, the system does provide safeguards so that abuses of the mental health system do not occur. Patients in New York State, for instance, can request legal counsel through the Mental Hygiene Legal Service, and thus fight for a say in their treatment and hospitalization. (Each locality will have its own service; check with your local government for yours.)

The entries below reflect the "Notice of Status and Rights" given to each patient upon admission to the hospital (though some wording has been changed here):

· Based upon the certificates of two examining physicians, whose findings have been confirmed by a member of the psychiatric staff of this hospital, you have been admitted as an involuntary-status patient to this hospital which provides care and treatment for persons with mental illness. You may be kept in the hospital for a period of up to sixty days from the date of your admission, unless you have had a court hearing. During this sixty-day period you may be released, or converted to voluntary or informal status, if you are willing to continue inpatient care and treatment and are suitable for such status.

· You, and anyone acting on your behalf, should feel free to ask hospital staff about your condition, your status, and your rights under the Mental Hygiene Law, and the rules and regulations of this hospital.

· If you, or those acting on your behalf, believe that you do not need involuntary care and treatment, you or they may make a written request for a court hearing. Copies of such a request will be forwarded by the hospital director to the appropriate court and the Mental Hygiene Legal Service.

· The Mental Hygiene Legal Service, a court agency independent of this hospital, can provide you and your family with protective legal services, advice, and assistance, including representation, with regard to your hospitalization. You are entitled to be informed of your rights regarding hospitalization and treatment, and have a right to a court hearing, to be represented by a lawyer and to seek independent medical opinion.

Chapter 12

Trauma!: Emergency Care for the Gravely Injured

T he haunting story of John Lennon's assassination on December 8, 1980, has become a national legend, a tale told and retold for its deeper meaning—for the shadow it casts on us all. But as many times as you've heard the story, how many times have you heard it from the vantage point of John Lennon's doctor, the emergency physician who struggled to bring him back to life? That doctor was Stephan Lynn, MD, director of the Department of Emergency Medicine at Roosevelt Hospital the night John Lennon died.

"It was about two minutes of eleven when I got the call that a shooting to the chest had come in and they thought it was John Lennon," recalls Lynn, who arrived at the emergency department within minutes. "The emergency staff and surgical staff were already poised and ready to roll. Fortunately, Dr. Richard Marks, one of our cardiovascular surgeons, lived across the street from John Lennon. He saw the shooting on his way home from the hospital, while still in his car. He just turned around and came back."

Evaluating the patient, Lynn, Marks, and the surgical chief resident in the ED, David Halloran, found four gunshot wounds to the chest and no breathing, no pulse, no blood pressure. The bleeding was profuse. "We performed an emergency thoracotomy in an effort to stop the bleeding," says Lynn. It was his only chance. But it was just too late. His injuries were too significant and he had already bled to death.

"The staff did not initially recognize John Lennon in death," recalls Lynn, whose physician's eye duly noted the signs of fatal trauma. "He had no color, he was gaunt and thin. And then, as a doctor, you don't expect to see people you know in the ED. In fact, we weren't sure it was really John Lennon until Yoko Ono walked in."

For the public, the story had the stamp of modern tragedy, in which the random arm of fate can smite even our icons. For Yoko Ono, the loss was uniquely personal. For Steve Lynn, emergency physician, there was another meaning as well: Once the body has been violently assaulted by traumatic injury, once a knife rips the major arteries or several bullets rocket through the heart, he understood again that day, as on other days, that even the best of medical science may be too little, too late.

Lynn's announcement of the tragedy to the public is forever captured in a two-page picture in *Rolling Stone* magazine. But for him, the most indelible image came from breaking the news to the family. "Yoko Ono refused to accept it at first," recalls Lynn. "We had to tell her again and again. Like the rest of us, she couldn't believe it was true. And when the realization finally sank in, she had only one request—to go home and tell her son, Sean, before he saw it on TV."

Even when heroic efforts do not succeed, trauma specialists fending off the inevitable push their abilities to the brink. When lives are saved, it is because these persistent, hyperfocused, never-say-die specialists push the outside of the medical envelope. Sometimes they are unable to save a life; but often, especially today, given technical advances in the field, lives are saved. A decade after Lennon was shot, for instance, another deranged gunman walked into a New York City bus-repair depot in Manhattan and attempted to drive off with a bus. When police intervened, the angry man pulled out a gun. He fired in the direction of police, but hit an unsuspecting bus mechanic instead.

Sustaining an injury to his chest, much like Lennon, the mechanic was rushed by ambulance to the St. Luke's emergency department. Doctors quickly intubated him so he could breathe, inserted a chest tube to drain the blood and fluids seeping into the chest cavity, and rushed him to the operating room in the nick of time.

Here the ending was a happy one: The mechanic's wife came to the ED along with New York City Mayor Rudolph Giuliani, Lynn recalls. It was an uplifting experience. The mayor and the patient's wife exchanged Italian recipes, and the patient did well.

Guns, of course, constitute just one cause of traumatic injury regularly treated at Roosevelt and its sister institution, St. Luke's. To understand the nature of trauma, says Lynn, it's instructive to state what multiple trauma is *not*. It is not slipping on the ice and spraining an ankle or an arm, or even breaking a leg. Nor is it a series of bruises sustained while falling down a flight of steps, no matter how painful, or a laceration to the face, even if thirty-five stitches are required to repair the wound. Instead, multiple trauma generally occurs during an automobile accident at significant speed; during a fall from a height; or in an assault with a knife or a gun. It may include a head injury so severe that the victim loses consciousness; devastating injury to vital organs like the heart, kidneys, lungs, or brain; or the shattering of several bones throughout the body, especially those of the neck or spine.

When it comes to multiple trauma, injuries are not simply additive: There's a process of synergy in which the whole is vastly greater than the sum of the parts. The person who breaks two arms is in more than twice the danger, medically speaking, than the person who breaks just one. As more of your body is injured, you put more of the basics—the ABC's of airway, breathing, and circulation—at risk. And the risk increases geometrically with the number of injuries.

Trauma is best treated in a specialized trauma center designed, organized, and staffed to provide trauma care. Of course, all emergency departments can assess and stabilize the trauma patient—but *not* all can provide the specialized care these gravely injured patients need. A trauma center is not simply a supergood emergency department: It is the sort of soup-to-nuts facility that includes its own dedicated emergency staff, surgical staff, rehabilitative services, and even social workers with expertise in multiple trauma. In many regions, the trauma center includes a heliport as well as an ambulance port and the best in complex operating rooms and intensive care units. These facilities boast not just surgeons but also microsurgeons skilled at reattaching limbs; not just X-ray machines, but also CAT scans and MRI machines in-house.

In the best of all possible scenarios, trauma patients aboard the ambulance will be able to bypass the all-purpose, neighborhood emergency department and head directly to the designated trauma center. Sometimes that simply isn't possible: The patient is so badly injured that unless he is stabilized in a hospital within minutes, he will die. In that case, the ambulance may be forced to stop at the local ED to stabilize the patient. Then, once the patient is improved enough to make a longer journey, he will be moved.

The time constraints for lifesaving with singular killers like heart attack or shock are narrowed still more when it comes to multiple trauma. After all, if not just the heart or the circulatory system, but also the lungs and liver and a few bones are damaged, then the body has still fewer reserves, and can sustain itself for that much less time. When it comes to multiple trauma, the "golden hour" is absolutely ablaze with potential; but as the hour dwindles, the threat of death is high. If the patient gets to the hospital operating room in the first hour, chance of survival is dramatically increased. But since the system does not always work fast enough, many multiple-trauma victims die at the scene.

The first thing trauma specialists do is attend to the ABC's. "We basically resuscitate just as we resuscitate in cardiac arrest," explains Dr. Lynn. Following the tenets of basic life support, trauma specialists will first open the airway (if blocked), then restart breathing and stimulate circulation.

But though the principals of resuscitation are the same, when it comes to multiple trauma, the process is far more complex. For instance, the cervical spine might be broken; if so, opening the airway forcefully could jar the spine still more, possibly damaging the nerves running through the spine to the rest of the body, even causing paralysis. Until X-ray images have been obtained and the status of the spine determined, the patient may be moved only with cervical collar and backboard in place. And, such life-saving techniques as intubating or emergency tracheotomy—often performed with quick, rough movements—must instead be executed with gentleness and precision.

Finally, problems with circulation may be difficult to correct when the blood is flowing from so many ruptures and wounds, some clearly visible outside the body but others internal and completely invisible until the skilled hands of a surgeon have opened up the dying patient to hone in on the problem and attempt repair. Bleeding caused by pelvic injuries can be particularly deadly. Often injured in a fall, the pelvis sits in front of the bladder and next to the major vessels carrying blood from the abdomen to the legs; if crushed and not swiftly repaired, these ruptured organs and vessels can interrupt vital functions and empty the body of blood.

Anatomy of a Trauma

What actually happens to the trauma patient from the moment he or she enters the medical system until the time of release? For most of us, the answer seems murky.

Who wants to spend time preparing for traumatic injury, anyway? Just focusing on the possibility can seem like courting disaster, and life is hard enough without trying to figure out what would happen were we to be hit in the head with a bullet, struck by a train, or thrown off a roof. Odds are, we're almost as likely to win the lottery—and it's a lot more fun to focus on that.

Nonetheless, even a little preparation can go a long way toward handling yourself or advocating for a loved one should traumatic injury occur. The story below will not fit the particulars of every traumatic injury, but it should help explain what to expect when such injuries bring you to the ED.

It was one in the morning when the car crushed into a steel divider along the highway and came to a screeching halt. The driver, who had fallen asleep at the wheel for a microsecond, and her husband/passenger were both wearing seat belts. The air bags inflated. But that didn't stop the compact car, moving along at a clip of sixty-five miles an hour, from folding like an accordion, crushing those within. The car was so mangled, in fact, that paramedics and police on the scene had to remove the victims by cutting through the roof, windows, and doors with the metal-bending rescue tool called Jaws of Life. Due to the violent impact and the potential for crippling spinal injury, the victims were lifted out carefully, each one maintained in a fairly rigid position with cervical collar for the neck and a long board for the back.

On the side of the road, surrounded by paramedics, each victim was set up with an IV line and cardiac monitor. The first patient, the passenger, drifted in and out of consciousness, seemed to have a chest injury, and had broken his leg. Apparently in desperate need of care, he was flown to the trauma center via helicopter. The driver, wife of the passenger, seemed to be in better shape. Her leg, crushed in the accident, was set in a splint, but not much else seemed wrong. She was strapped to a backboard, loaded in an ambulance, and driven to the hospital over highways and city roads.

The helicopter arrived first, of course, and was greeted by a team of doctors and nurses specializing in trauma care. They ducked down, wind from the propellers still churning, and listened to the paramedics' report: "High-speed MVA [motor vehicle accident]; car struck the divider at the side of the road; both patients belted and air bags inflated; passenger has questionable LOC [loss of consciousness]; hit either ceiling or windshield, struck chest; significant pain, and obvious fracture, right leg. Vitals: 120 over 70; pulse 110 and respiration, 32."

The patient was quickly, but very carefully, passed from the stretcher aboard the copter to a hospital stretcher and rolled into the emergency department. The first thing the doctor did was ask the patient to describe the accident. The purpose was to decide whether or not the patient had suffered any head injury. Was he conscious and lucid? Was he neurologically impaired or intact? The physician also asked the patient whether he had lost consciousness. "I'm not sure," he answered.

Then the doctor asked, "Where does it hurt?" Now the patient was emphatic: "I have a headache, my chest hurts, and my right leg is killing me."

During this exchange, nurses placed the patient on the hospital's cardiac monitor, a machine sophisticated enough to track not just heart rate, but also other vital signs, including oxygen saturation of the blood. The physician assessed the ABC's—the openness of the airway, the ability to breathe, and the circulation of the blood, then watched the patient breathe, examining especially the up-and-down movement of the ribs, and listened to the chest—the sounds of lungs and heart.

Noticing a distinct muffling and quietness in place of normal beating heart sounds, the doctor ordered a central venous line—an IV line placed in a large vein of the body for rapid delivery of medicine directly to the heart. But the doctor wasn't concerned only about what seemed like an injury to the heart. Remembering the questionable loss of consciousness, the doctor began to worry that the patient may have been bleeding near the brain. Other serious injuries, including neck and pelvic fracture, remained possibilities as well. Compared to these life-threatening problems, the obvious leg fracture paled; treating the leg would come only after other, life-threatening possibilities had been resolved.

To check out the damage, the physician ordered X rays of the neck, chest, pelvis, and injured leg. The images, created by X-ray machines slung overhead on movable caddies right in the trauma room were reassuring: There was no spinal fracture, so the cervical collar and long backboard were removed. The pelvis was intact; ribs were intact, though there was a fracture of the sternum, or breastbone. An echocardiogram of the heart was ordered and, amazingly, the medical team discovered, the heart, though slightly bruised, was more or less fine.

During this time, trauma room nurses stood by the patient and, like scribes, continued to assess the patient and record the vital signs: pulse, blood pressure, and oxygenation of the blood. They also tended to the IV bags, which continued to deliver fluids, and to the patient's urine output dripping from a catheter into a bottle alongside the bed.

Now the doctor could get to the injured leg. A severe compound fracture with the bone jutting through the skin required that the doctor irrigate and cleanse the wound and set the bone back in place. Then he applied a temporary splint to hold it steady, and a dressing. Soon, an orthopedist arrived to set a permanent cast, and this patient, an extraordinarily lucky man, was released—not to go home, of course, but for observation in intensive care.

His wife, sent in by ambulance because her injuries seemed less severe, did not fare so well. Arriving at the emergency department ten minutes after her husband, she too was greeted by the medical team. They instantly realized her journey in the ambulance had been a downhill slide. During the drive, paramedics had realized that in addition to a leg injury, she had apparently struck her left shoulder, now throbbing with pain, and was complaining of pressure in the abdomen. The paramedics also discovered fractures in the left side of her chest. For this patient, the pulse had held steady, but blood pressure was plummeting fast.

As with the first patient, physicians asked questions to assess neurological damage. The patient insisted she had not lost consciousness, but indicated that her shoulder and left side hurt. Doctors went on to assess the ABC's—the basics of an open airway, breathing, and circulation. The airway was clear, but the patient was having trouble breathing because of significant injury to the left side of her chest. Not only was her chest bruised, it also moved up and down in irregular fashion, suggesting several broken ribs. Even more worrisome, the doctors listening to the sound of her breathing could not hear a thing on the left side of her chest, suggesting a collapsed lung. This patient, originally thought to have sustained just a broken leg, might not pull through.

The doctors decided to insert a chest tube on the left side, and when air and blood came out, they realized their hunch about the collapsed lung was correct. They also ordered X rays. As was obvious through visual exam, the lower right leg and upper right arm, just below the shoulder bone, were broken; there were multiple rib fractures as well. Fortunately, the pelvic film was normal, but X rays of the abdominal cavity suggested the area was fluid-filled. A low blood count indicated that liquid filling the cavity was most likely gushing blood.

These doctors had to work fast; here is where all that training, all that right-brain deftness acquired over many thousands of hours in emergency played a role. There was no time to reflect, no time to fumble around and cast for solutions like the untrained residents in hospitals on television. In this real-world, life-and-death situation, the ED doctors must act with speed, and nothing else would do.

To supplement the patient's labored breathing, which had now produced an oxygen deficit in the blood, a physician inserted an endoctracheal tube and then placed the patient on a ventilator. Next, to prove the theory that the body was bleeding inside, emptying blood into the abdominal cavity, the doctor made a tiny cut in the abdomen, just below the navel, and a clear-plastic tube was slipped through. The tube was filled with saline solution, and when that solution turned blood-red, the answer was clear. The blood flowing freely through the saline solution indicated extensive internal bleeding. The bleeding had to be stopped at once, or the patient would die.

The woman was rushed from emergency to the operating room for exploratory surgery to pinpoint the source of all that bleeding in her abdomen so that it could be repaired. After hearing the risks and benefits of surgery, the patient and her husband agreed to go ahead. The procedure began. The operation was difficult: Surgeons found the blood was due to a laceration of the liver, and were unable to stem the flow with straightforward sutures. Finally, after replacing almost all of the patient's blood through transfusion, they were able to control the bleeding with simple pressure and medicine to promote clotting. After the operation, a pulmonologist was called in to attend to the collapsed and badly bruised lung; that organ was so severely damaged, the patient had to remain in intensive care, where breathing could be aided with a respirator for the next two to three days. Finally, an orthopedist arrived to set and cast the broken leg and place the broken arm in a sling.

While all this was unfolding, relatives were notified: two children, three elderly parents, and a brother. Aware of these concerned family members, the trauma team, including a social worker, poked in and out of intensive care and the recovery room to explain the treatment and prognosis for their patients. Thankfully, both pulled through.

It's worth noting here how tricky multiple trauma can be. The patient deemed most injured at the outset was actually in better shape. The person diagnosed with a mere broken leg was bleeding to death inside. That's the nature of multiple trauma: The event itself is so shocking, so mind-numbing, that it's often simply not possible for the victim to identify all the areas of pain and discomfort, all the things within the body actually going awry. And paramedics, after all, are not psychic: Without the diagnostic tools of the emergency department, they are limited as to what they can see.

Though the above description has been lengthy, in real time such events go by in a flash. From the arrival in the emergency department of the first patient to the departure (to surgery) of the second patient, perhaps thirty minutes had passed. With some luck and much skill on the part of the ED and trauma staff, those patients would live. But for the trauma team at the hospital, this chapter was closed. Patients dismissed, the medical team left the trauma room in the hands of housecleaning for a while. Soon, the room looked as before: computerized cardiac monitors blinking at the ready; movable surgical lights for the moment turned off; and overhead X-ray equipment pushed to the side. All was set for the next trauma victim to come through the doors.

MULTIPLE TRAUMA: The Most Common Traumatic Injuries from Head to Foot

Head trauma: Resulting most often from a fall, a car accident, or a gunshot, head trauma is characterized by bleeding around the brain. Head injuries are so lethal because the skull, by design, is fixed in volume without the ability to expand. The brain, on the other hand, is very soft and easily damaged. Anytime an injury results in bleeding inside the skull—usually called subdural hematoma or epidural hematoma—there is pressure on and distortion of the brain. The pressure and distortion translate into brain damage. In order to prevent permanent brain damage or death, physicians must identify bleeding fast—usually by CAT scan. After diagnosis, urgent surgical intervention is a must: Physicians generally drill through the skull to drain the blood and relieve the pressure on the brain.

Facial injury: A large number of complex injuries may damage the bones of the face and jaw. There may be breaks or fractures of single bones or many bones on one or both sides of the face. Facial bones may be cracked or shattered, causing deformity to the eyes, nose, teeth, or face. The most life-threatening of these facial injuries is a break, swelling, or hemorrhage that causes blockage of the airway. To treat this, trauma experts generally insert a breathing tube through the mouth or perform a tracheotomy. CAT scans are required before surgeons can operate to correct the damage. Like the shell of an egg, facial bones can easily shatter but, unlike Humpty Dumpty, can be put back together relatively easily.

Broken neck: This is among the most potentially damaging of multiple traumas. If the spinal cord passing through the neck is damaged, sensory and motor function will vanish below that point, and the individual will become quadriplegic—unable to move arms or legs. Fractures to the bones of the neck may initially cause limited pain or dysfunction, but if the neck is subsequently pulled or twisted, injury can become crippling or life-threatening. As a result, the use of a cervical collar and backboard is critical. If the neck injury is associated with swelling or bruising that may obstruct the airway, emergency physicians will intubate the patient with the utmost gentleness and care.

Larynx injury (voicebox): Made out of cartilage, the larynx is rubbery and bendable, but easy to damage. The voicebox is generally injured as the result of direct trauma—for instance, when someone gets punched, shot, or stabbed in the neck. The patient with a damaged voicebox has difficulty speaking, of course, and may experience significant pain; but more important, this individual may experience swelling and bruising that can obstruct the airway. If doctors note the potential for airway obstruction, the patient will be intubated before anything else is done. Then physicians will attempt to hone in on the specific damage. If the patient has not been intubated, and if broken bones are suspected, the larynx will be examined through "flexible laryngoscopy," in which a thin tube is inserted into the larynx through the mouth. If the patient has been intubated, physicians will diagnose the extent and location of fractures through a CAT scan. Careful surgical reconstruction may be necessary.

Collapsed lung: Major trauma in the form of a blunt blow or penetrating injury to the chest can cause the lungs to collapse on one or both sides. If both lungs have collapsed, the untreated patient cannot survive, because collapsed lungs cannot ventilate or oxygenate the blood. And without oxygen in the blood, the body's cells and vital organs cannot ultimately prevail. In addition, since multiple trauma often results in internal hemorrhage, blood may accumulate inside the body where the intact lung used to be. The treatment of choice for the collapsed lung is insertion of clear-plastic chest tubes through the chest wall and under local anesthesia, removal of accumulated air, fluid, or blood, thus enabling the lung to re-expand.

Rib fractures: Though doctors do not generally set or wrap a single broken rib, numerous rib fractures can cause severe pain and difficulty breathing; in fact, patients with multiple adjacent fractured ribs may suffer respiratory failure. In the emergency department this condition can actually be seen in the form of what physicians call a flail chest—in which a segment of the chest wall actually becomes detached from the rest of the chest and appears to move in the "wrong" direction with breathing. Treatment will depend upon the patient's respiratory status. If the patient continues to breathe easily, emergency department doctors will keep that person comfortable and quiet and deliver some supplemental oxygen through a nasal cannula. However, if the patient is struggling to breathe, doctors will investigate the underlying condition of the lungs. Depending upon what they find, they may intubate to assist with respiration while pumping oxygen into the lungs in order to expand and stabilize the chest cavity.

Myocardial contusion: This is an injury to the heart caused by direct trauma such as a blow. In the emergency department, a myocardial contusion in the form of bruised heart muscle may be difficult to diagnose because the usual heart monitoring instruments, including the EKG, may not be that revealing. A special echocardiogram done with ultrasound may be helpful. The reason: Myocardial contusion does not necessarily result in irregular heartbeat or, in fact, compromise cardiac output. In treating this injury, physicians tend to treat the symptoms. Cardiac arrhythmia, for instance, will be treated with the corresponding protocol and medications.

Injured liver or spleen: The liver and spleen are most commonly injured as the result of blunt trauma. These two solid organs require a large blood supply for normal functioning. When they are injured, therefore, the bleeding that results can be profuse. The problem is complicated because, though potentially life-threatening, these injuries are not that painful. In liver injuries some pain will present in the right-upper quadrant of the abdomen, while in the case of an injured spleen, pain may present in the left-upper quadrant. In addition to the absence of intense pain, doctors simply cannot *see* the blood draining into the patient's peritoneal cavity, and thus, it may be difficult to make a diagnosis. These patients may be tested for abdominal bleeding with thin tubes inserted into the abdomen itself; if blood rises through the clear-plastic tubing, doctors assume abdominal bleeding. CAT scans or ultrasound may also document the presence of bleeding from an injured spleen or liver. In that case the patient may receive transfusions, and may be rushed into surgery for repair of the damage.

Penetrating injury to abdomen: In this type of injury, usually inflicted by a knife or bullet, the intestine may be pierced, spilling intestinal material into the abdominal cavity. This situation can be extremely painful, and must be discovered and surgically repaired as soon as possible.

Fractures: Fractures generally occur in the extremities. In traumatic accidents, long bones are most frequently broken and require splinting either by the emergency physician or an orthopedist. Sometimes broken bones pierce the skin in an "open fracture," creating the potential for infection. These wounds are carefully cleaned and the bones set before a cast is applied. The patient will receive intravenous antibiotics.

Fracture of the pelvis: In this critical injury, the pelvis is usually crushed or fractured in a fall. The injury may be life-threatening because of the vital structures next to the pelvis, and because of the blood vessels running through it. First of all, the bladder sits right behind the pelvis, and is subject to damage by pelvic bones. What's more, blood vessels running from the abdomen to the legs may be ruptured, and internal bleeding may result. If the pelvis has fractured without damaging adjacent organs and vessels, the primary treatment is bed rest. If blood is being lost, the patient may be rushed to surgery. If the pelvic break is so severe the body has been destabilized, surgeons will operate and hold the pelvis together with nuts and bolts.

OPERATION TRAUMA: **Three Lifesaving Techniques for Victims of Trauma**

When they are stable enough, trauma patients in need of surgery will almost always be rushed to the operating room, where surgeons will do the job for which they are trained. In a dedicated trauma center, where surgeons are part of the round-the-clock staff, they will generally be called in to stem internal bleeding or repair severe laceractions and shattered bones. When the victim of trauma is brought to the hospital's emergency department, physicians there use the following lifesaving surgical techniques to stabilize the patient.

Thoracotomy: This surgical procedure is performed in the emergency department on rare occasions, when severe injury to the chest or heart damages the associated blood vessels. There is enough room inside the chest cavity, on either side of the heart, to accommodate all the blood in the body—about ten pints for the average adult—should that much internal bleeding occur. If a traumatic injury creates a big enough hole in the heart, the individual will literally bleed to death internally. Every time the heart beats, blood will squirt out, and eventually, the tank will run dry. The result is something doctors call traumatic cardiac arrest—the situation in which the heart keeps beating until all the blood is gone, and then the patient dies. The same six to eight minutes that physicians have to respond to medical cardiac arrest applies here: If the bleeding isn't treated within six to eight minutes of onset, the patient will die. Enter the emergency thoracotomy: Emergency physicians will make an incision between the ribs on the left side of the chest below the nipple. Scouring the area for the source of bleeding, the doctors will literally put a finger inside the chest cavity and plug the flow like the proverbial boy plugging the dike. Then they will suture the wound closed with a special catheter. Once stabilized, the patient will be rushed to the operating room for a more definitive surgical solution.

Peritoneal lavage: To test for internal bleeding, emergency physicians will make a tiny nick in the skin or muscle below the belly button. They will then insert a catheter filled with a sterile saline solution. If the solution turns bloody, it's a sign of internal bleeding, and a trip to the operating room—where surgeons can find the source of the blood and stem the flow—is next.

External fixation of broken bones: Doctors will perform this procedure to hold shattered bones in place. Generally performed not by the emergency physician, but by an orthopedist, and usually performed in the operating room, the procedure involves insertion of a screw or pin through the bone above the point of the break, and another pin through the bone below the point of the break. The two pins, which run through the bones like skewers, are then attached to each other outside the leg or arm with an external bridging device, so that the bones fit back together and are held in place. An external fixation apparatus may stay in place for weeks or months, until the bone has healed. This procedure is used most often in instances where the fracture is open or infected.

How to Be an Advocate in the Event of Personal Multiple Trauma or on Behalf of Someone Else

The last thing most of us would think of doing in the event of a traumatic accident or injury is intervening in the ensuing medical care. After all, if ever you had to put your faith in the hands of a doctor or hospital, the time is now. What choice do you have? That airway must be cleared, that heart must be restarted, that bleeding must be stopped—and pronto—or you or the victim for whom you are advocate will die. When it comes to multiple trauma, time is of the essence. It's hardly in your best interest to demand a lot of small things from hospital staff when they are working frantically to save your life or the life of your dear friend or relative. In the case of multiple trauma, more than perhaps in any other situation, the patient as self-advocate, as consumer, must step back so the medical professional can act *now*.

Trauma is never expected, but before you ever suffer multiple trauma, there are some things you *can* do in the event of personal medical trauma to ensure that things go as smoothly as possible:

Make some decisions in advance. Decide whether or not you want to donate your organs. Decide whether or not you want to be resuscitated in the event you will not be able to communicate following an injury. Whatever your decision, make it known in the form of documentation—a living will—and in the knowledge base of relatives and friends (see Chapter 13). Since you won't necessarily have your living will with you at the hospital, if you have communicated your feelings to someone close to you and have let that individual know where your living will is, you can make your feelings known.

Make sure relevant information concerning medications, health history, and identification can be found easily in your wallet. Furthermore, putting such information on a Medic Alert bracelet may help you communicate even if no one is with you.

When the Accident Occurs

· Do not move the patient unless that person is in the line of an explosive or some other deadly situation or device; likewise, if you are the victim.

· Call 911 as quickly as possible.

· Describe (or have the patient describe) pain and discomfort as quickly and precisely as possible. The injured individual may lose consciousness and if that happens, will no longer be able to provide signposts to problems, especially those that cannot be readily seen.

When the Ambulance Arrives

· Ask paramedics if the injury is serious enough to qualify for a designated trauma center as opposed to the regular emergency department. Believe it or not, paramedics might not think of it.

· Have a relative or friend ask questions on your behalf if you cannot yourself. While no one wants to stop a paramedic from doing the job, it is important to keep track of which medical treatment is being delivered, and why—whether it's on your own behalf, or for the person you're helping.

At the Hospital

· If you are the patient, ask staff to notify friends and relatives on your behalf immediately. You may be put under anesthesia quickly, and then nurses or doctors will not know whom to call.

· If you are in pain, be sure to tell the staff.

· Have a relative or friend ask questions on your behalf if you cannot. While no one wants to stop a nurse or physician from doing the job, it is important to keep track of which medical treatment is being delivered, and why.

Chapter 13

Final Journeys: Death and Dying in the Emergency Department

It was just after midnight on a frigid day in February when the dying woman, age ninety, was rushed to the Roosevelt Hospital emergency department. Afflicted with a longstanding case of lung disease, she had recently been given codeine to ease the worsening pain. Now, with her younger sister by her side, the old woman hovered near death. Though paramedics had stabilized her during the ambulance trip to the hospital, she could barely breathe.

Evaluating the situation, emergency physicians on call at Roosevelt found the level of oxygen in the woman's blood to be dangerously low; she was in grave danger and without intervention would probably die within hours.

Of course, there *were* things they could do. To make the woman more comfortable, they could set up an IV line for delivering fluid and nutrients; and they could supplement her deficient blood with oxygen delivered by mask. These interventions would enable the patient to die within hours, in comfort and peace. To help her survive the crisis, however, would require more aggressive treatments, including a breathing tube and ventilation with machines.

The woman herself was unconscious but, given the choice, her sister didn't think for long. "My sister has told me she does not want to be resuscitated," she explained to the doctors. "Let her go in peace." At ease with the decision, the Roosevelt staff went about making the sick old woman as comfortable as they possibly could.

Within an hour, however, the sister had called other relatives, including the patient's son. Rushing into the emergency department, frantic and confused, the son insisted his mother be given every chance of survival. "That," he asserted, "is what she would want us to do."

Emergency physicians were at a loss. They, themselves, could not make philosophical or legal decisions regarding a patient. They had no way of knowing whether the son's version or the sister's reflected the patient's inner feelings—she was unconscious and had left no documentation in the form of a living will. Finally, the sister reversed herself, siding with the son, and doctors rolled out the heavy artillery. The patient survived the emergency department and was transferred to a room upstairs. The ED doctors gave her forty-eight hours to live, but word came down that she lasted just twenty-four.

"We couldn't have known the patient's wishes," explains emergency department director Stephan Lynn, "though we felt aggressive intervention would bring her nothing but pain. In the face of her silence, we found ourselves catering to what seemed like the family's fear and guilt. But legally, we had no recourse. We couldn't do anything else."

Like this old woman with lung disease, the gravely ill and injured face death in the emergency department every day. Death has many faces, but especially with the advent of sophisticated medical technology, so does life. There is life in the full flower of youth and vigor, and life that requires a slower pace with the help of drugs. There is life in a wheelchair, without the use of legs; life as a quadriplegic, using eye blinks to communicate; and life as a human vegetable, governed by no central consciousness at all. These distinctions assume special importance in the emergency department, because the grievously ill and dying, who arrive without advance warning, often have little input into decisions governing their fate—unless, of course, they have prepared in advance.

In this chapter, we will discuss the steps you can take to ensure that when it comes to the end, your wishes are honored. Would you like doctors to pull out all the stops and use every trick in the book to bring you back from the brink? Or, does the thought of languishing for weeks or years on a ventilator, inspire dread? When is it appropriate to expect that doctors will cease their efforts? And when, despite what seem like your explicit instructions, are they correct in extending your life—perhaps for years?

There are other questions as well: Should you die in the hospital, would you like to donate your organs? Should you lose consciousness, who has the authority to make decisions that will impact your care? When can a visit to the emergency department make dying less painful? And when is it appropriate, despite a terminal illness, to refuse to go to the hospital under any circumstance at all?

Final Wishes: How to Plan for Death

Contrary to popular opinion, there is a fate worse than death. Just ask the family of Nancy Cruzan. In 1982, a devastating car accident left the then-twenty-five-year-old

Missouri woman severely brain damaged, in what doctors called a "persistent vegetative state," her life sustained through nourishment from a feeding tube implanted in her stomach. Five years later, Cruzan's parents began their crusade to have their daughter taken off life support, claiming that Nancy herself would have wanted to die. The case went all the way to the Supreme Court. In June of 1990, in a five-to-four decision, the justices blocked the family from withholding food and water in the absence of "clear and convincing" evidence that Nancy would have wanted it that way. Eventually, former coworkers from a Missouri cheese plant testified they recalled her saying she would never want to live "like a vegetable." A state judge ruled that the evidence existed and gave permission, on December 14, 1990, to remove the tube. Nancy Cruzan lived for twelve more days and then, mercifully, she died.

Cruzan's hellish journey, and the landmark decision that released her from life, paved the way for a new level of choice in dying. The tools of that choice, now available to everyone, are what experts call "advance directives": documents that allow individuals to communicate wishes for their future medical care if, for some reason, they are unable to make them known themselves.

The first of these tools, known in New York State as the health care proxy, enables you to appoint someone you trust to make decisions about your medical care if you cannot make those decisions yourself. The appointee—your proxy—is authorized to deal with *all* medical decisions when you cannot speak for yourself, though the law holds this individual must make the same decisions you yourself would have made, if possible. If your wishes about a particular situation are unknown, your proxy must act in your best interest, using his or her own best judgment.

To make your wishes known, moreover, you may execute another advance directive: the "living will." Through the living will you may specify whether you want to be maintained on life support, under what circumstances, and for how long. If hospital authorities or a court of law should question your proxy's decision, your living will can set them straight.

Health care proxy requirements may vary from state to state. For St. Luke's–Roosevelt Hospital patients and all others treated in New York State, however, the nonprofit group Choice in Dying, Inc. suggests the form below. If you do not live in New York State, you may contact your state health department or Choice in Dying at (800) 989-WILL (9455) for the appropriate document.

THE HEALTH CARE PROXY

(1) I, _____hereby appoint
   (print name)

_____
   (name, address, and telephone number of proxy)

_____

as my health care agent to make any and all health care decisions for me, except to the extent that I state otherwise.

   This health care proxy shall take effect in the event I become unable to make my own health care decisions.

(2) Optional instructions: I direct my proxy to make health care decisions in accord with my wishes and limitations as stated below, or as he or she otherwise knows.

_____

_____

_____

_____

   (Unless your agent knows your wishes about artificial nutrition and hydration [feeding tubes], your agent will not be allowed to make decisions about artificial nutrition and hydration.)

(3) Name of substitute or fill-in proxy if the person I appoint above is unable or unwilling or unavailable to act as my health care agent.

_____

(name, home address, and telephone number of alternative proxy)

_____

(4) Unless I revoke it, this proxy shall remain in effect indefinitely, or until the date or condition I have stated below. This proxy shall expire (specific date or conditions, if desired): _____

_____

(5) Signature_____Date _____

Address

_____

Statement by witnesses (must be age 18 or older)

I declare that the person who signed this document is personally known to me and appears to be of sound mind and acting of his or her own free will. He or she signed (or asked another to sign for him or her) this document in my presence. I am not the person appointed as proxy by this document.

Witness 1 _____

Address _____

Witness 2 _____

Address _____

Living will requirements vary to some degree from state to state. For St. Luke's–Roosevelt Hospital patients and all others treated in New York State, the non-profit group Choice in Dying, Inc. suggests the form below. If you do not live in New York State, you may contact your state health department or Choice in Dying at (800) 989-WILL (9455) for the appropriate document.

THE LIVING WILL

I, _____ , being of sound mind, make this statement as a directive to be followed if I become permanently unable to participate in decisions regarding my medical care. These instructions reflect my firm and settled commitment to decline medical treatment under the circumstances indicated below:

I direct my attending physician to withhold or withdraw treatment that merely prolongs my dying, if I should be in an incurable or irreversible mental or physical condition with no reasonable expectation of recovery.

These instruments apply if I am (a) in a terminal condition; (b) permanently unconscious; or (c) if I am minimally conscious but have irreversible brain damage and will never regain the ability to make decisions and express my wishes.

I direct that my treatment be limited to measures to keep me comfortable and to relieve pain, including any pain that might occur by withholding or withdrawing treatment.

While I understand that I am not legally required to be specific about future treatments if I am in the condition(s) described above, I feel especially strongly about the following forms of treatment (Please cross out any statements with which you do not agree):

I do not want cardiac resuscitation.
I do not want mechanical resuscitation.
I do not want artificial nutrition and hydration.
I do not want antibiotics.

However, I do want maximum pain relief, even if it may hasten my death.

Other directions: (Add personal instructions).

_____

_____

_____

_____

These directions express my legal right to refuse treatment, under the law of New York. I intend my instructions to be carried out, unless I have rescinded them in a new writing or by clearly indicating that I have changed my mind.

Signature_____Date _____

Address

_____

Statement by witnesses (must be age 18 or older)

I declare that the person who signed this document is personally known to me and appears to be of sound mind and acting of his or her own free will. He or she signed (or asked another to sign for him or her) this document in my presence.

Witness 1 _____

Address _____

Witness 2 _____

Address _____

Who Should Utilize These Documents?

According to Anna Moretti, legal affairs coordinator for the New York City–based nonprofit group Choice in Dying, just about anyone who wishes to.

"About 80 percent of us will die in a medical facility such as a hospital or nursing home, where medical technology can now prolong life as never before," Moretti notes.

"The quality of that life, however, may be greatly reduced. As a result, many patients, families, and caregivers face difficult questions about how much technology to use when the patient cannot get better, but dying can be prolonged. That means that most of us will face a decision about whether to use life-sustaining medical treatments at the end of our lives. If we can't speak for ourselves at that point, and if we have not made our wishes known, other people will have to make that decision for us."

And remember, without clear evidence of your wishes, health care practitioners will often continue treatment—not only because they are trained to do so, but also to protect themselves from lawsuits.

WHAT TO DO AFTER YOU HAVE EXECUTED YOUR HEALTH CARE PROXY AND LIVING WILL

Keep the original signed documents in a secure, accessible place.

Give photocopies of the original documents to your health care proxy, alternate health care proxy, your doctors, family members, and close friends; in short, to anyone who might become involved in your health care.

Discuss your wishes with your health care proxy, alternate proxy, family, and physicians, so that they understand exactly what you want. Leave no room for interpretation of the written documents.

END GAME: **Why Extraordinary Intervention Can Hurt the Terminally Ill**

Ever wonder why the living will highlights certain treatments and not others? Here's the rundown on the most aggressive medical interventions, and why they may sometimes be undesirable for someone who is dying:

Tube feeding: Including artificial nutrition and hydration, tubes provide nutrition and fluid to the body. As temporary measures, they may simply keep a patient nourished while the body heals. Some patients depend on permanent feeding tubes for their sustenance, yet still have fulfilling lives. Problems with the use of artificial nutrition emerge when terminally ill patients have suffered irreversible brain damage. The feeding tube can stave off dying for years, but will not change the underlying condition, and may actually cause infections or pneumonia.

Artificial respiration: A respirator can deliver oxygen to the vital organs, keeping a patient alive. But the patient who has been deprived of oxygen for more than eight minutes will nonetheless suffer irreversible brain damage, something the respirator can never correct once the damage has occurred. Like a feeding tube, a respirator can stave off death for a long period of time, but will not cure the underlying problem.

Cardiopulmonary resuscitation: This procedure saves untold lives. But for the terminally ill, sudden cardiac arrest may be the easiest, least painful way to go. For the patient whose death is imminent, CPR will not save the person's life, just prolong the dying process and the pain.

Antibiotics: Antibiotics may cure an ancillary infection that would have killed the patient painlessly. But they will not cure a terminal illness like cancer. By preventing a painless death, antibiotics can prolong the agony of dying.

Crisis of Conscience: Will Your Advance Directives Be Honored in the Emergency Department?

Will emergency physicians honor your advance directives 100 percent of the time? No, nor would you want them to. Remember, the documents will be activated only when doctors have diagnosed you as terminal or irreversibly brain damaged, with zero chance of regaining consciousness or of survival. Obviously, in the event of emergency, physicians cannot make that diagnosis immediately. If you have been injured in a car accident or an explosion, emergency department doctors will not activate the provisions of your living will before they have exhausted every possible means of saving your life.

True, your living will may specify your aversion to the respirator. But the spirit of the document is clear: You would not want to languish on a respirator *if* you had no hope of recovery. However, since emergency physicians have not yet determined that you are terminal—and that you will die even with treatment—they may use all the tools at their disposal, including a respirator, to bring you around.

And who would want it any other way? You may be plagued by the memory of poor Uncle Max, whose last five weeks on the respirator were a torment to his family. But that was Max. For you, the respirator may be transitional—a temporary tool the doctors are using until you can breathe on your own. Likewise, if you have suffered a heart attack and your living will states no cardiopulmonary resuscitation, it's obviously with the understanding that CPR is to be avoided *only* if you are going to die anyway. Your heart attack may be quite treatable. You may have many more years of high-quality life before you. And therefore, no matter what your living will says, and no matter how hard your health care proxy argues to activate it, emergency physicians will usually perform the CPR.

The bottom line is this: Your health care agent, or proxy, will be able to act for you when you are no longer able to make health care decisions for yourself, no matter what your underlying medical problem. However, a *medical* determination of your capacity must be made by a doctor before the power of the proxy can be assumed; moreover, the proxy's decisions *must be* medically informed, necessitating an explanation of treatments and procedures *by a physician*. That is why the proxy cannot act in the ambulance, outside the hospital setting.

As far as your living will is concerned, it will be activated when a doctor finds you to be in whatever condition has been spelled out by the document, *and* when you are no longer able to make decisions for yourself.

If ED physicians do finally diagnose a patient as terminal, if they find irreversible brain damage or irrefutable evidence of an inevitable, agonizing death, they will honor that patient's wishes as spelled out in a living will.

Do Not Resuscitate: When Ambulance Workers Can Cease and Desist

While advance directives such as living wills and health care proxies will be honored in the emergency department of your hospital, EMTs and paramedics will not be able to comply on an ambulance. These workers have one mandate: to keep the patient alive until he reaches the emergency department. If you call paramedics and they find the patient's heart has stopped, they *must* perform CPR. It's the law.

There are good reasons for this rule. Emergency Medical Service workers are *not* physicians, and they cannot make medical diagnoses. Therefore, they cannot take the basic step of declaring the patient terminal. It would be too easy to make a mistake.

There is one exception: EMS workers may provide the dying with comfort but hold back on aggressive interventions when that patient has what is called a "Nonhospital Do Not Resuscitate Order," often referred to as the DNR by paramedics.

The story of one Ohio resident makes the need for this document clear. "My husband had a seizure and was gone before the paramedics arrived," the woman wrote to the Choice in Dying staff in New York. "As they came in I said he was no longer breathing and had no pulse, to which one of them agreed. I also said that we had living wills. They said something to the effect of, 'Oh, you do?' Nonetheless, they proceeded to give him CPR, including electric shock to the heart. They had him breathing, I could see that.

"They proceeded to the hospital, where they continued working on him. I immediately told the nurse about our living wills. She replied, 'I'm so glad you told me.' She spun on her heels and entered the cubicle in which they had my husband: shortly thereafter we were informed he was gone.

"My question is, what did I have to do, have my living will tattooed on my forehead? How can I be sure *I* will not be resuscitated?"

The answer is the DNR, currently available in about half the states, with more signing on each month. But this document should be obtained with caution. Notes Anna Moretti of Choice in Dying, "The Nonhospital 'Do Not Resuscitate' order is *not* something everyone should rush right out to get. It is meant for people whose frailty or ill health gives them little chance of surviving and recovering from CPR."

We offer one last point: Paramedics are legally bound to resuscitate unless they actually *see* the DNR on an official Department of Health form. Therefore, terminally ill patients who do not wish to be resuscitated are advised to carry the order with them at all times.

Gift of Life: How to Donate Organs in the Emergency Department

You never know when a tragic car accident, a sudden heart attack, or a random gunshot wound will rob you of life. But it is possible to leave a legacy. If you have prepared in advance, you can donate your tissue (including the cornea of the eyes and the skin) or organs to others who may use them to live.

If you wish to make this donation, you can indicate your intent easily, by signing an organ donor card that you carry with you at all times. Indeed, one is distributed to everyone who receives or renews a driver's license. You may also discuss your wish to donate with family members before an emergency occurs, because often, in the middle of a trauma, the last thing on family members' minds is donating a cornea, a heart, a liver or some bones. Yet the very act of donating organs or tissue can help in the grieving process, as family members see that at least some good has come from the tragedy, and that the individual's death has helped others live on.

Once family members have agreed to the donation, a team of experts will arrive promptly to recover the appropriate organs. If the deceased is donating tissue, including skin, corneas, heart muscle for valves, or bones, the procedures are performed within hours: Bones and valves must be removed within ten hours, and corneas and skin, within twenty-four.

Individuals donating organs like liver, kidney, heart, or lungs must be "maintained" on life support to nourish those organs and keep blood pressure stable, sometimes for days, until death is determined. The organs must be shipped immediately: Heart and lungs must be transplanted almost immediately; kidneys must be transplanted within twenty-four hours; and the pancreas and liver in less than twenty hours.

For the grieving, organ donation may be an act of closure—or a violation. For family members who have fought so hard to have a loved one removed from life support, the thought of sustaining that person through the transplant process may be too much to bear. Donating tissue and organs is a wonderful gift of life, but it is a decision that is personal. In considering this option, family members should, first and foremost, follow the wishes of the deceased. If those have not been clarified, advocates should simply act as they believe the individual would have wanted. One should never feel pressured to make this bequest by members of the hospital staff.

Last Rites: How to Advocate for the Dying and the Grieving in the Emergency Department

Even while dying, patients may benefit if a friend or relative can advocate for them in the emergency department. First and foremost, do make sure your dying relative or friend is comfortable. These days, doctors should have no problem providing the dying with as much medicine as they need to manage pain.

In addition, if you have been assigned the role of health care proxy, make sure you follow the wishes of the dying individual, in spirit, as specifically as you can. This means resisting pressure you may feel from other quarters—including friends, family members, or hospital staff—to veer from the course personally chosen by the patient.

For instance, if the dying individual has rejected the notion of a feeding tube, do not listen to comments like, "Don't you feel guilty about starving him to death?" If the dying patient has been placed on a ventilator in an effort to save her life but is now considered permanently unconscious, and if this patient has specified objections to such "body maintenance," do not be bullied by comments like, "By shutting off that ventilator you will be killing her." Remember, you were chosen as health care proxy because the dying patient had confidence that you would follow her wishes.

By the same token, do not insist that physicians follow instructions in a living will precisely if there is a substantial chance the patient can be saved, and restored to a quality of life that individual would find acceptable. Listen to what the doctors have to say. The patient may object to permanent hook-up to machines, but if doctors think they have a chance to help that person return to a life he or she would have wanted, give it a try. If there is a living will, the equipment can always be removed.

As the patient's proxy, you may find such decisions difficult to make. Any such decisions should *always* be based on the individual's instructions, values, and beliefs as well as the physician's diagnosis and prognosis, including an explanation of the benefits and burdens of the treatment being offered.

If the dying individual left no official documents or advance directives, you can still advocate on that person's behalf. To do so, think about anything the patient might have said about life-sustaining medical treatment. Try to remember whether there were any deaths or illnesses that made an impression on the patient and sparked discussion. Television shows and movies can also lead people to talk about what they would want. Such conversations, if presented in sufficient detail, will often compel the physician to do as the patient would have wished. In fact, recollection of such conversations are often considered evidence of the patient's true wishes in a court of law.

Sometimes, you will find that a hospital staff member feels uncomfortable—on personal or religious (but not medical) grounds—with the choices the dying individual has made. In that case, you should request that another staff member be assigned. If you are in a small emergency department where the entire staff seems at odds, on a personal level, with the dying patient's wishes, you may want to change hospitals altogether.

Those who work with living wills have found that sometimes, health care professionals simply are not acquainted with the law. In some facilities, staff members still believe that taking an individual off life support is against the law. It is not, if that individual would have wanted it that way. Depending upon where you are, you may need to educate the medical professionals in that setting.

If you find you cannot resolve differences with the staff or other family members on your own, remember that most large hospitals these days have social workers and ethics committees. Bring the conflict to their attention and ask for input. Sometimes, hospital personnel may be afraid to carry out last wishes for fear of a lawsuit. However, if the facility's legal or ethical department can give its stamp of approval, physicians will feel much more comfortable about letting go.

Only in extreme circumstances will you need to call in your own attorney or go to court. However, if you find your friend or relative placed in a situation he or she would not have wanted, that is what you may need to do.

Friends and family should request some time with the dying individual, if that is appropriate. And, they may even request a private room or space where last good-byes can be made. Depending upon the religious affiliation of the dying individual, a member of the clergy may pay a visit or a priest may be called to deliver last rites. (Some hospitals have full-time clergy on staff.)

After a death, most emergency departments will devote some resources to comforting grieving family members. Family members should expect the attending physician to meet with them, even if briefly, and explain the cause of death. If a grieving individual needs further comfort, a social worker may be available to lend a shoulder or an ear. Either way, hospitals will often accommodate the bereaved with a private room, if one is available, to collect themselves and make final plans and phone calls.

When It's Better to Stay Home

If a dying patient wishes to avoid aggressive intervention at life's end, and if he is not too uncomfortable, it may be better to skip the hospital and just stay home.

"If someone is clearly in a terminal situation, to bring them to the emergency department, where aggressive intervention is the philosophy, may really be unfair," says Dr. Harrison Bloom, chief of geriatric medicine at St. Luke's–Roosevelt Hospital. "We have not learned to let people die at home. When push comes to shove, friends and relatives get scared, they panic. They don't know how to handle death, so they bring the dying to professionals in the ED."

In fact, Bloom notes, there are just a few instances in which terminally ill individuals with no hope of recovery should be taken to the hospital to die: If they are in terrible, intractable pain; if they are suffering from intractable vomiting; or if they are hemorrhaging.

Says Bloom, "The idea is that you want to comfort someone, to provide them with every conceivable form of relief without necessarily prolonging their lives. Often, they can stay home. But sometimes comfort can be provided only at the ED."

It is hoped that friends and family will plan in advance, discussing with the dying individual what steps to take in a given situation. If possible, the tools and potions of comfort will be accessible at home.

Death Defying

We conclude this chapter and this book with a caveat: Unless the stricken individual has received an irrevocable death sentence, the emergency department is the place to be. Dying in the emergency department, surrounded by hulking, noisy medical equipment, the smell of isopropyl alcohol and the anonymous swirl of strangers is hardly ideal. One would prefer to pass away among familiar objects, scents, and sounds, the warmth of lifelong relatives and friends. But if you hope to cheat death, you should, as the mystic Ram Dass once said, "Be here now." Though you may seem doomed, the people in the emergency department may, depending upon the situation, stave off disaster. With the right mix of medicine and faith, that eerie tunnel of light will fade in the mist and you will survive.

Index

dental procedures, 35, 162, 209
depression, 94, 106, 114, 139, 299, 309, 312–314,
    331, 333–334
dermatologists, 162
dextrose, 120
diabetes mellitus, 9, 24, 33, 35, 38, 44, 183, 209
    childhood, 209, 234–235
    first aid treatment of, 98–100
    insulin treatment of, 98–100, 196
    signs of, 24, 47, 98–99
diagnosis, 3, 4, 134
    early, 21
    focus on symptom vs., 15–17, 20, 98–104
    mistakes in, 153–155
    relying on professionals for, 15–16, 20
    techniques of, 3, 15, 16, 182–186
diarrhea, 98, 143, 195, 209, 210, 228–229
diazepam (Valium), 120, 187, 308
Dilantin, 197, 256
dilation and curettage (D and C), 256–257
diphenhydramine hydrochloride (Benadryl), 120,
    179, 194, 204
diseases:
    blood-borne, 49
    chronic, 34
    communicable, 36, 49
    genetic, 36
    see also specific diseases
dislocations, 20, 87, 154–155, 210
disorientation, 9, 20, 27, 115, 318
    "times three," 24, 113, 125
disseminated intravascular coagulation (DIC),
    243, 245
diuretics, 191
diving, 305
dizziness, 5, 9, 14, 20, 51, 94, 98
    possible causes of, 8, 27, 98
    treatment of, 98–100
DNR (Do Not Resuscitate) orders, 127, 160, 355,
    365–366
documents:
    advance directive, 36, 38, 356, 357, 360–362,
        364–365
    holding copies of, 33, 34–39, 55, 127, 362
    see also specific documents
dogs, 64
    protective instincts of, 47, 114, 165
    rabid, 25, 180, 197
    restraining of, 47
domestic violence, 42, 242–243, 270–271

Do Not Resuscitate (DNR) orders, 127, 160, 355,
    365–366
dopamine, 120
driver's licenses, 38
drowning, 7, 44
drugs, 24, 183–197
    abuse and overdose of, 10, 26, 60, 114, 132,
        180, 314–317
    allergic reactions to, 25, 34, 35, 38, 192
    antidotes to, 26
    combinations of, 35
    dosage and frequency of, 35, 54
    failure to take, 113, 132
    illegal, 35, 185, 299–300, 315–317
    keeping records of, 34, 35, 55, 56
    over-the-counter, 16, 35, 142
    paramedics' supply of, 120–122
    prescription, 3, 22
    testing for, 185

Ear drum rupture, 11
ears, 93, 103
    infections of, 11, 138, 181–182
    objects stuck in, 236
eating disorders, 217
eclampsia, 255–256
E. coli bacteria, 143, 200
ectopic pregnancy, 22, 243–244, 257–258
ED director, 150, 154, 155, 157
edema, 31, 191
EDs, see emergency departments
elderly patients, 33, 55, 273–274
    advance preparation for emergencies by,
        282–283
    advocacy for, 283–285
    detecting emergencies of, 276–281
    fever in, 13–14, 26, 278
    prejudicial treatment and abuse of, 282,
        286–287
electrocardiogram (EKG), 8, 13, 21, 30, 116,
    118–119, 144, 174, 183
    copies of, 34, 38
electrolytes, 112, 184, 229
elevators, commandeering of, 47, 50
E-mail, 48–49
Emergency, 110, 115
emergency checklist, 56
emergency communication networks, 39–40,
    49–51
emergency contact sheets, 36–38, 57

indigestion, 21, 22
infants:
 coughing and choking in, 44, 213, 225–22
 CPR for, 63, 66, 71–72
 fever in, 14, 26
 jaundice in, 213
 lethargy in, 213–214
 neonatal emergencies of, 213–214
 skin tone of, 213, 214
infections, 279–280
 bacterial, 5–6, 11, 14, 18, 25, 77, 80, 183, 192–193, 278
 exposure to, 5, 12, 14, 25
 guarding against, 16, 17, 18, 23, 25, 85–86, 97, 211
 tetanus, 18, 25, 77, 167
 treatment of, 14, 25, 35
 viral, 12, 13–14, 22, 132
influenza, 12, 42, 181–182, 233
 symptoms of, 5, 14, 27, 183
injections, 25, 116
 intracardiac, 190–191
 tetanus, 18, 25, 36, 77, 180, 196–197, 204, 237
injuries, 32, 45
 force, 11, 137
 internal, 4, 10, 19, 20
 multiple, 20, 122, 171–172
 supporting of, see slings; splints
 workplace, 3, 4, 61
 see also specific injuries
insect bites, 12, 25, 95, 96–97, 103
insomnia, 4, 139
insulin, 98, 99, 196
insulin shock, 99, 106
intensivists, 163
internists, 31, 211
interns, 6, 16, 53, 132, 151, 154
intestines, 22
intravenous (IV) lines:
 central, 187–188
 for children, 54
 medication and fluids through, 31, 32, 112, 116, 118, 178, 187–188
intubation, see endotracheal intubation
Isoptin (verapamil), 122

Jaws of Life, 343
joints, 87
 dislocation of, 154–155
 pain in, 20, 170–171

Kaopectate, 195
Kaufman, Ilene, 203–205, 208–209, 218–220, 222–224
kidneys, 35, 83–84, 171, 184
 infections of, 176–177
kidney stones, 176
 passing of, 12, 22–23, 191
knee injuries, 87, 291
knife wounds, 4, 18–19, 76, 105, 139, 154, 349
Krasnoff, Ellen, 79, 80, 85, 92
Kroning, David, 200

Labor:
 contractions in, 26, 34
 difficulties in, 123
 inducement of, 242
 pain of, 26
 premature, 256
laboratory tests, 4, 32, 149, 158–159
lacerations, 137, 186, 211, 220, 236–237, 350; see also cuts
laryngoscopy, 117
larynx, 6, 348
Lasix (Furosemide), 121, 190
Legionnaires' disease, 27
legs:
 loss of movement and sensation in, 23
 twitching and flailing of, 24
Lennon, John, 339–341
lidocaine (Xylocaine), 35, 118, 121, 186
lifestyle, 33
life support machines, 84, 127, 356–357, 363
ligaments, 87
 injuries of, 11, 87, 291
limbs, 3–4, 23, 76
 amputation of, 19, 51
 crushing of, 4, 105
 fractures of, 3, 4, 11, 82, 107, 115, 144–146
 frozen, 93–94, 103
 reattachment of, 105
liver injuries, 349
living wills, 36, 38, 356, 357, 360–362, 364–365, 368
lungs, 115, 355–356
 blood in, 22, 31, 191
 collapse of, 171, 173, 187, 348
 oxygen deprivation of, 6, 8, 9, 83
 testing capacity of, 175
 water on, 31, 191
lupus, 35

Lynn, Stephen G., 12, 15, 16, 30–32, 41, 123, 126,
134, 138, 142, 154, 156–157, 165, 262,
270–271, 289, 339–341, 356

Maalox, 16, 194
magnesium sulfate, 121, 256
magnetic resonance imaging (MRI), 148, 182
malnutrition, 285
manic depression, 309, 311
marijuana, 317
Marks, Richard, 339
Marsella, Richard, 49–51
martial arts, 305–306
masks:
  face-eye, 131
  nasal cannula, 117, 174
  nebulizer, 132
  oxygen, 117
  pocket CPR, 49, 63, 73–74
mastitis, 255
Mathisen, Dan, 107, 115
medical emergencies:
  ABCs of survival in, 6–9, 22, 25, 26, 62, 76, 84,
    93, 94, 98, 100, 116
  age factors in, 4, 5, 13–14, 17, 19, 33, 45
  assessment of, see triage
  communicating information in, 13, 29–30, 32,
    34–51, 98, 99, 106, 137–139, 141–144,
    153–154
  consideration of complete medical picture in,
    13–17, 33, 34–40, 142
  danger of delay in, 5–6, 10, 13, 29–30, 31, 34,
    45, 47, 48, 50, 76, 108, 123–125
  determining seriousness and urgency of,
    30–32, 136–144
  erring on side of caution in, 15–16, 18, 20, 21
  follow-up care in, 149, 168, 182, 221, 225–239
  "golden hour" window of opportunity in, 20,
    30, 76, 108, 124, 341
  insurance coverage of, 15, 36, 38, 55, 56,
    149
  legal aspects of, 49, 51, 75, 126, 159
  life-threatening, 1, 6–9, 20–22, 29–30, 32, 45, 54,
    145
  patient demands and requests in, 3, 24,
    123–127, 132
  preparing for, 6, 14, 29–57
Medical Emergency Services Reform Act of 1983,
  159
Medic Alert Foundation, 39

Medic Alert information bracelet, 38–39
medical guardians, 205–207
medical histories, 13, 15, 40, 115
  anticipating emergencies based on, 33, 34
  carrying copies of, 33, 34–39, 55, 56
  family, 13, 34, 36
  key points for inclusion in, 33, 35–36
  permanent, 35, 39
  reviewing of, 33, 34–36
  updating of, 34, 36
medical information cards, 38
medical records, 161
medical schools, 16, 52
medical students, 16, 150–151, 154
medications, see drugs
memory loss, 3, 38
meningitis, 14, 27, 181, 229, 230
menopause, premature, 33
Men's Health, 38
menstruation, 13
Mental Hygiene Legal Service, 337–338
microsurgery, 51, 77, 82, 105, 169
milk of magnesia, 15
Miller, Jack, 48–49
miscarriage, 10, 256–257
Moretti, Anna, 361–362, 365–366
morphine, 118, 192
morphine sulfate, 121
mouth sores, 19
MRI (magnetic resonance imaging), 148, 182
Mr. Jones, 309
Mulligan, Eleanor, 152–153, 165
multiple sclerosis, 326
muscles, 87
  injuries to, 19–20, 87–88, 297
  spasm of, 94, 297
  straining of, 11, 17, 21, 176
myasthenia gravis, 43
myocardial contusion, 349
myocardial infarction (MI), 53–116, 142; see also
  heart attack
myocardial ischemia, 174

Naloxone (Narcan), 121
Napoleonic Wars, 136
narcotics, 192, 315–316
nasal cannulas, 117, 174
nausea, 4, 8, 9, 17, 21, 23, 51, 94, 98
  treatment of, 99, 195
nebulizing devices, 116, 175, 188, 225

neck, 11
  broken, 21, 347
  injuries to, 10, 21, 91, 173
  stabilizing of, 106, 118
  stiffness of, 24, 178, 230
neck collars, 106, 118, 173
Neosporin, 85
neurological dysfunction, 23, 24
neurosurgery, 53, 108, 162, 170, 172, 199
New York City Marathon, 289–290, 298
New York City Regional Poison Control Center,
  26, 43, 95, 210
New York *Daily News,* 48
New York State Health Department, 161
911 emergency, 41–44, 48, 60, 75, 76, 107, 110, 127
  enhanced technology of, 44
  inappropriate use of, 43
  operators of, 111
nitroglycerine, 146, 174, 195
nitrous oxide (Nitronox), 121
nonsteroidal anti-inflammatory drugs, 35,
  191–192
nose, 92
  bleeding from, 18, 45, 189, 236
  objects stuck in, 236
  packing of, 189
numbness, 14, 23, 29, 100
nurses, 52, 131
  charge, 151, 155
  company, 49
  ED, 3, 4, 15, 30, 34, 53, 132, 134, 135, 151
  head, 55, 151, 155
  registered, 53, 111
  training and experience of, 53, 152, 153
  triage, 133, 136–139, 141–144, 147, 178,
    211–212, 218
  visiting, 307
nurses aides, 151
nursing homes, 42

Obstetrician/gynecologists, 53, 55, 133, 162, 181,
  255–256
odors, 61, 95
offices, 41
  emergency communication networks in, 49–51
  first aid and CPR training in, 49–50
  medical emergencies in, 48–51
  notification systems in, 50
  preestablished response protocol in, 49–51
Ono, Yoko, 339–340

operations, 52, 154
  keeping records of, 34, 35
  medical descriptions of, 35
ophthalmology, 53, 147, 239
oral airway device, 118
oral surgeons, 162
orderlies, 151
organs, 19
  donation of, 366–367
  oxygen deprivation to, 7, 8–9, 83–84
  protection of, 30
orthopedics, 20, 53, 55, 138, 147, 162, 351
osteoporosis, 276, 278
otolaryngologists, 163
ovarian cysts, 250
oxygen:
  deprivation of, 6–9, 29, 59–60, 69–70, 83–84,
    108, 207
  supplemental, 29, 31, 32, 106, 108, 114, 116,
    117–118, 121, 126, 171, 188
oxygenation, 116–117
oxygen masks, 117
oxygen saturation, 140, 141

Pacemakers, 38
  temporary, 190
pain, 15, 134
  reduction of, 1, 12, 23, 87, 355
  severe, 10, 11–12, 20, 22–23,126–127, 136, 138,
    143–144
  stress of, 3, 11–12
  see also specific sites
pancreas, 99
Pappas, Gus, 108–109
paralysis, 23, 356
paramedics, 3, 15, 20, 26, 38, 39, 51
  authorized procedures of, 112, 115–119, 151
  "big black bag" of, 107
  heroic actions of, 105–106, 110
  job-related stress of, 114–115
  providing vital information to, 43–48, 106–107
  slang and humor of, 128–130
  specialized precautions of, 21, 29
  summoning of, 29–30, 31, 51, 60
  training of, 42, 107, 112, 122
  typical daily shifts of, 113, 115
patient representatives, 151, 155–156
patients:
  accompanying of, 50
  comforting of, 1, 84, 98, 115, 131